THETAHEALING®
DISEASES & DISORDERS

Vianna Stibal

HAY HOUSE, INC.
Carlsbad, California • New York City
London • Sydney • Johannesburg
Vancouver • Hong Kong • New Delhi

Published and distributed in the United States by: Hay House, Inc.

Compiled from the teachings of Vianna by Guy Stibal of Rolling Thunder Publishing.

The trademarks ThetaHealing® and Orian Technique™ are owned by Vianna Stibal, owner of Vianna's Natural Path. Any unauthorized use of these marks is prohibited.

Special thanks to the ThetaHealing Teachers, Dixie Schulz Nowell, Debbie Cavette, and David L. Lowe for their assistance in compiling this text.

ISBN: 978-1-4019-3497-2

Printed in the United States of America

CONTENTS

Acknowledgements

I must thank all the wonderful clients who gave me the opportunity to learn the information that has finally come to rest in this book for posterity. May this knowledge be a gift for all those brave souls out there who dare to believe.

From the Editor: To our readers in the U.S. and Canada, please note that for the most part, we have maintained the British style of spelling, grammar (including noun/pronoun agreement), punctuation, and syntax of the initial printing of this book, which was published in the United Kingdom.

PROLOGUE

ThetaHealing Diseases and Disorders is the companion to the books *ThetaHealing* and *Advanced ThetaHealing*. In *ThetaHealing*, I explain the processes of the reading, the healing, the belief work, the feeling work, the digging and gene work, and offer additional knowledge for the beginner. *Advanced ThetaHealing* gives the reader an in-depth guide to belief, feeling and digging work, and insights into the planes of existence and the beliefs that I believe are essential for spiritual evolution.

This book does not include the specific step-by-step processes that proliferate in *ThetaHealing* and *Advanced ThetaHealing*, so it is necessary to reach an understanding of these processes first. In this book are the intuitive insights, intuitive remedies, belief work and supplements that I have found to be of value as they pertain to certain diseases and disorders. It is the result of experiences with diseases and disorders from over 47,000 sessions.

THE ROLE OF CONVENTIONAL MEDICINE

The reader will notice that I have drawn upon the knowledge of modern conventional medicine. The reason for this is that unlike some in the alternative field, I do not see doctors and prescription drugs as the enemy. I believe that we all benefit from conventional medicine. I believe that the essence of conventional medicine has its own powerful spiritual vibration and it is up to us to use it wisely. I will say, however, that it does have its drawbacks.

One of the problems with conventional medicine is that of specialization. Medical specialists often fail to recognize the synchronistic attributes of the human body. For instance, medicine that is prescribed by a heart specialist might help the heart but have an adverse effect on the rest of the body.

Another oversight of many medical practitioners is that they fail to see that each person is different, each person is special, and so each person will have their own reactions to medicines.

In Western society, we also give a lot of power to our doctors. We wait with bated breath on every word the doctor says and believe what we are told. Proper discernment of what we are told by our doctor is important, as well as the knowledge that there are always other opinions and other doctors. Doctors are like us, with positive and negative attributes, and in the end it is our decision whether or not to accept their suggestions. Be careful of accepting negative statements from a doctor as the ultimate truth.

On the flip side, there have been incredible advances in conventional medicine that we all benefit from. Antibiotics, for example, help us fight infection. They do not kill the infection but are designed to work with the immune system. There is a great deal of hype in the alternative field that antibiotics are bad for you because they deplete the immune system. The truth is antibiotics can do several things to the system. They can cause the die-off of good bacteria in the intestinal tract. They also have a tendency to push the immune system into overdrive. However, when you have a client who is using an antibiotic, you have to work with the antibiotic. You cannot tell your client to discontinue its use. The full course of antibiotics must be taken, otherwise the bacteria will have time to mutate and cause an even worse infection. In addition, there are times when an antibiotic is beneficial, such as when truly nasty bacteria get into the system. And yet I have seen people who refused to take antibiotics even though they had terrible infections.

I am and always have been an advocate for what works. If it is an antibiotic that is needed, fine. If it is a healing that is called for, fine. All things are equal under the eyes of the Creator.

It may surprise you when you hear the Creator specifically tell you that a person should use an antibiotic. But this simply means that on some level the person is not ready to release the bacteria any other way. Some people believe everything the doctor says, so the thought that the antibiotic will work is the healing essence. Keep your ego and belief systems out of the equation.

Many of us in fact owe our very lives to conventional medicine. But in the field of medicine, conventional or alternative, humans have not been able to copy the life-force that suffuses all things. Our body consists of more than just matter, or cells running around with autonomic responses, communicating with each other like a 'biological machine'. Feelings, emotions, beliefs and programmes influence how we behave and have dramatic effects on the body's well-being, even on a cellular level. The cells are very aware of the environment both inside and outside the body and have individual intelligence, while still remaining connected to the whole. The concept of interconnected wholeness, from the smallest particle in our bodies to the farthest reaches of creation, inspires me when I witness the Creator heal.

THETAHEALING®

ThetaHealing is designed to open up your psychic abilities to heal. Being psychic and being a healer are two different skills. Putting the two together is the key.

As a body psychic, you are expected to recognize different viruses, bacteria, parasites and heavy metals in the body. The client will expect you to identify these influences with accuracy.

As a healer, you are put on the spot in a different way: you do not have to know what the disease is to have the Creator heal it, but you do have to put yourself in a deep enough Theta state to witness the healing being done. And the client will often come to you expecting to be instantly healed.

So, both being psychic and being a healer have their pressures. The healer is expected to heal and the psychic is expected to see inside the body and validate what they see. This is what a ThetaHealer® is – a healer who uses psychic abilities to witness a healing through a connection to the Creator.

THE MECHANICS OF A HEALING

Who can say what the mysterious mechanics of a healing are? Who knows what secrets lie in the depths of the brain?

Each healing is different. It might be that once the connection to the Creator is reached, the automatic response of the brain is to release a special chemical messenger to heal the body. However, will this chemical be accepted by the body or rejected out of hand simply because the receptors only know how to accept negative responses? These negative receptors in the brain could be blocking messages that tell the body to heal itself.

The belief and feeling work are designed to change the way we send and receive messages in the body. When we remove and replace enough programmes in a person's brain, the right chemical messengers are released, and the receptors accept the message as valid.

For many years I observed people and asked myself why some would heal and some would not. I have found that for the most part, just the basic healing – just going up to the Creator of All That Is and commanding the body to heal – can do amazing things. When someone comes to me with a sickness, this is the first thing I do. In many instances, their body miraculously heals.

When I experienced instant healing for the first time, I asked myself: 'What made my leg heal so fast?' Years later, when I was diagnosed with congestive heart failure and found another way to heal incredibly fast, once again I asked: 'What made my body heal so fast?' Perhaps the question should have been: 'Why did I have to get sick in the first place?' I will do my best to answer these questions throughout this book. And as always, the Creator answered me patiently. I was told, 'Vianna, you have a resilient body. You should bless your body. Encourage your body, and don't discourage it.'

As a healer using energy, you should never underestimate the power of the simple healing. Some people will receive an instant healing, while others will not be prepared to receive one. These people might require multiple healings, belief work, the use of herbs or, according to their beliefs, conventional medicine.

Each person is different with respect to their beliefs, but the overall patterns of emotions that attract a specific disease to a person and are created by a specific disease within a person tend to be the same from client to client.

The supplements, beliefs and downloads in this book are what I have found have made a difference in my sessions with clients. This text is a compilation of what I do for the different diseases and what I have seen actually work.

When I ask the Creator to change what is wrong in a person's body, amazingly the body always responds in some way. At this point I can sense whether it is reacting negatively or positively to the healing. If the person is apathetic, or if they're using a chemical such as morphine, the healing seems to sputter through the body, achieving some results, but not the instant healing we are after. I've discovered that certain drugs may inhibit intuitive healings. We will discuss this aspect of healing later. For the most part, however, I'm amazed by the number of people who benefit from intuitive healings. No matter what the disease, it is still what we believe inside that makes the difference. And if we believe healing is possible, the body will respond.

STAY OPEN

The problem can be the healer. If they believe that one illness is worse than another or that a healing is going to be difficult or even impossible, then the healing will be stopped then and there. Throughout this book, as we look at diseases and their associated belief systems, consider how you feel towards certain diseases. You may harbour fears, doubts and beliefs that will block the healing process. It is paramount that you believe that it is possible for a person to heal.

It may help you to know that the majority of people who come to me for a healing improve immediately. Some actually heal instantly, in many instances from diseases that you would never have imagined could be resolved so easily. This is why it is important to stay open to all possibilities.

SELF-HEALING

ThetaHealing is designed to empower the individual to bring the Creator into themselves in order to release beliefs, instil feelings and witness healings. For some people, self-healing in this way works better than working with another person. It allows them to feel that they are taking control of their disease.

THE DISEASE SPEAKS

With regard to the healer–client relationship, it is valuable to understand that you have to determine whether it is the sickness that is talking to you or the actual person. People don't always change their personality when they are ill, but I have found that diseases have a tendency to match the personalities of the people who have them. So you need to work out who is speaking at any given time.

CLEANSES AND COMMON SENSE

As an intuitive, you cannot give good advice unless you have a decent grasp of nutrition, supplements and medication. One of the biggest mistakes I see health practitioners make is suggesting the *Candida* cleanse without giving something to help with the die-off of the *Candida*. Another mistake is putting people on cleanses when the body is too weak to handle them. Some people need to be strengthened with vitamins and minerals before they perform any kind of cleanse.

I have even seen people become compulsive about cleanses to the point that their immune system is exhausted. Their electrolytes, vitamins and minerals are depleted from too many cleanses!

Building the body up before and after a cleanse is a good suggestion.

REACTIONS TO HEALING

There are many reactions to healing.

Even if a person experiences a perfect instant healing, they may go away and five months later deny the existence of the Creator. People are strange that way.

Then there is the person who becomes so comfortable with the healer–client relationship that they do not want it to end.

It has been my experience that some people create sickness to get attention, nurturing and love. They become dependent on the healer and are afraid that they will die without them. There have been times when I have considered refusing readings and healings on someone because they expected me to live their life for them. The trick is to give them back their own power, a power that they may never have known.

Endorphins are released into the system of the client each time they experience a reading or healing and this may be why they come back.

I am careful to honour everyone who comes to be worked on, even when I do not agree with why they came to me.

It is also the responsibility of the practitioner to make the client aware that they may experience a healing crisis, i.e., relive a past sickness to a lesser degree, as a result of memories being released into their body during the healing.

MASSAGE

Sometimes, a person doesn't need any form of healing other than a good massage. This can stimulate the lymphatic system, relax the muscles and just plain make the person feel pampered.

However, if the person has cancer, it can spread rather quickly through the body because of the massage. With other people, a massage can cause their body to detoxify. It is always best to ask the Creator if the person can handle a massage. If the Creator says they will be fine or they will only detoxify a little bit, this means that they will be ill for about a day. If the Creator tells you, 'Absolutely not!' to a massage, listen to what you are told!

AFTER THE ILLNESS

More often than not, when people have finished with an illness, they will look at me and say, 'Now what?' They have spent so many years working on their illness that they have no idea what to do next.

So I have found that anyone who has a long-term injury or illness needs to write down what they are going to do afterwards. Having that goal will enable them to look forward.

Always encourage people to plan for life after the disease.

Also, when you have done a healing session with a person, you need to get them to go to their doctor and be checked to make sure they are improving. This is a very important facet of the healing process.

CARE FOR HEALERS/PSYCHICS

Healers themselves should look for people who are of like mind to be in partnership with. Healers will often stay in relationships to allow their partner time to change, and this may not be beneficial for them. It is easier to work with like-minded people from the start.

A healer will use up many minerals when they are doing intuitive work, as you do with any physical activity. Make sure to keep up on vitamins and minerals, at least at first.

With some people who are intuitive, scans of the brain show shadows on the frontal lobes. This is due to the high-frequency electrical currents caused by intuitive activity.

Healers may be prone to asthma and adrenal problems because they overwork themselves. To avoid this, regularly pull any resentment programmes.

Touch and love are very important parts of healing. The healer opens people's heart chakras and then works on their issues. So take regular salt baths to clear overwhelming emotions and make a psychic break from clients.

Downloads

Healers and psychics will benefit from the following downloads:

'I know what it feels like to live without taking on other people's issues.'

'I know what it feels like to live without taking on other people's emotions.'

'I know what it feels like to live without taking on other people's curses.'

'I know what it feels like to live without taking on other people's programmes and beliefs.'

'I know what it feels like to live without taking on people's sickness.'

'I know how to convert sickness, emotions, programmes and beliefs into love and light, which are sent to the Creator and returned to me.'

'I know what it feels like to be of service to others and be appreciated for it.'

'I know how to be of service without being taken advantage of.'

'I know how to permit others to know they are important to the Creator.'

'I know what it feels like to be at peace with myself.'

'I know what it feels like to enjoy the breath of life.'

'I know what it feels like to enjoy every moment.'

'I know what it feels like to be connected to everything, always.'

'I know what it feels like to discern between the feelings of others and my own.'

'I know how to work with others in the highest and best way.'

'I know how to accept others for the way they are.'

'I know how to live my life in acceptance without resenting others.'

'I know what it feels like to live without the negative thoughts of others affecting my life.'

'The most important thing in my life is my connection to the Creator.'

'I know how to tap into the Creator of All That Is of the Seventh Plane of Existence easily and effortlessly.'

'I know how to stand in my truth.'

'I know how to be accountable for my words.'

'I know how to live my life without unreasonable fear.'

'I know how to create a kingdom of heaven within myself.'

'I know how to create a heaven on Earth.'

'I know what it feels like to appreciate and love people who are close to me.'

'I know it is possible to have peace, happiness and joy without being bored.'

'I know it is possible to use my experiences with wisdom.'

'I know it is possible to be thankful for every experience in my life.'

MICROBES

This is an A to Z book of disorders. In order to address these disorders, there needs to be an understanding of microbes and their energetic influences. So we will begin by exploring the influences of microbes and heavy metals in our daily lives.

Microbes are living things that are simply too small to be seen with the naked eye. This group includes bacteria, fungi, protozoa and microscopic algae. It also includes viruses.

We tend to associate small organisms with things that make us feel uncomfortable, like infections or diseases, but the majority of micro-organisms are crucial to the welfare of this world. Without them we simply could not live. Some microbes help us to break down water, incorporate nitrogen from the air, digest food, absorb vitamins and create useful chemicals in our body. Most of the microbes on Earth are actually good. Only a small number are considered pathogenic, meaning 'disease producing'.

There is much more than we realize to bacteria, viruses, heavy metals, fungi, yeast and parasites. This section goes beyond the physical aspects of microbes to illuminate the emotional and subconscious components of microbial infections and infestations. We will show how to prevail over these influences by changing beliefs and instilling feelings.

There are basic rules that apply to every infectious disease:

- A harmful bacterium is attached to emotions of guilt.
- Harmful fungi are attached to the emotions of resentment.
- Harmful viruses are attached to worthiness issues.
- Mycoplasmas are attached to worthiness issues and guilt.

Knowing these basic tenets will give you an idea of how to deal with these different disease-causing toxins.

Today we understand that micro-organisms are found almost everywhere, but it wasn't very long ago, before the invention of the microscope, that thousands of people died in epidemics from food spoilage and other related aspects because there were no antibiotics. In fact, people would die simply because they didn't understand the need to wash their hands while delivering a baby. Germ theories were difficult to prove, because people didn't believe that something could exist if you couldn't see it.

Every single day during my readings I do see microbes, bacteria and fungi causing people to become extremely ill.

One thing that many people who are interested in metaphysics seem to believe is that if they are ill, it means they have done something wrong. This seems to be a genetic belief that dates back to medieval times, before the discovery of micro-organisms. Please understand that not everything is based on karma. Whether you lead a good life or a bad one, exposure to pathogenic microbes can still make you sick. It would be accurate to say that if our minds and bodies were in true sequence with one another, if we were balanced emotionally and if we lived in a clean environment, we could resist many illnesses. However, the truth is that some diseases are caused by exposure to radiation, toxins, mercury and microbes.

So, when you look inside someone's body and see disease, it may not be because the person has been unkind to their loved ones, but because they have been drinking water that is contaminated with microbes. The key is to uncover the belief that inspired them to drink the water in the first place. The following downloads may be helpful:

'I have the Creator's definition of how and when to say no.'

'I know what it feels like to be listened to.'

'I understand what it feels like to be heard.'

'I know what it feels like to live without being constantly angry.'

'I know what it feels like to live without allowing people to suck me dry.'

'I know how to live without allowing people I love to take advantage of me.'

'I understand what it feels like to live without being overwhelmed.'

'I know how to live without being miserable.'

'I know how to interact with others.'

Always follow up this list by doing further belief and feeling work with the digging work.

These are just ideas to work on. Remember, every individual is different, so ask the Creator of All That Is what the person you're working with needs to help them heal.

BACTERIA

Bacteria are relatively simple single-celled organisms. They are unicellular (one-celled) and may have spherical (coccus), rod-like (bacillus) or curved (vibrio, spirillum or spirochete) bodies. Their genetic material is not enclosed in a nuclear membrane, i.e., they are prokaryotic (*prokaryote* is Greek for 'pre-nucleus'). They have a collective consciousness, so work together.

Understand that you cannot command all of the bacteria in the body to disappear. When you make a command like this, you will hear laughter. This is the amusement of the universe. You see, the body needs some of the bacteria that are present.

You can, however, be very specific about what bacteria you want removed from the body and you can command that the body be balanced. When the body is alkaline balanced, the bacteria that cause challenges in the body will transform into beneficial bacteria. Bacteria are only detrimental when the body is out of balance.

When I go up and ask the Creator to change a person's belief system, I am sure to witness it change in every cell in the body. I make sure that every cell knows what is going on. This creates a condition in which harmful bacteria cannot live in the body anymore, and so they transform.

I know that you have to experience both the negative and the positive in life to understand what duality is. It's a question of balance. Most of you will already have experienced sadness, sorrow, depression and other negative emotions. This is because sometimes our spirit chooses to experience the negative first and then the positive. However, the more positive information we put into our body, the faster it will heal. If you pull belief systems like 'I have to be lonely' or 'I have to be sad' and replace them with new beliefs, then harmful bacteria can't stay and will transform.

We must not forget, however, that positive feelings and programmes can also cause disease. An example would be: 'I have to be ill to bring my family together.' This is why the digging work is so important.

Bacteria and Emotions

One of the reasons why bacteria are able to enter into the system is because of unbalanced emotions. If you are angry or fearful all the time, your immune system works harder. Anger and fear can be beneficial as survival reflexes. This is what they were designed for. However, they were not designed for continual, compulsive use. If overused in this way, they have a tendency to exhaust the immune system. This is how emotions deplete the body.

These 'negative' emotions become positive, however, if kept in balance. It can make you sick if you never express your anger and hold it inside. The ability to express your anger in a positive fashion is beneficial.

Intuitive Remedies

Bacteria are easy to get rid of intuitively. Make the command: *'Creator, change this and show me.'* Witness the healing as done.

Belief Work

Guilt issues hold bacteria in the body, so download:

> 'I know what it feels like to live without guilt.'
>
> 'I know how to live without holding on to guilt.'
>
> 'I know how to live without feeling guilty for who I am.'
>
> 'I know how to live without feeling guilty for the way my body looks.'
>
> 'I know how to live without feeling guilty for everything my parents have taught me.'
>
> 'I know what a friend is.'
>
> 'I know how to have friends.'
>
> 'I know how to be a friend.'

'I know how to be a friend without feeling guilty.'

'I know how to be accountable for my actions.'

'I make decisions easily.'

FUNGUS

Fungus grows in acidic low-moisture aerobic environments. It can grow on the skin, hair or nails, or inside the body. Its gender will change according to the environmental temperature.

Fungus infections can affect all organs of the body. People are getting more of them now than ever before. Fungus is becoming one of the leading causes of infection in hospitals. People who have been on antibiotics for extended periods of time are especially susceptible.

If a person has a fungus infection, they should consider removing white flour and sugar from their diet and consider an alkaline diet. Some sinus infections are caused by fungus. Mould problems are common. Black mould in houses is only now beginning to get attention from public officials for the health hazard that it is.

Intuitive Insights

When seen intuitively in the body, fungus has a range of colours, depending on what type it is. It is seen as a cloudy colour in the lungs (bacterial and viral infections look different). Dead and dying fungus is seen as a black cloudy substance.

Fungus projects programmes of 'I'll do it later' and the person thinks these feelings are their own.

Since all fungus is tied to resentment issues, you should clear these issues and then the fungus will go away.

Intuitive Remedies

The best way to deal with fungus is to change it into a harmless form. You can do this just by saying, 'Creator, show me what needs to be done and change this now.' However, you must first find and release the beliefs that are holding it in place. If you find the bottom belief, it will change in just seconds. If you make the command to change the fungus without finding the bottom belief, the client could go through a healing crisis as a result of the terrible die-off of the fungus.

Beliefs associated with fungus usually have to do with resentment. The person must find out how this resentment is serving them.

Downloads

'I know what it feels like to live without resentment.'

'I know how to live without resenting my body.'

'I know how to live without resenting my parents.'

'I know how to live without resenting my friends.'

'I know how to live without resenting my mate.'

'I know it is possible to live without resenting the people around me.'

Supplements

- calcium–magnesium (this helps to ward off fungus)
- eucalyptus (use topically only)
- noni
- olive-leaf extract
- pau d'arco
- tea tree oil (use topically only)

HEAVY METALS

The body is made up of heavy metals such as calcium, magnesium and zinc, but some metals are not meant for the human body, such as aluminium and mercury. These are poisonous and may be the source of many diseases. Also, viruses and bacteria are drawn to heavy metals because of the weakness they cause in the body.

If you are in a person's space and you see shiny flecks in their body, it may mean that they have toxic heavy metals there.

Types

Aluminium: There are many different kinds of aluminium. It can be a cause of Alzheimer's disease and Parkinson's disease.

Fluoride: Fluoride makes a person age quicker and leaves deposits in the body.

Iron: Too much iron naturally oxidizes in the body. High levels are poisonous.

Lead: Causes depression, insanity, cancer and immunological diseases. It is as easily absorbed as calcium; the receptors that absorb calcium will just as easily absorb lead.

Manganese: Manganese is needed to regulate sugars in the body, but too much can make you go crazy. Psychopathic killers have very high levels of it in their brain. It can be found in well water and also comes from pesticides and herbicides.

Mercury: Mercury can cause depression and many cancers. It may bind to other heavy metals in the body. Any amount is poisonous. In many people, an over-abundance of mercury may block the intuitive abilities.

Silver: Silver naturally oxidizes in the body. High levels are poisonous. Overuse of colloidal silver will turn the skin blue.

Intuitive Insights

Many people absorb heavy metals based on their feelings and programmes, for example:

- Lead is absorbed by the innocent and unsuspecting and most easily by children, particularly those who do not have proper emotional structure in their family life. Fake Love: When someone hurts and abuses you they often say it is because they love you. Generally, they also lack vitamins and proper minerals.

- Manganese is more readily absorbed by those who have more anger and stress around them.

- Mercury seems to be absorbed by unsuspecting victims, those who are very naïve and innocent. These people may be unaware that they are being taken advantage of by their friends and family; they are gullible. Gullible people want to believe everything they are told.

I also believe that many learning disabilities are due to heavy-metal poisoning.

Intuitive Remedies

The healer should not command all heavy metals from the body to be gone since heavy metals such as calcium and zinc are a vital part of our molecular structure. It is best to ask the Creator of All That Is what to do, since everyone is different and toxins should be pulled out of the body at a rate tailored to the individual. Ask the Creator how to clear them in the highest and best way.

When you pull out heavy-metal toxins, you pull out old memories attached to them, so be aware that the person may act out these emotional memories. For these feelings, do belief work.

A good way to release the heavy metals from the body is to teach the person that they have a good emotional foundation and they have emotional structure.

Supplements

To remove toxic heavy metals from the body, take:

- ALA
- blue-green algae
- calcium
- CoQ10
- lots of greens
- magnesium
- omega 3
- zinc

MIASMS

It is believed that a miasm is caused by a marker in the DNA left from a disease suffered by an ancestor. The disease disrupts the genetic code and the change is passed down. For instance, it is thought that syphilis mutates in the DNA to produce a predisposition for psoriasis or psoriatic arthritis that is passed down from generation to generation.

So, to heal a client, go back in time to work on the ancestor and then watch the energy being brought through the generations into the present.

Once I have made these genetic changes in the client, I work to clear the residual energies that are left over. I think the miasm mutates to a fungal energy that goes into the DNA and invades the liver.

PARASITES

Many things in our environment expose us to parasites. One of the most common ways to pick them up is to get worms from pets (especially indoor pets). Other major causes of infestation are eating uncooked meat, fish and raw vegetables, walking barefoot in warm climates and poor hygiene in the company of infested people. The risk of parasitic infection is increased by travel to places with poor public sanitation.

The broad range of parasite-induced health problems is evident once the nature and extent of parasitic infection is understood. A general misconception about parasites is that they inhabit only the intestines of the host. In fact there are parasites that live in the blood, lymph system, vital organs and/or other body tissues. Some parasites may affect the whole body. Yeasts often proliferate first in the intestines and then spread throughout the body, becoming septic. Other parasites attack specific organs. For example, hookworms enter the body through the skin, travel through the blood and eventually inhabit the lungs and small intestines. Left untreated, they can remain in these organs for years, causing a variety of symptoms.

Types of Parasite

Over 650,000 different kinds of parasite are associated with the human body, including:

Cestoda: This is a tapeworm that inhabits beef, pork, dogs and fish. People come into contact with these worms when eating red meat or simply by walking barefoot outside. Once in the body, they attach to the sides of the colon and steal nutrients. The first indications are that the host becomes very thin and then gains weight. They will feel hungry all the time. The body thinks it is starving and holds on to fat reserves.

A *heminath* is a flatworm or roundworm.

Nematodes, including roundworms and hookworms, are unhealthy to humans. They infect the body with their eggs. Flatworms will lay their eggs in the digestive system. Pinworms, hookworms and roundworms enter the heart, intestines, liver, lungs, lymphatic system and pancreas. They vary in size from 0.078 to 13.78 inches. Children easily transmit this group of parasites.

Patyhelminths are a class of worms, such as flukes and flatworms, which infect the human body. Tapeworms in this class will actually eat other tapeworms in the human body. Humans serve as suitable hosts for beef, pork, fox and dog tapeworms.

Protozoa can be parasitic and harmful to the human body. *Cryptosporidium*, *Endolimax nana*, *Giardia lamblia* and *Trichomonas* are microscopic organisms that travel through the bloodstream and infect all body parts.

Trematoda: This is a fluke parasite that is in the bladder, blood, intestinal tract, kidneys, liver and lungs. Flukes are approx. 0.4–1 inch in length and look like snails or leeches in the liver.

There are some parasites that are transferred during sexual intercourse, called *Triginos vaevadinalis*, which are carried in body fluids.

Symptoms

The following are some of the most common symptoms of parasites:

- a voracious appetite
- a withered yellow look
- anal itching (especially at night)
- bluish or purplish specks in the whites of the eyes
- cravings for sweets, dried food, raw rice, dirt (usually in children), charcoal and/or burned food
- emaciation
- facial pallor
- fretful sleep
- general weakness
- grinding the teeth while asleep
- nose picking
- white coin-sized blotches on the face

Intuitive Insights

It is necessary to recognize that the person infested with parasites is influenced on more than a physical level. Parasites are drawn to thought processes that block our development on all levels: physically, emotionally, mentally and spiritually. Once inside us, they relay feelings to us to ensure their own survival.

A person is more susceptible to parasites if their belief systems permit other people to take advantage of them. People with parasites may not know how to say no and may allow themselves to get sucked dry. Feelings such as 'I must allow others to take advantage of me' and 'I must allow people to suck me dry' are a magnet to parasites. People with parasites have self-esteem issues.

If a person has heavy-metal poisoning, they seem to have an abundance of parasites.

All vegetables and meats have some parasites. Regardless, the more balanced your beliefs systems, the fewer parasites you pick up. Remember, some of these belief systems are genetic, deep within us.

When we do belief work and feeling work, we are freed from the programmes that attract parasites.

The next step in the process is to free ourselves from parasites of all kinds, such as certain people in our lives. As we remove, replace and add feelings from the Creator with the belief work, we will gain the strength to expel parasites from the inner body as well as from the outer body. Parasites cannot survive in or around a body that doesn't have programmes that will attract them. The fewer limiting beliefs you have, the more balanced your pH is, creating a healthier body.

Intuitive Remedies

Some parasitical bacteria help digest food and it is normal to have them in the body. For this reason, we do not intuitively command that all parasites leave the body. Also avoid killing parasites using ThetaHealing. The die-off will create an over-abundance of waste products and dead parasites, which will cause the person to be ill.

Be sure to use belief and feeling work to release beliefs that draw parasites to a person. This in itself can be enough to pass the parasites from the system and will not cause a die-off.

You can also suggest an herbal parasite cleanse. Truly, both belief work and a cleanse may be in order. As an herbal parasite cleanse is done, feelings and emotions will come up to be cleared.

Ridding yourself of parasites also helps you to let go of 'emotional parasites' (people who suck you dry) and 'energetic parasites' such as waywards, spiritual hooks, etc.

Parasite Cleanses

Use an herbal parasite cleanse in the spring (not in winter because the body is in a rest period). Doing many herbal parasite cleanses in succession is very hard on the body, so proper discernment of one's health is in order.

If it is found that an herbal cleanse is needed, follow this process: ten days on, five days off, ten days on, five days off, ten days on, five days off. That way you can destroy all the eggs laid by the parasite.

Suggested parasite cleanses for tapeworms and flukes:

- clove
- ionic copper (a very good parasite cleanse, good for tapeworms, but you cannot use it if you have Wilson's disease)
- noni juice or seeds
- oregano oil (which can be hard on the stomach, so put two drops in capsules)
- walnut/wormwood combination (this should not be used by a diabetic)

Herbs and minerals for a parasite cleanse:

Cascara sagrada

cayenne pepper

chamomile

charcoal (kills *Giardia* and other parasites)

Echinacea root

garlic

ginger

noni or ionized copper for pets (10 days on, 5 days off)

olive leaf (kills yeast as well)

platinum (is said to kill all kinds of parasites and yeast)

Colloidal silver kills all kinds of parasites and yeast, but taking it all the time is not a good idea.

Thyme kills parasites in drinking water, as well as *Salmonella* (in very small quantities).

To keep yourself clear of parasites, make up a fresh juice with 2 carrots, 1 stick of celery, half a beetroot, a little garlic and a pinch of ginger.

In the cleansing process, a healing crisis can manifest and bring up the memory of any number of past challenges, such as old infections, toxins, trauma from accidents, and so on. Be aware that these emotions and physical symptoms may feel real, but are only phantoms of the past.

Also, as parasites die off in a cleanse, they can transmit feelings of 'I am dying' to the host, causing the host to believe that they are dying.

It is best to balance a parasite cleanse with an alkaline diet so that the process is not so emotional. If the body has an alkaline balance of 7.2 to 7.4, parasites will have a difficult time surviving.

Belief Work

Do belief work before beginning a cleanse, as this will make the process smoother. Download:

'I know how to live without being sucked dry.'

'I know how to say no.'

'I know when to say no.'

'I know I am connected to the Creator at all times.'

'I know what it feels like to live without parasitical people in my life.'

'I know how to say no to parasitical people with grace and ease.'

'I understand what it feels like to deal with the Earth's vast variety of people without drama.'

'I know the difference between the feelings of my parasites and my own feelings.'

'I know when I am too tired to do something.'

'I know I can live my life without having to be a martyr.'

'I know how to live without giving up all my time and effort to please someone else.'

'I know the person I have to please is the Creator of All That Is.'

'I know how to put good food in my body.'

'I know how to command my body to have the proper pH balance.'

'I know how to live without attracting parasitical people to me.'

See also Worms, below.

VIRUSES

A virus is an infectious agent, small in size and of simple composition, which can multiply only in the living cells of animals, plants or bacteria. The name is from a Latin word meaning simply 'liquid' or 'poison'.

A virus has either RNA or DNA but not both. It uses its host to reproduce itself. For this reason, it is very difficult to destroy a virus. One thing that the body will create to fight off a virus is interferon. This is actually an antiviral protein. It is created in the cell and is designed to interfere with the multiplication process. The human body creates three different types of interferon, alpha, beta and gamma, according to the types of cell that are infected.

Viruses can cause many serious diseases, including several forms of cancer, but on the other hand can remain in a host for long periods of time before actually producing a disease. Some people may never display symptoms. An example would be the herpes virus. Although many people carry this virus, only around 15 percent will ever display symptoms.

Every virus has the ability to quickly mutate to something different in order to survive.

Intuitive Insights

I believe that worthiness issues hold viruses in the body, and some viruses have fear issues associated with them as well. Many people are immune to viral and other sexual diseases, for example, when they feel good about themselves and refuse to accept the disease. This may not have anything to do with how they feel about sex, but rather with how they feel about themselves at the time.

We attract diseases to us in the same way that we draw other people to us, through parallel belief systems. When we have the same belief system as a virus, bacterium, yeast or fungus, it will be attracted to us and attach itself to us. Take a good look at yourself. Do you attract the human equivalent of parasitic energies?

Viruses are drawn to a particular person because they share the same programmes. They have four levels of belief systems, much as humans. They are drawn to the negative attributes of a person, because negativity makes a person weak on all levels, physically, mentally and spiritually. In some instances, they are held and hidden on different belief levels. When you are in a belief work session with a client, there may be a signal that they have a virus.

A virus goes through the cell wall and uses our DNA or RNA to replicate itself so it can get to the nucleus of the cell. I have made a discovery here: I believe there is a kind of micro-plasma organism that attacks the mitochondria and causes disease. It is present in everyone I have seen who has muscular dystrophy. The mitochondria have their own DNA and this must be worked on as well.

Remember that a virus is an alien invader in every cell. Herpes and hepatitis look like little robots when seen intuitively, so it is good to remember that you are not seeing aliens, but viruses, a different type of invader.

The older a virus is, the smarter it is. Younger viruses, such as AIDS, are not very developed, since they kill their host.

Through the symbiosis between host and virus, the virus will learn to send thought forms to the host in an attempt to control it and prolong its own life, for example persuading the person to stop taking the medication that is killing it. Once again, ask the Creator what is truly going on in the situation.

Intuitive Remedies

At one time, I used a tone or vibration from the Sixth Plane to destroy viruses. But I learned that to guard ourselves against them we have to change the beliefs that are drawing them to us and mutate them with belief work at the same time. As viruses are drawn to us because we have the same negative programmes, if you work on your beliefs, the beliefs of the virus will change, too. Changing the belief system of a virus means it does not have to attack us to survive and is thus transmuted into a life form that is harmless to us. We do not want to make viruses our enemy and command that they all be gone, since they could be to our benefit. Rather, we should witness them changed to a form that is harmless.

If a person comes to you with a virus, check to see whether they believe that illness is a punishment or that they should be ill. Ask the Creator of All That Is what feelings to work on so that the virus will change to a form harmless to the host.

Downloads

'I know what it feels like to live being worthy of the Creator's love.'

'I know I am worthy of the Creator's love.'

'I know I am worthy of having a compatible soul mate.'

'I know it is possible to be worthy of the love of a compatible soul mate.'

'I know what it feels like to see truth.'

'I know what the Creator's power is.'

'I know what it feels like to be totally connected to the Creator.'

'I know what it feels like to live without panic.'

'I know what it feels like to trust myself.'

'I know how to live without panic.'

'I know that with the Creator anything is possible.'

'I know that I am worthy and deserve a good life.'

'I know the difference between my feelings and someone else's.'

'I know the difference between my thoughts and someone else's.'

WORMS

When I first began doing body readings, I did a reading on a woman who was very sick. By the time she came in to see me, her hair was a red colour and stiff like wire. She had so many worms coming out of her body that she could pull them from the skin on her arm. They were about a quarter of an inch long. This was one of the most repulsive things I had ever seen.

Her story came out as we talked. It seems that she had become very sick with the infestation and had gone to the doctor. Numerous tests had been carried out, including X-rays. The X-rays of her back had shown dark masses around her spine. The doctor had recommended that exploratory surgery be performed to find out what these anomalies were. The surgeons had found masses of worms wrapped around her spine, obviously a massive parasitical infection of some kind. They had not known what to do for her. They had left the parasites alone, sewed her back up and used radiation and antibiotics in an attempt to kill them. Sadly, this still had not stopped the infestation. So the doctors had sent her home and told her that it was not likely she was going to live.

Enter the last hope for her: alternative medicine.

At this point in time, I was only doing readings and had not begun to do healings, so I made an appointment for her with a naturopath for a parasite cleanse. I did not want to touch her as I was afraid of what I was seeing.

Four to five months later I saw her working as a waitress in a restaurant. Her hair was brown again and her skin was clear. She had used a parasite cleanse and was better. However I did not eat the food she served me.

Though this was an extreme case, worms are more common than most people suppose and they can be the underlying cause of many illnesses. They are more common in children than in adults and are prevalent in people with AIDS, *Candida*, chronic fatigue syndrome and many other disorders.

Worm infestations can cause poor absorption of essential nutrients and loss of blood from the gastrointestinal tract and lead to such deficiency-related disorders as anaemia or growth problems. They can be contracted through a variety of mechanisms, including improper disposal of human or animal waste, walking barefoot on contaminated soil and ingestion of eggs or larvae from uncooked or partially cooked meat. In some instances, eggs may become airborne and be inhaled.

Types

The most common types are hookworms, pinworms, roundworms, tape-worms and threadworms.

Symptoms

Depending upon the worm involved and the severity of infestation, there may be a variety of symptoms:

- *Hookworms* can cause itching on the soles of the feet and in some instances, bloody sputum, fever, rash and loss of appetite.
- *Pinworms* are white threadlike worms about one third of an inch long. They cause severe anal itching, insomnia and restlessness.
- *Roundworms* are shaped like earthworms, only smaller in size. They can easily be seen by the naked eye. Trichinosis is a disease caused by a microscopic roundworm and, if left untreated, can lead to muscle damage and cardiac or neurological complications.
- *Tapeworms* vary in length from an inch to up to 30 feet and can survive for up to 25 years in the body. Small tapeworms can cause abdominal pain, appetite loss, diarrhoea, vomiting and weight loss. Large tapeworms can cause similar symptoms, but usually without weight loss.
- *Threadworms* can cause abdominal pain, bronchitis, coughing, diarrhoea and wind.

Doctors treat most types of worms with pharmaceutical drugs. They do not, however, normally check for parasitical infections. This is why it is up to you to take the initiative and do a parasite cleanse once a year.

Intuitive Insights

People who are infested with worms will sometimes have the irrational fear that should they use herbal cleanses, the herbs will poison them and kill them. This is not the person talking, but rather the parasite projecting its emotions to the host. It should be made clear to the infested person that the parasite is attempting to control them and the feelings that they are experiencing will pass as soon as the worms are gone.

Belief Work

Worms are drawn to people with belief systems that are to do with being taken advantage of. Energy test for:

'I let people take advantage of me.'

'People take advantage of me.'

Replace with:

>'I know how to assert myself.'

>'I know how to say no.'

Downloads

>'I know how to live my life without people taking advantage of me.'

>'I know what it feels like to live my life without allowing others to take my energy.'

>'I know what it feels like to say no in the highest and best way.'

>'I know what it feels like to uplift people when I interact with them.'

>'I know what it feels like to live my life in joy, happiness and spiritual generosity.'

>'I know when I should give and when I should receive.'

Supplements and Other Nutritional Recommendations

* *Aloe vera* juice taken twice daily can stop a worm infestation.
* Black walnut extract destroys many types of worms. Use it on an empty stomach three times per day. Avoid if diabetic.
* Bromelain is a good expectorant of worms, so a regimen of raw pineapple can expel parasites.
* For a severe infestation, a colonic irrigation is said to be beneficial. A professional usually performs this procedure. I am not a fan of this.
* Hanna Kroeger's Wormwood or Rascal cleanses are great! Suggested use is 10 days on, 5 days off, 10 days on, 5 days off again. This cleanse is particularly good for tapeworms. Do not use wormwood during pregnancy or if you have sugar problems.
* If you know you have a worm infestation, good vitamins such as a multivitamin–multimineral combination are important, because the worms are stealing essential nutrients from the body. (Avoid commanding that vital minerals and vitamins be created by the Creator out of air. Without practice, the body does not understand how to assimilate minerals and vitamins in this way; it already absorbs them from food.)
* Pumpkin seeds will kill many different types of worms.
* Remember to have your pets dewormed regularly, as this can be a source of infestation. Noni works on pets.

- Some sushi has been found to be contaminated with a worm-like parasite called antisakis, which can cause illness similar to Crohn's disease if ingested. This parasite is a tightly coiled, clear worm about an inch in length. It is commonly found in herring and other fish. Fortunately, an experienced sushi chef can spot it easily. Wasabi kills it.
- Vitamin B complex is good to strengthen the immune system.
- Wormwood and clove work very well for American worms.
- Zinc clears the waste products left from the die-off of the worms.

YEAST

Yeast requires special mention. It can cause illnesses such as asthma, fatigue, headaches and weakness. It also creates acetaldehyde, which is its waste product. Unable to be broken down by the body, this is simply stored and eventually becomes toxic. Molybdenum will break it down and may need to be taken in small doses.

Yeast craves sugars, as it needs these to survive in the body.

Antibiotics can cause yeast infections.

Intuitive Insights

Intuitively, yeast looks like a dusty, misty or cloudy energy in the body. It is a problem when a person is too critical or resentful towards themselves or others.

An over-abundance of yeast in the body can cause weight gain.

Yeast in the colon affects the sinuses.

Intuitive Remedies

It is not advised to intuitively command all the yeast in a person's body to die. The body needs a certain amount of yeast to function. Alkaline diets are good to control yeast.

Belief Work

Yeast is attracted to and held by anger and resentment issues. Download:

'I know what it feels like to be in a loving environment.'

'I know what it feels like to be appreciated.'

'I know how to live my life without resenting myself and others.'

'I know what it feels like to understand what a person thinks and feels.'

'I know it is safe to see intuitively in the body.'

'I know what it feels like to witness intuitive changes in yeast and fungus.'

FOOD

There are literally thousands of books out there with ideas about food – books that tell you to eat raw meat, books that tell you not to eat sugar, books that tell you not to eat gluten, books that tell you to eat only fruit and books that tell you to eat only vegetables. All these books are based upon an individual person's opinion and what has worked for them. As you explore these opinions, you have to use good common sense. Any diet, herbal supplement or medication must pertain to the individual, because we are all different in our reactions to these substances.

The best thing to do is to go up and ask God what to eat. Ask what is good for your body. When you go out to a restaurant, ask what food on the menu would be most beneficial for you.

Salad bars at restaurants can be dangerous, because fruit and vegetables set out in the open air can accumulate bacteria. Ask the Creator if the salad bar is safe.

CONCERNING FATS AND OILS

Fat is the most abundant substance in the body after water. More than 70 percent of your brain and nerve cells are made of fat, and the membrane of every cell in your body is 30 percent fat. There are about two dozen total fats (lipids) in the body and two, called essential fatty acids, or EFAs, must come from your diet. These two are omega 6 and omega 3. Your cells use EFAs for energy production, your glands use them to make healthy secretions and your immune system is helped by them. They also nourish your skin, hair, mucous membranes and the myelin sheath surrounding your nerves.

Bad Fats
Bad fats are those that are rancid, imbalanced, overly saturated, over-cooked or modified by modern food processing. These include:

- chips
- crisps
- dairy products
- fried food

- margarine
- pastries
- red meat
- shortening

Good Fats

Good fats are those that contain a healthy balance of EFAs and are fresh, unheated and unprocessed. These include:

- beans
- canola oil
- flaxseed
- fresh fish
- fresh vegetables
- lean meats
- olive oil
- pumpkin oil
- seaweed
- seeds
- wholegrains

All fats are needed, even the bad ones, as long as there are more of the good ones. Now that we have gained some background knowledge, we will move on to the diseases and disorders that I have worked with.

ThetaHealing®
Diseases, Disorders and
Associated Beliefs,
A to Z

THE BODY SINGS

The thing to realize about the systems of the body is that they sing to one another. From the smallest cell to the largest organ, the systems of the body are wonderful, even magical, in the way that they work together in an interconnected synchronicity.

When you look into the body and see a single cell, you should listen to how it sings its tiny song of harmony with the rest of the body. When there is something wrong with an organ, you will hear that it doesn't sing true and sends the wrong signals to the other organs. Learn to listen to these vibrations and their signals. Perhaps the body is out of tune or an organ has a challenge in it. You should investigate what is amiss.

Each of the systems of the body must work in harmony with the others for us to function properly. This is why it is so important to realize that if there are diseases and disorders present, it is an indication that there are likely to be mental, emotional or spiritual components that may be factors in the healing process, and that harmony in the body must be restored.

Each system can have beliefs attached. The belief systems that are outlined in the following text are what I have found that people are likely to have, but they are not necessarily the same from person to person. They are an overview from my 47,000 readings with clients and students.

The following list of diseases and disorders includes conventional medical information, intuitive insights, intuitive remedies, associated beliefs, programmes, feelings, supplements and herbal remedies as they pertain to ThetaHealing. I am not diagnosing in any way, only sharing with you what I have witnessed. I do not prescribe medicine or offer a medical diagnosis.

ABUSE – *See the Digestive System and the Reproductive System/Sexual System.*

ADDISON'S DISEASE – *See Adrenal Disorders.*

ADRENAL DISORDERS

The adrenal glands are a pair of triangular-shaped organs that rest on top of the kidneys. The cortex, or outer section, is responsible for the production of hormones called aldosterone, androstenedione, cortisol, cortisone and dehydroepiandrosterone (DHEA). The medulla, or central section, secretes another hormone called adrenaline, also called epinephrine or norepinephrine, which functions both as a hormone and neurotransmitter. Adrenaline, cortisol, DHEA and norepinephrine are the body's major stress hormones. Cortisol is also involved in the metabolism of carbohydrates and the regulation of blood sugar. Aldosterone regulates the salt balance in the body. DHEA and androstenedione are androgens, hormones that are similar to and that can be converted into testosterone.

The adrenals speed up the metabolism to produce other physiologic changes designed to help the body cope with danger. In situations of great stress, excessive amounts of cortisone are released, which can lead to many health problems.

One of these is called Addison's disease. This develops when the adrenals are weak and exhausted. Symptoms include dizziness or fainting, fatigue and loss of appetite. The tissues of the adrenals are attacked and slowly destroyed.

The most common problem associated with Addison's is an underactive thyroid. Addison's disease that is associated with hypothyroidism is called Schmidt's syndrome. Addison's can also occur together with insulin-dependent diabetes mellitus or insufficiencies in the parathyroid glands or pernicious anaemia.

Another adrenal dysfunction is called Cushing's syndrome. This is a rare disorder caused by the excessive production of cortisol or by the excessive use of cortisol (glucocorticoid steroid hormones). A person with Cushing's syndrome is generally heavy in the abdomen and buttocks but has very thin limbs and a rounded 'moon' face. They generally have deep circles under their eyes with round red marks that mimic acne. Other symptoms include depression, fatigue, increased thirst, mood swings and, in women, the absence of menstrual periods. It is not uncommon for people to flip back and forth between Addison's disease and Cushing's syndrome. The over-use of cortisone (prednisone) can cause Cushing's disease.

Intuitive Insights

People who generally have problems with their adrenals will not know how to stop and rest. They try to push themselves too far, believing that they have to save the world.

Issues with the adrenals are generally focused on resentments and regrets. These programmes cycle through the adrenals and possibly cause the beginnings of disease.

Problems with the adrenals start a chain reaction in the body. If the adrenals aren't working right, then the lungs aren't working right. If the lungs aren't working right, then the heart isn't working right. So you may have to work on the lungs at the same time as the adrenals, depending on the severity of the case.

When you're working with Addison's and Cushing's, you need to intuitively check the person to see if there are associated diseases such as diabetes.

Belief Work

Pull any resentment of people, situations and of the self – 'I resent my body', 'I resent my mother', etc. Replace with forgiveness, unconditional love or whatever the Creator says. Dig for the bottom belief and then see how it is serving them; reference advanced digging tape if needed.

Work on issues of fetal stress.

Energy test for these programmes:

'I resent myself for not doing better.'

'I regret that I have not accomplished all my goals.'

'I have to work all the time.'

'I have no time to rest.'

'I am not worthy of rest.'

'I fear resting.'

Download:

'I am worthy of rest.'

'I am worthy of making quick decisions effortlessly.'

'I stand by my word.'

'I live without fear of making decisions.'

'I am allowed to make decisions and change my mind if necessary.'

'I know when I am giving too much of myself.'

'I know when to set boundaries so I can rest.'

'I know what it feels like to be completely healthy and strong.'

'I know when to trust someone.'

'I know when I am too tired to make a good decision.'

'I know I am in charge of my own life and my fate.'

'I know how to control my temper.'

'I know what it feels like to be able to control my temper.'

'I can live without creating extra fear in my life.'

'I know how to live without creating regrets.'

'I know how to stand by my truth.'

'I know what it feels like to have fun.'

'I know what I say is important.'

'I know what it feels like to live without being exhausted.'

'I know what it feels like to be safe.'

For Healers

With many healers, the adrenals are very tired, because they hold the energy of:

'I must save the world.'

'I try to make everyone happy.'

'I have to want to help other people.'

'I have to work myself into a frenzy.'

'For people to love me, I have to take care of them.'

'The world is a cold and harsh place because I have the need
to serve.'

Change these to 'I *choose* to change the world', 'I choose to help other
people', etc. Cradle the adrenals with unconditional love and energy from
the Creator. Download:

'I know what it feels like to be happy.'

'I know what it feels like to rest.'

'I know what it feels like to know I am getting stronger.'

'It's OK to be happy.'

'I can live without regret.'

'I can create and stand by my truth.'

'I can do better, but I understand that I have done my best.'

'I know what it feels like to live without feeling the world is harsh.'

'I know what it feels like to live without feeling that I cannot go on.'

'I know what it feels like to be happy to be alive.'

'Every breath is filled with energy.'

'Every breath is filled with love for myself and others.'

'I know how to live in this moment and in this day with happiness.'

'I know how to hold on to this happiness.'

'I know how to hold onto my connection to the Creator.'

'I know what it feels like to live without others taking all my energy.'

'It is easy for me to send love and energy to people without feeling
drained.'

'I know what it feels like to make decisions quickly and effortlessly.'

'I can follow through.'

'I know what it feels like to change my mind if I need to.'

'I know how to stand by my decisions.'

'I know what it feels like to stand by my word.'

Supplements and Other Nutritional Recommendations

For exhausted adrenals, DHEA and pregnenolone are suggested, unless you have or have had breast cancer or any other type of reproductive cancer. Many doctors prescribe DHEA to help the adrenals recover. The suggested dose is 50 milligrams (mg) for a woman and 100 milligrams for a man. It is best to slowly taper off DHEA, so that the body starts producing it again. In most instances, it will begin to have an effect in about two weeks, unless you are using cortisone.

It is also important to alkalize the body.

Also useful:

- ALA, 300–600 mg
- fresh fruit and vegetables, particularly onions
- omega 3s
- salmon and fish – anything with naturally occurring omega 3s
- spirulina

Liquorice Root

An important thing to remember with people using glucocorticoid steroids is that you should never suggest that they use liquorice root to stimulate the adrenals. This can cause a reaction such as adrenal failure, a heart attack, high blood pressure or a stroke. You should tell the person the dangers of using these substances together.

AGE SPOTS

Age spots are generally caused by lack of exercise or problems in the liver. If you have problems in the liver, they will show up on your skin within three months. So if you have age spots on your skin, there is something going on inside. In fact, most of the difficulties with the skin begin with beliefs that are held in the liver.

Belief Work

The Theta practitioner can do healing work to clean up the age spots, but it is important to clean up the liver. The liver holds old anger. If it is diseased with cirrhosis, the person will anger quickly. It also has old programmes of stored hate. People with liver diseases need to let go of hate in order to be well.

Enegy test for issues of anger, fear, guilt, old abuse, resentment and the inability to accept love. Download:

'I know how to live without fear.'

'I know what it feels like to live without fear.'

'I know how to live without resentment.'

'I know the Creator's definition of what it feels like to be safe.'

· 'I know the Creator's definition of what it feels like to be protected.'

'I know the Creator's definition of what it feels like to be secure.'

Supplements

It is suggested that you begin to clean up the liver using ALA, milk thistle and a little bit of selenium.

See also the Liver.

AGING

There are many wonderful books about aging telling you that your body is programmed to age because of free radicals in the environment. Many people are unsure what a free radical is, so let me explain.

Inside your cells you have mitochondria, which hold ATP, the energy for the cells. Any time that the cells release ATP, they also release an extra oxygen molecule called a free radical. This is a waste product. It can float around and actually cause destruction inside the cell, unless there is an antioxidant present. If so, the antioxidant will attach to the oxygen molecule/free radical and make it harmless.

If, on the other hand, the free radical bumps into the DNA several times, it can cause permanent destruction. If the DNA has any major damage, the cell will not be able to reproduce successfully and it will self-destruct. This is one way that people get older.

Many of the cells in our body self-destruct because of free radical damage. There are other ways that the cells are damaged (such as heavy-metal poisoning), but the key to preventing cell damage and thus aging is to take as many antioxidants as possible.

In the following exercise we will send a message to the receptors of the cells to constantly regenerate and to stop aging.

The Process for Changing Genetic Programmes for Aging

1   Centre yourself in your heart and visualize going down into Mother Earth, which is a part of All That Is. Visualize bringing up the energy through your feet, opening each chakra to the crown chakra. In a beautiful ball of light, go out to the universe.

2   Go beyond the universe, past the white lights, past the dark light, past the white light, through the gold light, past the jelly-like substance that is the Laws, into a pearly iridescent white light, into the Seventh Plane of Existence.

3   Go into the person's space into the pineal gland, to the central cell.

4   Make the command: *'Creator of All That Is, it is commanded that all genetic programmes in* [name person] *for aging be pulled and cancelled, sent to the Creator's light, replaced with the programme of "I am young and ageless, forever regenerating", for all present and future bodies, to be replaced all through the body. Thank you! It is done. It is done. It is done. Show me.'*

5   Witness the process. Stay in the person's space until the process is finished.

6   Rinse yourself off and put yourself back into your space. Go into the Earth, pull the Earth energy up through all your chakras to your crown chakra and make an energy break, or remain in the Seventh Plane of Existence where you are in perfect balance.

After this exercise, the person may feel unwell for a few days, as the body will go through a detoxification process. To avoid this, use calcium–magnesium and chelated zinc.

Belief Work

Check for:

'I will get old.'

'No one will need me.'

'Retirement means that I am old.'

Download:

> 'I am forever young.'
>
> 'My body is young.'
>
> 'My body is beautiful.'
>
> 'I regenerate easily.'
>
> 'I live without regret.'
>
> 'I am rested.'
>
> 'I care about my body.'
>
> 'I know what it feels like for my body to regenerate easily.'
>
> 'It's easy to see myself as young and beautiful.'
>
> 'I am happy with the way I look.'
>
> 'I am attractive.'

Supplements and Other Nutritional Recommendations

- ALA
- an amino-acid complex
- glutathione
- noni, five days on and two days off
- vitamin B complex

***

- Avoid smoking, because smoking destroys cells.
- Following *The Complete System of Self-Healing: Internal Exercises* by Dr Stephen T. Chang (Atlantic Books, 1986) will promote youthfulness.
- Omega 3s, 6s and 9s are very important to repair the skin. Omega 3s create serotonin and omega 6s create oestrogen. Omega 3s, 6s and 9s are good for the function of the brain and the whole body.
- Also, remember to bless your food when you eat. And don't waste your life and the precious moments of pleasure eating things you don't like. Natural, live foods are always better, but understand that if you are compulsively fussing about every little thing that you eat, you are not living. Eat wholesome foods that bring you joy.

AIDS–HIV

The AIDS and HIV virus diminishes the immune system so that the person dies from viral and bacterial infections or possible cancers.

What happens is the virus starts out as HIV. HIV gets into the T-cells, forcing the body to make new T-cells to keep the immune system going. Eventually it is completely exhausted and is no longer able to defend itself.

There are many risks for people who have HIV. They have to be very careful of colds and 'flu, for example, because a bad cold or 'flu can be detrimental to their body.

For the most part, HIV–AIDS is transferred by sex, contact with bodily fluids, open wounds, drug use and, in the past, blood transfusion. The healer needs to understand that there are only certain conditions in which they can catch HIV–AIDS. However, it is important to take precautions. You need to be extremely careful whenever there is blood present.

Symptoms

Some of the symptoms a person is going to have when they first get HIV are:

- a persistent cough
- *Candida* problems
- diarrhoea-constipation
- fatigue
- fevers that last up to 10 days
- headaches
- swollen lymphatic glands
- weight loss

Other more pronounced diseases caused by advanced AIDS are:

- Candidial oesophagitis
- cryptosporidiosis
- herpes simplex
- Kaposi's sarcoma
- lymphoma
- pneumonia
- toxoplasmosis of the brain

Intuitive Insights

HIV is like a caterpillar chrysalis, and AIDS is the full-blown vampiric butterfly. When HIV changes into AIDS, even its DNA is different. When it turns into AIDS you are playing with a mean, nasty virus. It's very rude, by the way. So don't go in and expect to chat to AIDS. HIV, on the other hand, will talk to you. AIDS will broadcast thought forms like 'This is where I am.'

HIV is a young virus. If it were an old virus, it would know that it wasn't supposed to kill the people it infected. Old viruses have this kind of wisdom. They might make a person sick, but on the whole do not attempt to kill them. The young ones, they're renegades. Hanta virus is a young virus as well. It's evolved enough not to kill mice, but not enough not to kill the human carriers. The older that HIV–AIDS gets, the better our bodies will learn how to fight it. They will learn how to stop HIV from turning into AIDS.

What is happening now is that children are developing an immunity to HIV and their systems are killing the virus. So in my view it will not be that much longer before AIDS is not a problem anymore. I think the reason that it got out of control was that it was a man-made virus. So it evolved and spread faster than if it had started naturally.

It is interesting to note how many people actually do have HIV–AIDS.

When you go into the body of a client with HIV in a reading, you will notice that it is very quiet. One of the indications that HIV is present is that the blood appears to be milky. Most of the clients will already know they have HIV. They will come out and tell you so.

Intuitive Remedies

I find that AIDS responds to healings very quickly. HIV responds to healings quickly, too, but if you don't get results with it, you have to find out what belief systems are being held there. You can command the virus to be gone from the person's body, but they still have to feel they are worthy of accepting the healing. They may have many punishment issues. But a lot of it is the desperation of wanting to live. They are so desperate that they are clinging onto life like a drowning person clutching at straws.

In fact, HIV–AIDS comes with so much fear attached to it that the healer can become afraid. If you find that you have a fear of HIV–AIDS, you need to release it and replace it.

I don't claim to have healed people of HIV or AIDS. But if they have been clear of the virus for five years and had a clean bill of health for five years, then the Creator has healed them. Avoid taking credit for what God does.

In the early years I devised an intuitive technique through observing that every living thing had its own vibration and emitted a certain tone. After listening to the organs singing to one another, I began to listen to the cells to see if they did the same thing. What I found out was that they *did* sing to one another. This led me to believe that perhaps viruses, bacteria and fungi might do the same thing. I began to listen to the tones that they sang to the body. Then I came up with the idea that if I went out of my space to bring a matching tone into the body and then played the exact opposite tone, I would be able to kill the virus. For the time, this was a great idea and I began to use this technique on people with HIV–AIDS. It raised the T-cell count in almost every person, but the AIDS virus did not completely go away.

One day, in a moment of frustration when I found out that one of my clients with AIDS still had the virus, I heard the Creator say, 'Why didn't you ask me what needed to be done?'

It took a moment to adjust to this because I had thought I had come up with the best conclusion. I swallowed my pride and asked, 'OK, God, what needs to be done?'

I was told that diseases such as herpes and AIDS were held by a symbiotic relationship because of the matching belief systems of both the host and the virus. If the person were ready to let the virus go, they would heal immediately.

I began to ask the Creator to heal people with HIV and AIDS and witnessed them healing immediately. Then I worked on the belief systems that were associated with the disease. We had people who were dying of AIDS, unable to get up out of bed, planting flowers in their garden the next day.

I started listening to the belief systems that came up in sessions that related to HIV–AIDS and this is what I found: people hold on to their HIV. You would think that would be because of the partner who gave it to them, and with a small percentage this is the case, but what I found was that the majority thought HIV was serving them in some way. Specifically, it was teaching them *spirituality*. It was teaching them to appreciate everything in life. They had actually become so dependent on the virus that they were afraid that if it were gone, they would go back to their old ways.

Resentment can also be a factor. For instance, I worked on HIV in a man who had contracted the disease from his sweetheart. He definitely had a great deal of resentment toward that person. Even though his viral load was low and his T-cell count was good, the virus had not gone completely. So we worked on resentment issues.

Here's the other key: the disease was broadcasting thought forms to him. It was telling him, 'Without me, you wouldn't be this spiritual. Without me, you wouldn't be a good person. Look at all that I have done for you!' It was making him feel that it was truly his friend.

So I asked him, 'What will you do when you're free of this?'

He said, 'I am afraid that I'll go back to the way that I was.'

At that point I knew I had to pull the 'I have to have this disease in order to get close to God' programme.

What was amazing was what he said next: 'I'm really comfortable with this disease. It doesn't bother me. I have it under control and as long as I know that I have to keep it under control, that's good for me.'

With HIV–AIDS, be aware that it is possible the client will fight you to keep the disease.

Belief Work

You need to ask every single person that you work on with HIV the important question: 'What has HIV done for you?' Amazingly enough, you will often hear them say:

'I am a better person.'

'I take better care of myself.'

'I'm more conscious.'

'Without HIV, I will go back to the way I was.'

It is the disease itself that is telling them that they need it. Some of the things that HIV tells the host are:

'Because of me, your life has changed.'

'Because of me, you are a better person.'

'Because of me, you take better care of yourself.'

'I'm here to help you.'

'I'm here to be with you.'

'I'm here for your own good.'

So, ask the person what the disease is doing to serve them. They will come up with some really good reasons!

If you don't pull the belief that they have to have HIV–AIDS and the associated programmes, that it will make them a better person or enable them to have a better life, then you are missing the belief system that holds the disease to them.

Releasing the programmes . . .

'I am afraid that without HIV I will become reckless.'

'Without HIV, I will destroy myself.'

'I am being punished with AIDS.'

. . . will often drop the viral load in the body. But HIV–AIDS is an incredibly intelligent virus. It realizes that if the person believes they need it, their body-mind and spirit will not fight it as much. So download:

'I can live without HIV.'

'I can still be a good person without HIV.'

'I can be good to my body without HIV.'

'I can appreciate my body without HIV.'

'I can make a difference without HIV.'

'I know what it feels like to appreciate what HIV has done to serve me.'

'I am now ready to learn the spiritual lessons of life without the HIV virus.'

'With good thoughts, I thank HIV and send it away.'

'I know I can take good care of my body without HIV.'

'I know what it feels like to be strong, healthy and full of energy.'

'I know what it feels like to put good things in my body.'

'I know how to live without using illegal drugs.'

'I know what it feels like to live without the shame of having HIV.'

'I know it is possible to be completely cured of HIV.'

'I know what it feels like to live and know that my body is getting stronger every day.'

'I know what it feels like to know I am a good person.'

'I am accountable for my body without HIV.'

'I know what it feels like to have a relationship based on love.'

'I know what it feels like to know I have no viral load.'

'I know what it feels like to live without this disease.'

'I know how to get close to the Creator without HIV.'

'I know I am worthy of a complete healing.'

'I know my family believes I am worthy of a complete healing.'

'I know to live without having to suffer to please my family.'

'I know how to live without guilt in relationships.'

'I know how to forgive myself and allow myself to move forward.'

'I know how to forgive myself for not loving my body.'

'I know it's possible to love my body.'

'I know it's possible to be happy.'

Make sure the person knows they can live without the disease and still be close to God:

'I understand how to be close to God without HIV–AIDS.'

'I know what it feels like to live close to God without HIV–AIDS.'

Remove the group consciousness that HIV–AIDS is incurable. Pull the belief 'I need you for spiritual growth' from both the person and virus.

HIV in little children is easy to heal, but if they comprehend that they have HIV–AIDS, they may think they have contracted the disease because they have to take on the 'sins of the father or mother'. You may have to work on this belief system.

At no time do we ever discourage anyone with HIV–AIDS from going to the doctor to be checked. We want them to go to the doctor to see results.

Also, never discourage anyone with HIV–AIDS from using a drug that may help their immune system.

Supplements

A person who has AIDS should keep up on all their vitamins and minerals. Other important supplements are:

- ALA, 600–1,200 mg
- cat's claw
- DHEA
- Echinacea (high doses have been shown to lower viral loads)
- mixtures of amino acids
- proflavanols
- selenium, 250 mcg

- vitamin B complex
- vitamin C

ALCOHOLISM

Once alcohol gets through the blood–brain barrier, it causes the brain to release endorphins and dopamine. In normal situations it's very important that the pleasure centres of the brain reward us. For example, when we are hungry, we get pleasure from eating food. However, alcohol abuse can have toxic effects.

Up until recently, alcohol abuse was thought to create these effects by dissolving the brain tissue. It does have this effect, but not the way we once thought it did. It dissolves both water and fat, the two components of brain cells, forcing these cells to produce emotions ranging from euphoria to depression or from calmness to aggression.

We know that there is not one alcoholism gene, but there are some disturbances in mutated genes that make people more prone to alcoholism. The tendency is definitely present when there is a low level of serotonin in the body.

There are some good things alcohol does. If you're an occasional drinker, it can lower your cholesterol. Small doses can prevent clogging of your arteries, prevent blood clots and actually ease menopause and reduce the risk of heart disease. If you drink just a small amount each day, it can stimulate your brain to function better.

However, drinking to excess can cause enormous brain damage. It can cause the brain to shut down millions and millions of neurons, and this can have a devastating effect. Russian men, for instance, drink the equivalent of three and a half bottles of vodka a week, and their life expectancy is about 55 years.

Alcoholics also have a tendency toward malnutrition and do not absorb their folic acid correctly. Long-term alcohol abuse can create pancreatic difficulties, liver dysfunction and diabetes. Alcoholics do not get enough REM sleep.

Intuitive Insights

Too much drug use of any sort will cause various changes in the brain. When you go into the brain to repair these changes, you will start changing the neurons around and command the serotonin levels to change. This will create a difference in the need for the particular substance the person is addicted to.

One thing that is important to understand about alcoholics is that so many receptors are being turned off and turned on with the use of alcohol that when it is no longer used the serotonin levels will fluctuate a great deal. People who have been alcoholics for many years will go back to how they were before. So, if they began drinking at 18 and quit at 40, in certain ways their brain will go back to that of an 18-year-old, making them a little immature until their brain catches up with itself. This is why sometimes people who have had great addictions and have recovered from them find life a little more difficult.

The fact that alcohol can make people depressed is also something to consider.

Intuitive Remedies

When working with an alcoholic, it is important that they want to get better. You cannot work with an alcoholic who does not genuinely want to recover. To balance the brain chemicals, go into the brain and witness the serotonin and the dopamine levels being balanced with the following process:

The Process for Normalizing Brain Chemicals

1   Centre yourself in your heart and visualize going down into Mother Earth, which is a part of All That Is.

2   Visualize bringing up the energy through your feet, opening each chakra to the crown chakra. In a beautiful ball of light, go out to the universe.

3   Go beyond the universe, past the white lights, through the gold light, past the dark light, past the white light, past the jelly-like substance that is the Laws, into a pearly iridescent white light, into the Seventh Plane of Existence.

4   Make the command, 'Creator of All That Is, it is commanded that [name the person]'s noradrenaline, serotonin and hormone levels be balanced in the highest and best way, as is appropriate at this time. Thank you! It is done. It is done. It is done.'

5   Move your consciousness over to the person's space. Go into the brain and witness the noradrenaline/serotonin levels as a graph. Witness the levels becoming balanced as is proper for the person.

6   As soon as the process is finished, rinse yourself off and put yourself back into your space. Go into the Earth and pull the Earth energy up through all your chakras to your crown chakra and make an energy break.

Release the programme of 'I am addicted to alcohol' and replace it with what the Creator tells you. Ask the Creator what to do.

When the person stops their use of alcohol, there is the need to prepare for some kind of withdrawal, because the brain receptors that were quieted down from the overuse of alcohol are suddenly awakened. It takes a while for the brain to adjust. For a full recovery, it is important that the alcoholic has a support team to help them through the first stages.

Alcoholics have a tendency to lose soul fragments during heavy abuse. It can be beneficial to call back any lost soul fragments, washed and cleaned, to them.

The Process for Retrieving Soul Fragments

1   Centre yourself in your heart and visualize yourself going down into Mother Earth, which is part of All That Is.

2   Visualize bringing up energy through your feet, opening up all of your chakras as you go. Continue going up out of your crown chakra in a beautiful ball of light, out to the universe.

3   Go beyond the universe, past the white lights, past the dark light, past the white light, past the gold light, past the jelly-like substance that is the Laws, into a pearly iridescent white light, into the Seventh Plane of Existence.

4   Make the command: *'Creator of All That Is, it is commanded that the history programme of "I love myself, no" be pulled from [person's name], resolved and sent to God's light, and that all soul fragments be washed and cleaned and replaced with "I love myself". Thank you! It is done. It is done. It is done.'*

5   To witness this, you must command to be taken to the history level by saying, *'Creator of All That Is, it is commanded to be taken to the history level of* [person's name].' You will be taken to a place that is a little above the person's head and shoulders and you will actually see memories of their past lives, or humankind's history, flash before you. This is the auric

field around the body, where the energy is resolved. It is very important when working on this level to remember what issues you are working on. This level is seductive in its beauty. When going into past-life memories, there will be visions and an incredible amount of information. It is easy to be overwhelmed and forget why you are there. Stay focused upon the issue at hand.

6   Witness the energy of the programme of 'I love myself, no' being pulled, resolved and sent to God's light and all soul fragments being washed, cleaned and replaced with the new programme 'I love myself.'

7   As soon as you envision the process as finished, rinse yourself off. Put yourself back into your space, ground to the Earth, draw Earth energy up to your crown chakra and make an energy break.

Alcoholics are also prone to free-floating memories.

The Process to Pull All Free-Floating Memories

1   Centre yourself in your heart and visualize yourself going down into Mother Earth, which is part of All That Is.

2   Visualize bringing up energy through your feet, opening up all of your chakras as you go. Continue going up out of your crown chakra in a beautiful ball of light, out to the universe.

3   Go beyond the universe, past the white lights, past the dark light, past the white light, past the gold light, past the jelly-like substance that is the Laws, into a pearly iridescent white light, into the Seventh Plane of Existence.

4   Gather unconditional love and make the command: *'Creator of All That Is, it is commanded that any free-floating memory that no longer serves this person be pulled, cancelled and sent to your light in the highest and best way and replaced with your love. Thank you. It is done. It is done. It is done.'*

5   Move your consciousness over to the head of the client and witness the healing taking place. Watch as the old memories are sent to the Creator's light and the new energy from the Creator replaces the old.

6   As soon as you envision the process as finished, rinse yourself off. Put yourself back into your space, ground to the Earth, draw Earth energy up to your crown chakra and make an energy break.

Also use the following exercises with an alcoholic:

*   'Healing the Broken Soul' (*see Cancer*)
*   'Sending Love to the Baby in the Womb' (*see Cancer*)
*   'The Heart Song' (*see Cardiovascular Disease*)

You may see the spirits flying to God's light when you do the 'Healing the Broken Soul' exercise.

Belief Work

Check for:

'I want to feel numb.'

'The pain of life is too much to bear.'

'The world is too difficult.'

'I avoid responsibility.'

'I am not good enough.'

Download:

'I understand how to live without alcohol.'

'I know it's possible to live without alcohol.'

'Every day in every way I grow better and stronger.'

'Every day in every way I take care of my body, mind and spirit.'

'I can get close to God without having to suffer.'

'I know what it feels like to be alcohol-free.'

'I know it is possible to have a good time without alcohol.'

'I know what it feels like to express my feelings without alcohol.'

'I know what it feels like to live without using alcohol as a crutch.'

'I know what it feels like to have friends without alcohol.'

'I know how to live my day-to-day life without alcohol.'

'I know how to enjoy life.'

'I have my spirit back.'

Supplements

- ALA
- amino acids
- folic acid
- glutathione
- oxygen therapy
- vitamin B complex
- vitamin C

See also Drug Abuse.

ALLERGIES

An allergy refers to an exaggerated reaction by the immune system in response to contact with certain foreign substances. Allergy-producing substances are called allergens. Examples include dust mites, food, mould, pet dander and pollen. People who are prone to allergies are said to be allergic or atopic.

The immune system is the body's organized defence mechanism against foreign invaders, particularly infections, which are called antigens. The aim of the immune system is to mobilize its forces at the site of invasion and destroy the enemy. One of the ways it does this is to create protective proteins called antibodies that are specifically targeted against particular antigens. These antibodies attach to the surface of the foreign substance, thereby making it easier for other immune cells to destroy it. The allergic person, however, develops a specific type of antibody in response to a normally harmless foreign substance and creates an over-abundance of this antibody, causing the overproduction of histamine and other chemicals. These chemicals in turn cause inflammation and the typical allergic symptoms. This is how the immune system becomes primed to cause an allergic reaction when stimulated by an allergen.

The person suffering from allergies should experiment with their diet because they may have a food allergy. Some people are even allergic to meat. Red and yellow dyes are two of the most prevalent allergens in our environment because they are in our food. Food preservatives can also be the cause of allergies.

Some people are allergic to aspirin, but on the other hand, taking small amounts of aspirin can clear allergies.

The best way to prevent the formation of allergies is to permit your children to play in the dirt. Let them get used to their environment. One of the ways in which people develop allergies is by moving to a completely different environment that the body is not used to.

Allergies seem to be more prevalent in people with a high level of *Candida* in their body.

Allergic reactions can be very dangerous. Some people can go into what is called anaphylactic shock, where, as well as other symptoms, swelling in the throat can block their airways. They should be taken immediately to hospital. Do healings on them all the way there.

Belief Work

For people with allergies, I work on resentment and anger issues. These are yeast related.

A good intuitive guideline is to go up and ask if something is offending the person. Then you should begin to test for the things in their everyday life such as 'I am offended by cats' (to be replaced with 'It is safe to be around cats').

Place the allergen in the person's hand and energy test them to see if it offends them. Then go to the Creator of All That Is and teach them what it feels like to be able to live with it.

Allergies seem to be closely connected to the past life or history level. Trace back though the person's timeline to find out when the symptoms first began. Ask what they were feeling and what was happening when they began to have allergic symptoms and explore the related beliefs from these incidents.

Teach the person what it feels like to live in their environment.

Supplements

- Acidophilus and ALA (to break down and digest food) are useful supplements for someone who has allergies.
- Ephedra (Chinese Ma Huang) can help allergies in some situations, but you must be very careful using it, particularly with those with heart problems.
- If the person is taking conventional medication, this should be supported by certain vitamins because most of the allergy medications have side-effects that strip vital minerals and vitamins. Vitamin A

and vitamin C are very important to help with allergies. Too much vitamin C is bad for the kidneys, but 5,000–7,000 mg daily is good for someone with allergies and can stop a runny nose. Take at intervals throughout the day, as the body will not break down more than 2,000 mg of vitamin C at a time.

- Quercetin helps in some situations, but only if the person is not taking allergy medication.
- Stinging nettle is one of the best things that I have found for allergies.
- Zinc is beneficial in doses recommended on the bottle.

Hay Fever

Hay fever is an allergic response to pollen or mould that affects the mucous membranes of the nose, eyes and air passages. Animal hair, dust, feathers, fungus and spores can also trigger the symptoms.

There are three different hay-fever seasons. Tree pollens come first, between February and May in the northern hemisphere. Weed and grass pollens are next, later in the spring and summer. In the autumn, ragweed pollen is prevalent.

People who suffer from hay fever can also have disorders such as asthma and dermatitis. Those who suffer from hay fever throughout the year are said to have perennial rhinitis.

Symptoms

Symptoms include:

- fatigue
- itchy eyes
- nervous irritability
- sneezing
- watery discharge from the nose

Symptoms differ from those of the common cold in that a clear thin nasal discharge is typical with allergies, as opposed to the thick yellow-green discharge of bacterial infections.

Remedies

- A study at the University of California found that eating yogurt every day reduced the incidence of hay-fever attacks.

- Antihistamines are the most commonly recommended conventional treatment for hay fever. They can reduce itching in the eyes, ears and throat and dry up a runny nose. However, they also cause drowsiness and depression and have other side-effects. It is not advisable to use antihistamines with grapefruit juice, as this could cause a reaction.
- Avoid alcohol and cigarette smoke.
- Keep the windows closed during the day with the air conditioner on to filter the air.
- Use an air purifier in your home.

Supplements

- Noni is a good supplement for hay fever, but you should use it only by itself, as it will inhibit other herbs.
- Simply taking molybdenum and using a yeast cleanse can help with hay fever.

ALZHEIMER'S DISEASE

Alzheimer's disease (AD) is a slowly progressive disease of the brain that is characterized by impairment of memory and eventually by disturbances in reasoning, planning, language and perception. Many scientists believe that it results from an increase in the production or accumulation of beta-amyloid protein in the brain, leading to nerve-cell death.

Intuitive Insights

More than a few people who come in to see me thinking they have Alzheimer's really only have a lack of magnesium or other minerals. I know that dementia can be caused by a lack of magnesium.

I believe Alzheimer's is caused by heavy-metal poisoning, so the more you cleanse the person of heavy metals, the clearer their mind is going to get. Some people believe that Alzheimer's is a gift from the gods to take them back to times when life was easier. I say it's a gift of heavy metals and that you should pull it out.

I believe that one of the causes of Alzheimer's is aluminium poisoning from containers and cooking implements, not to mention poisoning from over-the-counter medicines such as antacids. The aluminium interferes with the dopamine receptors. There has been scientific evidence that supports this view.

With Alzheimer's, I also know that you have to work with the family. By the time a person has Alzheimer's, the disorder will be causing a lot of stress in the family, so you may have to work with everyone involved.

Belief Work

When you start working with Alzheimer's, you are going to experience a lot of odd opinions about it, so you may need to convince the children that 'It's OK to take care of my parent in the highest and best way.'

Some parents with Alzheimer's have treated their children badly in the past. When the children are stuck with the responsibility of taking care of the parent, it pushes them right over the edge, since they never had a decent relationship with them in the first place. Even when there is a good relationship, when older people become ill, the stress can make their children ill too. They are totally overwhelmed. You are usually dealing with two or three illnesses by the time you get a client with Alzheimer's – in the children and the parent.

In some instances the person with Alzheimer's is simply afraid of being helpless and having to have someone take care of them and they draw that set of circumstances right to them.

Before you start working on these people, you need to make sure that they have really good vitamins and minerals, especially when it comes to the brain, because their symptoms may not be due to Alzheimer's at all but vitamin and mineral deficiency.

Belief Work

Check for:

'The best part of my life is over.'

'The past is better than the present.'

'I live in the past.'

'The future is too much to bear.'

Download:

'I know what it feels like to be healthy and strong.'

'I know what it feels like to live my life without being trapped.'

'I know what it feels like to live my life being responsible for everything I do.'

'I know what it feels like to take responsibility for myself.'

'I know what it feels like to allow others to take care of me in a good way.'

'I know what it feels like to have my physical independence.'

'I know what it feels like to live without the fear of this disease.'

'I know what it feels like to witness this disease as it disappears.'

'I know what it feels like to live without the stereotype of this disease.'

'I know what it feels like for my brain to work perfectly.'

Supplements and Other Nutritional Recommendations

- ALA
- amino acids such as tyrosine and creatine
- beta carotene (for memory loss)
- calcium–magnesium
- CoQ10
- DHEA
- magnesium (for memory loss)
- vitamin B complex
- vitamin C, 3,000 units a day
- vitamin E

- Glutathione injections and alpha-lipoic acid are suggested. These clean up heavy metals fast and pull toxins out of the brain.
- Do three to four liver cleanses (*see the Liver*) to pull out heavy metals.

ANAEMIA

In and of itself, anaemia, insufficient red blood cells, is not a disease but a symptom of other diseases, including bone-marrow diseases, Crohn's disease, dietary deficiencies, haemorrhoids, hereditary disorders, hormonal disorders, rheumatoid arthritis and ulcers.

Anaemia can also result from B12 levels in the body being depleted. Most anaemia is caused by iron deficiency, which is most prevalent in women.

Generally speaking, men need to be careful if they use iron as a supplement, because their liver does not process it in the same way that a woman's does. I don't usually suggest someone use iron unless they have checked with their doctor first. I usually work with the diseases that cause the anaemia.

Intuitive Remedies

Some of the beliefs associated with the blood have to do with communication. The person will have a difficult time communicating with you, or with anyone for that matter. They will be in denial and tell you that everything in their life is fine.
Download:

'I know that life is joyful and fun.'

'I understand how to communicate well.'

I understand what it feels like to communicate well.'

Supplements

- B-complex vitamins are important.
- Many herbal books suggest the use of goldenseal for anaemia, but you need to be very careful with it and cannot use it for very long. Only one week of use is recommended, and people who are diabetic should not use it at all.
- Stinging nettle is very good for those with anaemia since it has many vitamins and minerals that they need.

Sickle-Cell Anaemia

Sickle-cell anaemia is an inherited blood disorder that mostly affects people of African ancestry, but also occurs in other ethnic groups, including people of Mediterranean and Middle Eastern descent.

The disease affects haemoglobin, the protein found in red blood cells that helps carry oxygen throughout the body, and occurs when a person inherits two abnormal genes (one from each parent) that cause their red blood cells to change shape. Instead of being flexible and disc-shaped, these cells are stiffer and curved in the shape of the old farm tool known as a sickle. This is where the disease gets its name. It is an inability to create a specific amino-acid chain.

If both parents are born with this genetic tendency, they will pass sickle cell on to one out of four children, but the other three will be immune to malaria.

Intuitive Remedies

Ask the Creator if gene work needs to be done. If so, command it to be done and witness the Creator making the changes. Sickle-cell anaemia is easy to repair. Because blood changes quickly in a healing, you can see the immediate effects of the work. The changes in the brain cells and the blood happen almost instantly. The deeper you are in Theta, the better the healing. Be sure to connect to the Seventh Plane.

Belief Work

With sickle-cell anaemia, generally little belief work needs doing. When there is belief work to be done, it will be related to hereditary issues, such as how the person feels about their parents and their ancestors.

ANOREXIA NERVOSA/BULIMIA

Anorexia nervosa is characterized as a psychological disorder. People with it have an intense fear of becoming obese. In many instances they will eat food, only to go to the bathroom afterwards and induce vomiting. This is bulimia.

In extreme cases, the person refuses to eat at all. They have negative feelings about the way they look, are obsessed with exercise and begin to lose their hair due to vitamin and mineral loss.

A person who has anorexia nervosa and bulimia is very good at hiding their disease from the world. In fact, hiding the disease is part of the disease.

Intuitive Remedies

I found that most people who have anorexia have a lack of magnesium. It seems that they need to have magnesium before a healing can be done on them.

Convincing the person that they need vitamins and minerals is one of the biggest challenges you face. One of the best ways that I have found to get nutrition into their bodies is to convince them to use protein drinks that have vitamins, minerals and amino acids in combination. Since it is a drink, it is more likely that they will use it and less likely that they will throw it up afterwards.

Belief Work

It is important that the person genuinely wants to be helped. It is very difficult to help someone with anorexia who is dragged to see you by another person. If they do not want help, you can work on their belief systems for hours and not accomplish a single thing.

Most of their beliefs are associated with 'beauty' and how the world sees them, but also with the way that they absorb life and the way that they feel about life.

People with this disease have a tendency to blame their parents, their healer, their doctors or anyone else it is possible for them to blame for the way that they are.

If the parent is too controlling, the individual with anorexia nervosa will develop the disorder as a last stand to maintain their own power. Energy test for this and replace it with what the Creator tells you.

ARTHRITIS

A woman once came into my office because of large calcium deposits on her knees that were causing her to have arthritis-like symptoms. She was an incredible woman. She told me that she had never eaten processed sugar or white flour and had been healthy all her life. She had recently gone to a chiropractor and he had given her oyster-shell calcium. After taking this for a while, she had begun to develop large calcium deposits.

When I went into her space, I felt that this was because her body was not properly breaking down the supplement. I suggested that she discontinue her use of the oyster-shell calcium and instead use the carrot juice she had been drinking all her life.

Within two weeks, the nodules she had developed were gone. The usable calcium in the carrot juice had broken down the unobtainable calcium caused by the oyster-shell calcium.

As you can see, the woman never really had arthritis at all, but arthritis-like symptoms. Other conditions can create arthritis-like symptoms too, so it is better to not assume anything because of outward appearances.

Types

The three main types of arthritis that I have worked with are osteoarthritis, rheumatoid arthritis and psoriatic arthritis.

- Osteoarthritis is mostly the result of wear and tear on the joints of the body. It reacts well to healings.
- Psoriatic arthritis and rheumatoid arthritis are auto-immune disorders.

Intuitive Insights

When you are doing a body scan on a person with rheumatoid arthritis, you will see that there are tiny little cells moving at high speeds inside the joints. You will sense that there is something inside the joints and that the immune system is after it. It is my opinion that there is a micro-organism inside the joints and the immune system is going crazy to stop it. Doctors know that with rheumatoid arthritis the immune system is attacking the cartilage in the joints, but they don't know exactly why.

Rheumatoid arthritis is an inherited disease and I believe the defective DNA is caused by micro-plasma or bacteria. This gives the person the predisposition for rheumatoid arthritis. This predisposition has been transferred in the genes and the micro-plasma or bacteria has then been contracted at some point in the person's life. This means that you may have the tendency for the disease, but without the micro-plasma, there will be no symptoms. It is the micro-plasma that is the culprit. This is why it is possible to heal the affliction by stopping the micro-plasma with a healing.

Intuitive Remedies

The best results that I have had with rheumatoid arthritis have come from doing a healing and witnessing the micro-plasma debris inside the joint being released and made into a substance that is harmless to the body. If you have a difficult time visualizing these tiny cells in the joint, ask the Creator to show them to you until you get a sense of what they look like in the body.

You probably only have one or two sessions working with someone who has rheumatoid arthritis to convince them that your healing is helping them. This is because the micro-plasma and the micro-organisms will be broadcasting guilt, sorrow and resentment. The disease will be making them feel that they have to fight you over everything you're trying to tell them.

Belief Work

People who have arthritis have the fear of moving forward, are very stubborn and do not want to change. They feel that they have to be right all the time. They feel that they have to carry everyone.

The more stress they are under, the more the arthritis affects the body, so we work on the things that are causing the stress. How we do this depends on where the arthritis is in the body. For instance, if it were in the leg, we would work on issues of moving forward.

As rheumatoid arthritis is an inherited disease, you have to remember that what you are working on are ancestral programmes. Energy test for the following beliefs:

'I always have to be right.'

'I fear having to depend on other people.'

Look for programmes of criticizing others too.
Download:

'I know what it feels like to live without always having to be right.'

'I know what it feels like to live without fearing change.'

'I know what it feels like to live without having to resent everything.'

'I know what it feels like to listen to the words of another without rejection.'

'I know what it feels like to listen to others.'

'I know how to live without criticizing others.'

'I know how to live without thinking rigidly.'

'I know what it feels like to be able to release the crying inside.'

'I know what it feels like to release the pain easily and effortlessly.'

'I know what it feels like to live without others driving me crazy.'

'I know what it feels like to move easily and effortlessly.'

'I know what it feels like to live without fighting everyone and everything.'

'I know what it feels like to move without pain.'

'I know how to live without permitting the thoughts, emotions and beliefs of others to interfere with my thoughts, emotions and beliefs.'

'I know that I am allowed my own thoughts, feelings and emotions.'

'I know how to live without my thoughts, feelings and emotions making me ill.'

'I know it is possible to get stronger every day.'

'I know what it feels like to live without the fear of this disease destroying me.'

'I know what it feels like to know that my body can and will heal.'

'I know what it feels like to live each day enjoying every breath I take.'

Feeling Work

Check for feelings of:

- anger
- crying inside
- fear
- guilt
- hostility
- resentment
- rigid thinking
- sorrow

Supplements and Other Nutritional Recommendations

- ALA
- calcium
- carrot juice
- garlic
- grapeseed extract
- magnesium
- MSM
- omega 3s, 6s and 9s
- phosphorus
- silica
- vitamin B complex
- vitamin C
- vitamin E

Pasteurized Milk
One of the first things I do for people who have osteoarthritis and rheumatoid arthritis is to tell them, 'If I were you I would increase my bran intake, reduce my salt and tobacco intake, go off red meat and quit milk.'

It is strange, but when you suggest that people stop using milk, they want to walk out of the door. This is because their bodies crave calcium, but even though milk has a great deal of calcium in it, it is not in an obtainable form for people with arthritis. It is important to note that in order to be absorbed from the intestine into the body, calcium must break down in the stomach in eight minutes. Otherwise, it is flushed though the digestive system.

Next I suggest that people with arthritis use a good absorbable calcium supplement such as carrot juice. This helps the joints to stop swelling.

People with arthritis should feel free to use butter, cottage cheese and yogurt. But if they are serious about getting better, they will stop using milk and start taking the supplements.

ASTHMA

Asthma is a lung disease that causes obstruction of the airways. During an asthma attack, there is a restriction that stops the outward flow of air from the lungs. The person with asthma feels as though they are starving for air. They are not getting the old air out of the chest to bring in the new. These attacks can last a few minutes to several hours.

Asthma is very dangerous and people can die from it. In fact, this happens all the time. If the attack is bad enough, the person isn't getting any air in the lungs at all and in a sense is suffocating.

Many children develop asthma and grow out of it as they get older, only to have it return later in life.

If a person uses an inhaler more than twice a day, it is likely that they have a serious asthma problem. It is important that they consult a doctor.

Types

There are two forms of asthma, allergic and non-allergic, although these can be related.

Allergic Asthma
Common allergies include animal dander, chemicals, dust mites, environmental pollutants, feathers, food additives and so on.

Asthma can also be triggered by high amounts of fungus in the body. If a person lives in an environment that has fungus in it, they will be constantly inundated with it. You can do healings on them, but if they live in a contaminated environment, it is likely that they will be reinfected.

Many people with asthma are sensitive to food additives such as sulphites.

These are put on foods such as fruit and shellfish to keep them from turning different colours.

If the asthma is caused by natural allergens, such as grasses and pollens, it is likely that the person was not permitted to play in the dirt as a child and have contact with the very thing that would have stimulated their immune system and enabled them to develop antibodies to combat the allergens. When we are children, lack of exposure to the natural world can actually create an asthmatic condition.

Non-allergic Asthma

Asthma is a modern-day crisis because of the pollution in the air. It is especially prevalent in children and old people.

Respiratory infections such as bronchitis and pneumonia have a tendency to bring about asthma. Intrinsic asthma is associated with other respiratory diseases such as sinusitis and bronchitis.

Another type of non-allergic asthma is cardiac asthma, which is a condition that results in the same symptoms but is caused by heart failure. It is therefore important to check if the heart of a person with asthma is beating correctly. If not, they may not be pumping out the fluids from their lungs and this can cause asthma attacks. In this instance, asthma medicine will only make things worse. It is important for the person to follow up with a visit to both an asthma doctor and a heart doctor.

Emphysema, too, is associated with asthma. This is generally caused by toxins going into the lungs from coal mines, steel mills and other dusty environments. Emphysema responds very well to healings and in some cases is cleared with only one healing.

Stress is a huge trigger for asthma. A person who has chronic panic attacks can have a panic attack at the same time as an asthma attack and make the asthma much worse.

Causes

As well as the causes mentioned above:

- Asthma is often caused by fungus.
- Chlamydia during pregnancy can give the baby asthma.
- Too much stress in pregnancy can cause a baby to have asthma.
- Asthma may be caused by parasites in the lungs or by Lyme disease.
- Lack of water can trigger asthma attacks and so can the use of aspirin.
- Attacks can even be triggered by cold air.

Children with Asthma

Studies have proven that children can develop asthma because of tension. The lungs are very sensitive to emotions.

Little children with asthma have a tendency to be fearful; they are afraid of standing up for themselves and often of playing with other children. This is because people who have asthma are always incredibly sensitive. In ancient cultures it was accepted that these individuals had natural healing abilities. They may have had breathing problems, but they could help others heal. Many Native American medicine men had asthma.

Some parents take their children to allergy specialists for shots to help with their asthma. This can be an effective method of treatment; however, removing processed flour, white sugar and artificial sweeteners from their diet is also extremely beneficial. Increasing the daily dosage of vitamin B and the different mineral supplements helps, as do blue-green algae and chlorophyll. Both of these stimulate the adrenals.

Intuitive Remedies

With asthma, the first priority is to give the person healings in the adrenals, heart and lungs.

Asthma has the associated belief systems of heartache. If it is the heart that is causing the asthma, use 'The Heart Song' exercise (*see Cardiovascular Diseases*).

Sorrow influences the lungs. When someone you love deeply dies, every cell in your body grieves. If a person with a shared DNA connection dies, suddenly your DNA cannot connect to the person on a physical level. Because of this, your body will go through a mourning process. In some instances, this grieving process will play itself out in the lungs. This can be prevalent in men more so than in women. Men carry programmes that will not permit them to grieve and release the pain held by the body. Often they have the belief that they must be the strong one.

When grief is stored in the lungs in this way, it is known as silent crying. In most instances, it is released by tears. If the person does not allow themselves to grieve, this stored sorrow can cause physical issues and weaken the immune system.

If a person has sinus problems, it may mean that they need to cry to release the emotions that have built up.

Lungs are so connected to the Creator that as you release sadness, your connection to the Creator will become stronger.

Loneliness can also be an emotion that is found in the lungs.

When healing a person with asthma, it is important to understand the problem you are working on: is it the asthma itself or the side-effects, including emotions, of the medication that the person is on? Asthma medication can make people jumpy, depressed and nervous and strip them of calcium and potassium, not to mention making them just downright nasty if they are on prednisone. It is important to realize that you may not be talking to the person or the sickness, but the emotions and programmes generated by the medication. Never suggest that anyone stops taking their medication; rather work with the medication and release the beliefs. Let the doctor take the person off their medication slowly.

Some of the best results that we've witnessed with asthma have come about from changing the diet and level of exercise. Moderate exercise is one of the best things for asthma. However, over-stimulation of the lungs can cause an asthma attack. It is best to begin exercise gently and gradually.

In our society we have so many pollutants that actually attack the membrane of the lungs. Relocating to a place where the air is clean and pure would be ideal, but in any event removing flour and sugar from the diet seems to have a positive effect.

Belief Work

Always begin the session exploring with the digging work for issues that pertain to when the asthma attacks first started. Look for issues pertaining to moving forward, exhaustion, fear and old sorrow.

With many asthmatics, there is a direct connection with the adrenals. Most of the belief systems that are associated with the adrenals are also connected to programmes and beliefs surrounding asthma.

Many beliefs are held in the lungs. Not only do the lungs carry sorrow but they also carry deep amounts of regret. Work on the person's issues of sorrow and beliefs that they must carry everyone.

If the person with asthma had a lot of stress and sorrow as child, changing the beliefs that 'Life is sad', 'Life is sorrowful' and 'Life is hard' can help a great deal.

People who have asthma and emphysema have a tendency to let people take advantage of them, because it is almost too much effort to fight for themselves. Most of them do not have the energy to take a stand.

Download:

'I know what it feels like to take a breath easily and effortlessly.'

'I know what it feels like to live my life without having anxiety attacks.'

'I know what it feels like to live my life without stress.'

'I know what it feels like to live my life without controlling everything.'

'I know what it feels like to live my life without getting caught up in my own paranoid delusions.'

'I know what it feels like to live my life without the panic of not taking a breath.'

'I can breathe easily and effortlessly.'

'I know what it feels like to be secure and strong in every situation.'

'I know what it feels like to be allowed to use my medication.'

'I know what it feels like to allow my body to grow stronger.'

'I know what it feels like to want to exercise.'

'I know how much to exercise without overdoing it.'

'I build my body gradually to become strong.'

'I know what it feels like to not take on other people's sorrow.'

'I know what it feels like to not take on other people's drama.'

'I know how to live without other people taking advantage of me.'

'I know what it feels like to live without my family draining me.'

'I know what it feels like to live without resentment.'

'I know what it feels like to live without being discouraged.'

'I know what it feels like to live without being moody.'

'I know how to be consistent and show my love easily to those I love.'

'I know what it feels like to live without my mother controlling me.'

'I know what it feels like to live without my father controlling me.'

'I know it's possible for my lungs to heal.'

'I know it's possible to live without resenting my body.'

'I know what it feels like to have my body work in harmony.'

'I know how to have patience with my breathing and exercise.'

'I am determined.'

'I am allowed optimal health.'

Downloads for the Lungs

'I know what it feels like to live without being a victim.'

'I have the Creator's definition of what it is to cry.'

'I know what it feels like to live without regret.'

'I know the Creator's definition of what forgiveness feels like.'

'I know how to live in joy.'

The person may have a foetal memory of the mother's transferred anxiety. This may be the real cause of their disease. Instill:

'I forgive myself.'

'I know how to live without asthma.'

'I know how to breathe.'

'I understand how to breathe the breath of life.'

Supplements and Other Nutritional Recommendations

- noni
- olive-leaf extract
- pau d'arco

***

- Build the person's strength so the doctor will slowly wean them off their medication.
- DHEA is helpful in some cases of acute asthma.
- In adults, use myrtle, oregano and a product called Fungi Cleanse. This will help kill any fungus that may be causing the asthma and thus clean out the body.
- In some instances, an alkaline diet will clear asthma.
- Infra-red saunas are beneficial for asthmatics.
- One of the things that is very helpful is to take the person off all processed flour and white sugar. This makes a huge difference almost immediately.
- People with asthma will likely need vitamin A, the B vitamins, especially B6, and a little copper, magnesium, calcium, potassium and iron (for women).
- Proper hydration is also very important. Drinking lots of water makes a significant difference.

- Research has shown that people who drink coffee or other caffeine-containing drinks generally have reduced instances of asthma attacks.
- Sibu berry drink is an amazing supplement drink that can help with asthma.
- Spirulina and a product called Green Magic are beneficial for asthma.
- There is recent contention among some scientists that the amino acid tryptophan helps in people with asthma. I support these findings in my practice with clients.
- Vitamin B complex is good, as are stinging nettle, magnesium and calcium.
- With children, starting them on good vitamin and mineral supplements helps. You need to be careful with the vitamins and administer them according to the children's age, but a good mineral supplement seems to make a huge difference.
- Zinc is a phenomenal mineral that can be used as an aid for asthma.

See also the Respiratory System.

ASTIGMATISM

See the Eyes.

ATTENTION DEFICIT DISORDER/ATTENTION DEFICIT HYPERACTIVITY DISORDER (ADD/ADHD)

Attention deficit hyperactivity disorder (ADHD) is a biological brain-based condition that is characterized by poor attention and distractibility and/ or hyperactive and impulsive behaviour. It is one of the most common mental disorders that develop in children. Symptoms can continue into adolescence and adulthood. If left untreated, ADHD can lead to poor school/work performance, poor social relationships and a general feeling of low self-esteem.

ADD or attention deficit disorder is a general term frequently used to describe individuals who have attention deficit hyperactivity disorder without the hyperactive and impulsive behaviour. The terms are often used interchangeably for both those who do and those who do not have symptoms of hyperactivity and impulsiveness.

Causes

ADD and ADHD are more prevalent in people than anyone realizes. In many instances, they are caused by red and yellow dye in our food. The use and abuse of too much sugar can also be a cause, as can food allergies. Allergies can trigger ADD and ADHD. Studies have shown that children with ADD and ADHD have high levels of harmful bacteria and yeast in their urine.

Symptoms

Symptoms include self-destructive behaviour, tantrums, being quickly frustrated and the inability to sit still. The parent needs to be very careful that the child is not misdiagnosed, as many of these symptoms are normal for a child. Children have the tendency to want to wriggle and move around a lot.

It is a great source of amusement to me when a parent comes in completely distraught over the way their child is acting. In many instances, the child does not have ADD or ADHD at all; they are simply acting their age. Some parents have unreasonable expectations of children and want them to act like adults. They are children! They are not going to act as an adult would. As parents, we need to be able to tell whether our children have disorders or merely growing pains.

It is also possible that a child with ADD or ADHD is incredibly psychic and needs more stimulation.

Intuitive Remedies

The DNA activation seems to help with children who have ADD and ADHD. My recommendation is to put your hands on the child and command that their body and mind function like those of a perfectly normal child.

Belief Work

Very little belief work has to be done on a child. If you have to do belief work, it is likely to be the parents who need it. This can, however, make a great deal of difference to the child.

Most of the beliefs around a child have to do with feeling special.

'I am special.'

'I feel good about myself.'

'I am smart.'

'I am good enough.'

'I learn fast.'

'I am good.'

'I am lovable.'

Downloads

'I know what it feels like to be special.'

'I know what it feels like to feel good about myself.'

'I know how to be smart.'

'I know how to learn.'

'I know how to slow down so that I can learn.'

Supplements and Other Nutritional Recommendations

- Acidophilus is recommended to help the digestive system.
- Calm Child by Planetary Formulas may be good.
- Discontinue the use and abuse of sugar.
- Do not let the child eat fast food.
- Omega 3s, 6s and 9s are helpful.
- Remember that food allergies are a possible cause.
- The amino acid GABA has helped children who have a tendency towards violence.
- No red or yellow dyes that are found sometimes in certain foods.

AUTISM

Autism is not a disease, but a developmental brain disorder that affects a small percentage of the population. In spite of over 50 years of research, it is still little understood. Many of my clients from the eastern seaboard of the United States (particularly in New York and Boston) and the western state of Utah show a high incidence of autism in their children.

Autism usually manifests before the child is three years old. Signs include self-absorption, lack of reaction to other people, constantly rocking or sitting by themselves in silence. The child has a difficult time having conversations and making friends and can withdraw into themselves and be preoccupied by the details of an object.

The evidence indicates that autism is a disorder of the nervous system. It can be a genetic disorder and can be caused by a brain injury before or after birth. There is speculation that it can be caused by venereal diseases or viral infections.

Four times as many boys suffer from autism as girls. This is likely to be due to the fact that boys are more vulnerable to influences in the womb.

It is my opinion that there is a direct connection between autism and vaccinations.

There are varying degrees of autism. Children with mild autism can become very high achievers when they grow up. Those with more severe autism avoid physical contact and show no signs of understanding. Many of them do not attempt to communicate, but some of them will make gestures and sounds.

Medical science currently believes there is no cure for autism. Doctors take the view that children with autism should be assessed by an experienced psychologist and placed in programmes that might help them.

Intuitive Remedies

There are two kinds of autism that I see in children. The first is caused by trauma during birth. It is as if the spirit has pulled a little bit away from the body. Going in and asking the Creator to put the spirit back into the person's space does help. It seems that part of their spirit is trying to depart, or came very close to leaving and hasn't quite been put back into their space.

We have also found that the inability to communicate can be changed by commanding the body to go back to fetal memory and to develop as a normal child.

The other form of autism that I've observed seems to be caused by too much mercury in the system. I believe this is coming from vaccinations as well as from the mother's milk. With this form of autism, no matter how many times you put energy back into the body, it will not hold that energy because mercury is constantly being reintroduced into the system. Giving the child extra apple juice will help pull out the mercury, and commanding the Creator to change the mercury into a harmless substance may heal them.

Never command all of the heavy metals to be completely pulled out of the body, however, because our body is made up of metals. If you command too much of the mercury to be pulled out all at once, it will also make the body very sick, even if you change it to another energy that isn't mercury.

The response to healings has been extremely successful with autism. One of my past students did healings with his two autistic nephews who had never spoken and within three days both of them were speaking coherently. One of the boys walked up to his mother and said, 'Mommy, I love you.'

The child with autism can be trapped in a bubble that they can't get out of. Making sure that they feel constantly loved will break through that barrier. They are often very brilliant children.

Downloads

'I am special.'

'I am important.'

'I enjoy being around other people.'

'I feel safe around other people.'

'I know how to live without other people and children making me irritable.'

'I know how to live without noise making me stressed and irritable.'

'I know it's possible to feel smarter every day.'

'I love to interact with other children.'

'I love to interact with my mother.'

'I love to learn.'

'I understand what it feels like to be strong.'

'It is easy for me to be accepted.'

'I know what it feels like to receive love from another person.'

With autism, it is important to work on the belief systems of the parents, too. Ensure they know it is possible for the child to get better.

Supplements and Other Nutritional Recommendations

- Apple juice will pull mercury out of the body. Use it for several months.
- Limit the use of wheat products.
- Making sure that the child has good vitamins and minerals is very important, especially vitamin B complex, vitamin C and vitamin E.
- No processed sugar.
- No red and yellow dyes (in food).
- No soft drinks of any kind.

BACKACHE

I've had a great deal of success clearing backache by simply going into Theta, commanding that the back goes back into place and witnessing it done. You have to command the vertebrae as well as the muscles. Most of the time the person is in pain for 15 minutes to an hour afterwards as the body readjusts itself, but then they are better.

What is interesting is that bones and muscles that have been out of place have a tendency to fall back into the same pattern again unless the healing is followed up with belief work.

Belief Work

With backache, the belief systems have to do with communication with the Creator and a higher relationship with the Creator, also with feeling supported and structured in life. If a person is not feeling supported, they are likely to get backache.

In many instances, however, backache is caused by simple calcium-magnesium deficiencies or picking up something too heavy without proper support.

Download:

'I know what it feels like to be completely loved by the Creator.'

'I understand the Creator's interpretation of love.'

'I understand the Creator's definition of the Creator.'

'I know what it feels like to be close to God.'

'I know how to live without regret.'

'I know how to live without fear.'

'I know the Creator's definition of truth.'

'I know how to hear the Creator's truth without imposing my own interpretation.'

'I know the Creator's definition of forgiveness and compassion.'

45

'I have compassion for myself.'

'I know what it feels like to be a success.'

'I know what it feels like to live without being a victim.'

'I know what it feels like to live without victimizing others.'

'I cherish myself.'

'I know what it feels like to live without unreasonable struggle.'

'I know how to live without the fear of the Creator abandoning me.'

'I know how to live without being a martyr.'

'I know what it feels like to live without the weight of the world on my shoulders.'

'I know what it feels like to grow and become strong.'

'I know what it feels like to have clear and decisive messages from the Creator.'

'I know what it feels like to live my life without blaming God for everything.'

'I know what it feels like to listen to the Creator's definition of what I need.'

BACTERIA

See Prologue.

BELL'S PALSY

Bell's palsy is a herpes virus that makes the affected area go numb due to neurological damage. Sometimes there is incredible damage to the face.

Belief Work

The first thing to do is to use belief work to remove and replace all worthiness issues. As with all herpes viruses, belief work is the key.

Ask the person what emotion was going on when they acquired the virus and use the digging work to find the bottom belief.

Change the beliefs that the virus and the host have in common.

Ask God to reconstruct the nerve endings in the face. Before you do this, however, you have to make sure that the person has the belief that it is possible, because by now their doctor will have told them that it is impossible.

See also Herpes.

BIPOLAR DISORDER/MANIC DEPRESSION

Bipolar disorder refers to mood swings from overly 'high' (manic) to overly 'low' (depressed). This refers to a person's mood alternating between 'poles' of mania and depression. Another name for the illness is manic depression. In the manic stage, the person has an abundance of serotonin and other hormones. In the depressed stage, they are low in serotonin and necessary hormones.

The symptoms of bipolar disorder are severe. They can result in damaged relationships, poor job or school performance and even suicide. But there is good news: bipolar disorder can be treated and people with this illness tend to be very creative and can lead full and productive lives.

Bipolar disorder typically develops in late adolescence or early adulthood. However, some people have their first symptoms during childhood and some develop them late in life. It is often not recognized as an illness and people may suffer for years before it is properly diagnosed and treated.

Symptoms of Mania

- a lasting period of behaviour that is different from usual
- an excessively 'high', overly good, euphoric mood
- abuse of drugs, particularly cocaine, alcohol and sleeping medication
- denial that anything is wrong
- distractibility; inability to concentrate well
- extreme irritability
- increased energy, activity and restlessness
- increased sex drive
- little need of sleep
- poor judgement
- provocative, intrusive or aggressive behaviour
- racing thoughts and very fast speech, jumping from one idea to another

- spending sprees
- unrealistic beliefs in one's abilities and powers

Symptoms of Depression

- a lasting sad, anxious or empty mood
- a change in appetite and/or unintended weight loss or gain
- chronic pain or other persistent bodily symptoms that are not caused by physical illness or injury
- decreased energy, a feeling of fatigue or of being 'slowed down'
- difficulty concentrating, remembering and making decisions
- feelings of guilt, worthlessness or helplessness
- feelings of hopelessness or pessimism
- loss of interest or pleasure in activities once enjoyed, including sex
- restlessness or irritability
- sleeping too much or being unable to sleep
- thoughts of death or suicide, or suicide attempts

The person with bipolar disorder will usually think it is everyone else's fault, not theirs. They think everyone else is out to get them. Their brain misfires with electrical pulses. The mother wants to push the child away because it is difficult to deal with the electrical pulses. Some people become very violent, and this can escalate until they abuse the people they love.

Manic depressant disorder can be aggravated by an over-growth of yeast in the intestinal tract. Food allergies can also make symptoms worse.

The use of the medication lithium can cause blurred vision, diarrhoea, frequent urination, hand tremors, kidney dysfunction, muscle twitching and thyroid enlargement.

Intuitive Remedies

When working with a person with bipolar disorder, you must ask if they want to change it and do as much belief work as can be done in one session. People with bipolar disorder have no idea what to do when they feel emotions. They are used to being very depressed and may not want you to fix it. They often want you to make them numb, rather than feel their emotions overwhelm them.

If they do want you to help, ask for the brain pulses to balance, clean out the liver and then ask for the hormones to balance. Teach the body what to do. High noradrenaline and low serotonin levels can be changed by sending the person an abundance of love. Witness it done. Say, *'Creator, show me.'* *For the process for normalizing brain chemicals, see Depression.*

Some children are not actually manic; they are just allergic to red dyes.

Belief Work

People who have bipolar disorder are excellent manipulators. It is difficult to use belief work on them because they will take you in circles with the digging process. They have to genuinely want to change before you can get anywhere with them.

Many people are misdiagnosed with bipolar disorder and believe that nothing can help them. This is when belief work can help them to have hope. Teach the client how to go to Theta and connect to the Creator. This will help them to balance the hemispheres of the brain.

'I am not good enough.'

'Nothing can help me.'

Download:

'I know what it feels like to have hope and energy.'

'I know how to stay in a balanced mood.'

'I know what it feels like to live without being irritable with others.'

'I know what it feels like to have good judgement.'

'I know how to make good decisions.'

'I see the possibilities in all things.'

'I live without feeling empty.'

'I live without feeling sad.'

'I know what it feels like to live without being over-aggressive.'

'I know how to live without taking a lot of medication.'

'I know what it feels like to take medication in a persistent and easy way.'

'I know what it feels like to have good judgement about the money I spend.'

'I know it what it feels like to live without taking my problems out on others.'

'I have control of my moods.'

'I have control of my feelings.'

'I have control of my life.'

'I feel totally connected to the Creator.'

'I know how to rest and benefit from sleep.'

'I know how to eat food that is good for me.'

'I know what it feels like to live without thoughts of death or suicide.'

'I know what it feels like to be appreciated.'

'I know I can connect to the Creator at any time.'

'I know how to live without explosive energy.'

'I know what it feels like to know I am safe.'

'I know how to appreciate all those who are in my life.'

'With every passing day, I think with more clarity.'

'I have good ideas.'

'I know how to listen to others.'

'I know what it feels like to be connected to the oneness of All That Is.'

'I know what it feels like to know there is always hope.'

Supplements and Other Nutritional Recommendations

- A balanced diet is important, with fruit and vegetables.
- Amino-acid complexes help to balance the system, especially tyrosine and taurine.
- Eat fish and take omega 3s.
- High doses of vitamin B and injections of vitamin B12 seem to help.
- Vitamin C is beneficial.
- Zinc is helpful.
- Avoid tryptophan, as it can cause a manic episode, and stay away from gluten (wheat).

BLADDER INFECTIONS

Bladder infections are some of the easiest to clear up psychically:

The Process of Clearing Bladder Infections

1   First find out who it is you're angry with and pull the energy of 'I am angry with [person's name]', replace it with 'I release this anger' and instil the feeling of forgiveness. (Other external energies may also cause bladder infections.)

2   A bladder infection can be easily fixed by going up to the Creator of All That is and making the command: *'It is commanded that this bladder infection be gone now, thank you. It is done, it is done, it is done.'*

3   Go down into the bladder and witness the infection cleared and sent to the light of the Creator.

Once you are able to clear up bladder infections, you will have a clientèle that will love you.
    See also Urinary Tract Infections.

BLOOD DISORDERS

The blood is the great communicator for the body. It carries nutrients, hormones and beliefs with it. If it is not flowing correctly, these vital nutrients and messages are not sent. Hormones sent through the bloodstream communicate to us the feeling that we are having a life experience. If we have poor communication skills, we have poor blood flow in our body and vice versa. For instance, when we cannot speak up and say no to someone, we will generally have poor blood flow.

Blood is also connected to how we perceive ourselves. If our self-perception is a healthy one, then our blood will flow evenly through our body and others will perceive us in a balanced fashion. The thoughts that are sent to us in return will be balanced, causing the blood to regulate evenly.

Seen under a microscope, a blood cell is yellow. It is iron that makes the blood red and if there is no oxygen in the blood, it will appear blue.

Bone marrow produces platelets and white and red blood cells. If you go into a person's space and meet the blood cells, they will be busy and in a big rush. Red and white blood cells have different roles. Red blood cells function as supply troops, delivering oxygen to cells and carrying away carbon dioxide waste, while white blood cells, called leukocytes, defend against attacks from invaders and clear away the debris for the blood. Five types of leukocytes are strategically deployed in the body:

- *Basophiles* release anti-coagulants and constrict and dilate to heal inflammation.
- *Eosinophils* combat certain allergic reactions and detoxify foreign substances.
- *Lymphocytes* battle disease microbes and accumulate at cancerous lesions.
- *Monocytes* swell up to become macrophages, able to swallow large particles whole.
- *Neutrophils* spearhead the fight at the site of an injury, engulfing bacteria and foreign particles.

Red blood cells do not have a nucleus. They destroy it after they are released into the bloodstream, so they have more room to carry oxygen to the cells. If a red blood cell fails to destroy its own nucleus, the spleen, in turn, destroys the cell.

Red cells live up to 90 days. Some white T-cells can live as long as the person does. T-cells can stay dormant until the virus they are programmed to fight comes into the system. You may only have one T-cell that knows how to fight a particular virus, but it will produce millions of other T-cells when it encounters that virus.

Blood Types

Humans have four types of blood: O, A, B and AB:

- *Type O* was the first to develop and was the type of our hunter-gatherer ancestors. It will only receive blood from a type O donor.
- An antigen is a substance with the ability to make an antibody that will fight off a disease. *Type A* blood has the protein antigen A and its plasma has antibody B. Type A blood can receive blood transfusions from both A types and O types.
- *Type B* blood has the antigen B and antibody A. It can receive blood from B and O types.

- *Type AB* has both antigens and no antibodies. It is compatible with all other blood types.

Intuitive Insights

Seen intuitively, the blood cells should look and feel happy, not angry or stubborn.

Black substances in the blood can be heavy metals. If brown particles are seen, then the kidneys or liver aren't cleaning the blood. There may also be brown particles if there are parasites or undigested nutrients present. If this is the case, the person needs more enzymes.

Belief Work

With blood disorders, the belief systems cycle around nurturing issues, receiving love and nourishment, co-dependence, the return of soul fragments, the fear of being alone, individuality, the fear of abandonment and the 'knowing' of what something feels like.

For more on beliefs, *see the Circulatory System.*

Supplements and Other Nutritional Recommendations

- cayenne pepper
- red clover
- vitamin B

***

- Echinacea is the queen of all blood purifiers.
- Niacin is also a blood purifier, but use it for only two weeks at a time.

See also Haemophilia, Heavy Metals, Kidney Disease and Leukaemia.

BONE FRACTURES

Fractures occur when a bone cannot withstand outside forces that are applied to it. 'Fracture', 'break' and 'crack' all mean the same thing in that the bone structure fails.

There are few bodily pains that can compare to that of a broken bone. Some people pass out from the pain, and people have even died from the shock of a large bone being broken. A broken bone hurts because the nerve endings that surround bones contain pain fibres. These fibres become irritated when a bone is broken. Also, broken bones bleed, and the blood and associated swelling cause pain. The muscles that surround the injured area may go into spasm when they try to hold the broken bone fragments in place, and these spasms too cause intense pain.

In many instances, a fracture is easy to detect, but it is not easily diagnosed if there is no obvious deformity.

Types

Fractures occur because of direct blows, twisting injuries or falls. The type of force on the bone determines what type of injury occurs.

Descriptions of fractures can be confusing. They are based on where in the bone the break has occurred, how the bone fragments are aligned and whether any complications exist.

The first step in describing a fracture is whether it is open or closed. If the skin over the break is disrupted, then it is an open fracture. If the skin is cut, torn or abraded, the potential exists for an infection to get into the bone. These injuries need to be thoroughly cleaned out and anaesthesia can be required to do the job effectively.

The next step is a description of the fracture line. Through an X-ray, a doctor will trace this to see if it goes across the bone (transverse), at an angle (oblique) or in a spiral. The fracture could also be in two pieces or comminuted, which means in multiple pieces.

Types of fracture:

Comminuted: Bones fractured into several pieces.

Complete: The bone snaps completely into two or more pieces.

Compound: The bone protrudes through the skin. This is also called an open fracture.

Incomplete: The bone cracks but does not separate.

Impacted: One fragment of bone is embedded into another fragment of bone.

Simple: A bone breaks into two pieces.

Stress: A hairline break that is often invisible on the X-ray for the first six weeks after the onset of pain.

Intuitive Insights

The bones and the spine align themselves when the muscles relax. It is tension in the muscles that prevents the bones from staying in alignment.

So, with a broken bone, it is necessary to do intuitive work on the muscles at the same time as the bones. Remember, the Creator of All That Is will take care of it.

Since the bones hold us up, they think they are the most important part of the body and it is true that everything is based on them: the ligaments, muscles and the nervous system. They are the core of all that we are. They are directly connected to the crown chakra and because of this they are the spiritual tuning fork, hence the saying, 'I feel it in my bones.'

Anytime you work with bones, you also work with cartilage. The front part of the rib is made out of cartilage so that we can breathe, while the back half is made out of bone. The sternum is cartilage.

Intuitive Remedies

In order to do a healing on any kind of fracture, go into Theta and command the bone to go back to before the time that the accident happened. Say, 'No, this did not happen,' and watch the change in the bone. The skeletal system is extremely easy to heal and happy to co-operate.

Bones that are broken and separated can be worked on by doing the basic healing technique, going up and commanding the bone to be completely healed, watching it heal and wrapping it in calcium.

When doing a healing on a bone, remember to bring in the creative energy of All That Is, otherwise the body will steal calcium from the other bones, especially the hip bones.

If you experience a person with a compound fracture, you will of course call the emergency services as well as do a healing on them. Never attempt to physically push a bone back into place.

Belief Work

If the bone does not heal immediately, go into a deeper Theta state. Be gentle with yourself. Consistency in the healings will come with practice. Remember that belief work might be necessary and it might be your beliefs that are blocking the healing. See if you fear injury or disease.

Injury can also be tied to subconscious beliefs pertaining to sacrifice and worthiness issues.

You must be very tactful with a client when there are emotional issues in the bones because they are generally about trust and having support in life. Many people have issues with God. They must trust that God supports them.

BONE SPURS

I have had an extensive number of people coming to me with bone spurs. These are caused by too much calcium. The problem could be that the parathyroid is not breaking down calcium. So calcium deposits are formed as the body's way of protecting itself.

Both spurs can also be caused by gout, lupus, muscle inflammation, nerve problems, obesity and physical injury.

Intuitive Remedies

Usually, all I have to suggest to a person with a bone spur is that they use a very good calcium–magnesium mixture and then I witness a simple healing. It usually does not take more than a quick healing to alleviate a bone spur. Go into the person's space and witness the calcium deposit being dissolved and absorbed by the body to be used for another purpose.

Belief Work

Check for hatred in relationships.

Supplements

- calcium–magnesium
- vitamin B
- vitamin C

Heel Spurs

The heel bone is the largest bone in the foot. It absorbs most of the shock and pressure from walking and running. A heel spur is an abnormal growth of the heel bone. Calcium deposits form when the plantar fascia pulls away from the heel area, causing a bony protrusion. The plantar fascia is a broad band of fibrous tissue located along the bottom surface of the foot running from the heel to the forefoot.

Stretching of the plantar fascia is usually the result of flat feet, but people with unusually high arches can also develop heel spurs. Women have a significantly higher incidence of heel spurs due to the types of footwear they wear.

Heel spurs can cause extreme pain in the rear foot, especially while standing or walking. They are common in people who have arthritis, neuritis and tendinitis.

Remedies

The key for the proper treatment of heel spurs and tendinitis is determining the cause of the excessive stretching of the plantar fascia. When the cause is flat feet, an orthotic with rear-foot posting and longitudinal arch support is an effective device to reduce the over-pronation and allows the condition to heal.

Other common treatments include stretching exercises, losing weight, wearing shoes that have a cushioned heel that absorbs shock and elevating the heel with the use of a heel cradle, heel cup or orthotic. Heel cradles and heel cups provide extra comfort and cushion to the heel and reduce the amount of shock and sheer forces experienced from everyday activities.

Heal as for bone spurs.

THE BRAIN

The brain is connected to and runs all the other systems. Neurons, the chemical messengers of the brain, communicate with the rest of the body and then messages are sent back from the body to the brain. All information is sorted out and registered and sent back for perception. You register much more information than you consciously perceive.

Each lobe of the brain has its function:

- The *brain stem* consists of the midbrain, the pons and the medulla oblongata. It is the message system between parts of the nervous system and has three functions:

  1. It produces autonomic behaviour in the body.
  2. It provides pathways for nerve fibres to neural centres.
  3. It is the origin of most of the cranial nerves.

- The *cerebellum* maintains muscle tone, muscle movement and body balance.

- The *cerebrum* has the nerve centre that controls sensory, motor activities and intelligence.

- The *diencephalon* consists of the thalamus and the hypothalamus. The thalamus is a relay station for all sensory stimuli and the hypothalamus controls autonomic functions.

- The *frontal lobe* influences abstract reasoning, judgement, language expression, movement (in the motor portion), personality and social behaviour.

- The *limbic system* has to do with the basic drives of aggression, emotions, hunger and sexual arousal.

- *Midbrain* is the brain's reflex centre for cranial nerves. It mediates eye movement.

- The *occipital lobe* mainly interprets visual stimuli.

- The *parietal lobe* interprets and integrates sensations, including pain, temperature and touch. It also interprets size, shape, distance and texture. The parietal lobe of the non-dominant hemisphere is especially important for the awareness of body shape.

- The *pons* connects the cerebrum to the cerebellum and links the midbrain to the medulla oblongata. It mediates chewing, equilibrium, hearing and taste and saliva secretions.

- The *reticular* is the activating system screening channelling to the right area of the brain.

- The *temporal lobe* controls hearing, language comprehension and storage and the recall of memories (although memories are stored throughout the brain).

Intuitive Insights

Every time you connect to the Creator and are in Theta, you activate the frontal lobe as well as other parts of the brain. Visualizing takes place in the frontal lobe. The inner knowing of intuition is in the heart chakra centre. Wake up the inner knowing with 'It is safe to see intuitively' and 'It is safe to know with intuition.' The more that you maintain a Theta wave in the brain, the more developed the intuitive abilities will become.

Accepting what is felt, sensed, heard or seen intuitively gives the ability to properly visualize inside the frontal lobe of the brain. Test yourself or your clients for blocks of intuition, trading for abilities and old obligations that prevent visualization.

Belief Work

If the brain is distracted or over-analyzes situations, you will not take appropriate action. Energy test for fear of action. Download:

'I know how to accept God's healing.'

'I know how to take action.'

'I know how to allow love.'

'I know how to live without over-analyzing.'

'I know how to receive a healing without resistance.'

'I know what it feels like to live without pain.'

'I know what it feels like to accept help from others without feeling weak.'

Brain Damage

Intuitive Remedies

To work on adults or children who have any kind of brain damage, simply go into the brain and command the brain cells to become whatever they need to become. Ask the Creator to show you the problem and command it to change.

If you are unfamiliar with different parts of the brain, all you have to do is ask the Creator to show you what needs to be done and witness it.

Working with children and teaching their brain what to do is simple. All you have to do is command it to be so and let the stem cells and the brilliance of an infant's mind and spirit go to work.

Belief Work

It is best to work on the beliefs of the parents to permit the child to heal. Never underestimate the power and influence of the DNA bond between parent and child. If the parent is broadcasting negative beliefs, the child will soak them up like a sponge.

BREAST IMPLANTS

Breast implants work fine for many women; however, in some women they may cause lupus, multiple sclerosis and other auto-immune disorders. It is now accepted in conventional medicine that the silicone and plastic in breast implants are toxic. Saline is presently used as the filler for the implants, and there is also concern about this.

I think that regardless of the substance, the bodies of some women simply begin to reject the implants.

Intuitive Remedies

Have you ever suggested that someone remove breast implants? Good luck!

Most women do not want to give up their breast implants. They feel beautiful with them and are afraid be without them.

If a woman is having problems but refuses to remove the breast implants, command that her body accepts the implants as though they were normal body tissue.

This may improve matters; however, in many instances a bacterium grows around the implant. Change this into a harmless substance and witness calcium encapsulating it so the person's body does not fight it. This goes for all implants, such as a femur or a hip implant. Then witness the Creator giving the message to the body to accept the implant.

Do not make the command that the breast implant evaporates, because when it actually disappears, the woman will get very upset. This has happened to me twice in my career.

Downloads

'I am beautiful with or without breast implants.'

'I know how to accept myself physically.'

'I accept my implant as part of my body.'

BRONCHITIS

It's a well-known fact that bronchitis and similar diseases are caused by infections in the lungs. When working with these types of diseases, I will sometimes wait and see if the immune system will take care of it. This is because it is important to let the immune system strengthen itself by destroying the disease. People will always come to me and wonder why I haven't worked on someone's flu or bronchitis. In many instances their immune system has already destroyed the bacteria or virus and their symptoms are due to the rapid die-off of the bacteria and virus and the damage they have caused, and the whole thing is a process the body has to go through.

Belief Work

For the most part, I first suggest that the person use herbal supplements and then I use belief work. If someone develops a cold or bronchitis, it usually means that they are fatigued or stressed. Many people will unconsciously permit a disease into their system just so they can stay at home and get some rest.

Belief systems associated with bronchitis are connected to sorrow.

Supplements

- colloidal silver (use judiciously and not all the time)
- CoQ10
- Echinacea
- mullin
- noni (use by itself, not with antibiotics, because the two will cancel each other out)
- pycnogenols
- Siberian ginseng
- vitamin A
- vitamin Bs

- Sibu-juice is wonderful!

BULIMIA

See Anorexia Nervosa.

BURNS

One day I accidentally poured hot tea over my arm that would have been likely to cause a third-degree burn. I did not look at it and covered it up. I said, 'No, this didn't happen.' When I uncovered it, the burn was completely gone.

On another occasion one of my students came to class with a burn and asked me to heal it. It was a third-degree burn and I did a healing on it. It did not heal instantly and I could see she was disappointed. However, it had healed completely within three days. The doctor that she went to said he'd never seen anything heal so quickly.

Intuitive Remedies

When a burn first occurs, don't look at it. Keep it covered and heal it before looking at it, so the conscious mind doesn't get in the way. Command, 'The pain is stopped now.' It's the pain in the nerve endings that makes the burn worse. The myelin sheaths are going crazy because of the burn and the neurons are screaming messages to the brain that make the situation worse. If you can dissolve the pain in the skin, you'll stop the burn from going in and burning more deeply. It will stop immediately and cause no skin damage.

Sometimes the shock of seeing a deep burn will frighten you into absolute panic, so be sure to put your hand over it or throw a towel over it (making sure it's clean and dry, especially if it's a deep burn) and say, 'No, this did not happen.'

Burns heal tremendously fast with small children. When the child is first burned, command that all the pain be gone.

Supplements and Other Nutritional Recommendations

- It is said honey heals burns because bacteria will not grow in it. Unpasteurized pure honey is said to be best.
- Light therapy: the colours to use are blue and magenta.
- Put only a first-degree burn under cold water.
- Third-degree burns: witness the Creator heal the burn and follow up with medical help. After treatment, apply a combination of unpasteurized pure honey, comfrey and vitamin E and the skin will grow back.

CADMIUM POISONING

Cadmium is an inorganic substance that is naturally present in the environment. However, with the advent of modern industry, it has become a health risk in areas where there is metal smelting, in plastics and in batteries. It is very toxic to the body. In the 1960s the British government conducted an experiment that involved spraying cadmium over the town of Norwich, causing untold health risks to the inhabitants.

Cadmium is present in paints, dyes and toys and can be present in lower levels in drinking water and fertilizers, and even in coffee, tea and soft drinks. Cigarettes have very high levels of cadmium and lead. This can cause high blood pressure, loss of smell and put a strain on the kidneys.

Intuitive Remedies

As with any toxic poisoning, cadmium poisoning responds well to healing. Witness the Creator release the toxins from the body and suggest supplements to rebuild the body.

Belief Work

The beliefs that draw cadmium involve:

- Being abused and told that it is love.
- Getting the promise of support and not receiving it.
- Not feeling enough love.
- Not getting enough support.

Download:

'I know the Creator's definition of love without abuse.'

'I know what real love is.'

'I know what love is without having to struggle or beg for it.'

Supplements

- alfalfa
- calcium–magnesium
- spirulina
- vitamin E
- zinc, 50 to 100 mg a day on a full stomach

CANCER

There are literally hundreds of different kinds of cancer. Science has put these illnesses in a nice little package and called them all cancer. This section is dedicated to all the different types of cancer that I have worked with over the years.

All cancers begin in cells that make up blood and other tissues. Normally, cells grow and divide to form new cells as the body needs them. When they grow old, they die and new cells take their place. Sometimes this orderly process goes wrong. New cells form when the body does not need them and old cells do not die when they should.

Types

Cancer falls into four broad categories, defined by conventional medicine as:

Carcinomas: Carcinomas are cancers that affect the skin, the mucous membranes and the glands in the internal organs.

Leukaemia: Leukaemia is cancer of the blood.

Lymphomas: Lymphomas are cancers that affect the lymph system.

Sarcomas: Sarcomas are cancers that affect muscles, the connective tissues and bone.

Causes

Modern researchers have found many causes of cancer. Poor diet is the cause of about 30 percent of all cancers; cigarette smoking causes 30 percent, genetics cause 10 percent, carcinogens in the workplace cause 5 percent, family history 5 percent, lack of exercise 5 percent, viruses 5 percent, alcohol 3 percent, reproductive factors 3 percent and environmental pollution 2 percent.

- Fluoride may be a risk factor for cancer.
- High-voltage power lines have been shown to be contributors to cancer.
- Obesity can be a cause of certain types of cancer.
- Oestrogen replacement is helpful in osteoporosis and Alzheimer's, but increases the risk of breast and uterine cancers.
- One of the most prevalent carcinogens known to man is tobacco. It is also the most avoidable cancer risk. Cigarette smoke is made up of over 4,000 chemicals, including 43 that are known to cause cancer. The cancerous effect of smoking is multiplied by alcohol consumption, as the two are frequently used in combination. It has been shown that women who smoke are at greater risk of developing lung cancer than men.
- Pesticide residues rank among the top three environmental cancer risks.
- The incidence of leukaemia has been found to be significantly lower among children who were breastfed.
- The risk of prostate cancer in men who have undergone a vasectomy is three times higher than those who have not had the operation.

Conventional and Alternative Therapies

Currently, there are many conventional and alternative therapies for cancer:

- herbal therapies
- immunological therapies
- metabolic therapies
- mind–body therapies
- nutritional recommendations

ThetaHealing uses mostly mind–body therapies. While I may tell you what vitamins, minerals and herbs work with cancer, these are merely suggestions to build up a body that is depleted by lack of nutrition because of the cancer. However, for the tumours to disappear, we use a healing.

Nutritional and Other Therapies
- DHEA is believed to prevent some forms of cancer by blocking an enzyme that promotes cancer-cell growth. However, it cannot be used for those with hormone-related cancers such as breast cancer.

- Evidence is growing that bee products may contain anti-cancer properties. Propolis, a substance bees produce to seal their hives, is rich in antioxidants.

- Hyperthermia, a procedure in which body tissue is exposed to extremely high temperatures, may be effective against tumour cells and can be used alone or accompanied by radiation therapy and other therapies. Researchers believe that it might damage tumour cells or deprive them of the nutrients they need to live.

- Max Gerson nutritional therapy works well for many people. This is a powerful natural treatment that boosts the body's own immune system to heal cancer, allergies, arthritis, heart disease and many other degenerative diseases. One aspect of the Gerson Therapy that sets it apart from most other treatment methods is its all-encompassing nature. An abundance of nutrients from 13 fresh organic juices is consumed every day, providing a super-dose of enzymes, minerals and nutrients. These substances then break down diseased tissue in the body, while enemas aid in eliminating the lifelong build-up of toxins from the liver.

- Research is under way regarding the anti-cancer effects of the melatonin hormone, which is involved in regulating the production of oestrogen and testosterone. However, it should not be used by anyone with leukaemia.

- Shark cartilage has been shown to be helpful for certain types of cancer, including cancer of the cervix, pancreas and prostate.

New treatments are coming out all the time, both in the conventional and alternative fields.

Chemotherapy

If the person is using chemotherapy, do not tell them that they should or should not use it. If they believe that they should, do not contradict them. My background is in naturopathic medicine, so I could definitely be an anti-chemo person, but I am not. Chemotherapy has come a long way since the 1990s.

With chemotherapy, doctors inject the patient with a chemical that stops all fast-growing cells, which unfortunately also means the beneficial cells in the oesophagus and stomach. This is why people get nauseated with chemotherapy. It will make you feel sick for a time, but it has the benefit of stopping the cancer cells growing. The medical profession has it down to such a science that some cancers, such as thyroid cancer, often respond immediately to it.

In some instances, it is permissible to suggest using CoQ10 with chemotherapy as long as the doctor clears this request. CoQ10 will help the person to keep their hair.

There are certain herbs, however, that are definitely not permissible to use with chemotherapy, such as Echinacea.

Intuitive Insights

Doctors used to believe that cells did not talk to each other and that was why cancer developed. Then they thought that since every cell in the body sent signals back and forth to each other, what was happening was that the cancer cells were making themselves invisible to the other cells; this was why the immune system did not destroy them. However, I believe that this is not strictly true. I believe that the body ignores cancer because it is taking on different toxins and serving a purpose that the body knows about. On some level, the brain knows it is there. If you talk to the cancer, it is quite friendly, polite, kind and sweet. If you tell it it's not supposed to be there, it will almost cry and say, 'I came to help!' It's telling the truth, because the body actually seems to be sending all the toxins right to it. The plan of the body is that the cancer will gather all the toxins and then the body will get rid of it later. The plan doesn't work, of course, if you keep putting toxins in the body.

One of the biggest toxins is hatred and stress. We are essentially animalistic, so we have to live with some stress in our life – that's how we are hard-wired. It stimulates our immune system, so sometimes we create it. It is also a natural response to stimuli, but sometimes we have too much and it can create heavy toxins in the body.

The cancer cell gathering all these toxins thinks it's quite the busy little cell. Cancer cells actually have special receptors that draw to them feelings of anger or hatred. This has been proven by a biochemist. Receptors are like little doorways that sit on the cell's surface and let hormones and other chemical messages in and out. Anger, hatred and sorrow are known to feed cancer. Cancer cells also pull high amounts of protein into their space and use it to grow. And people with cancer have low body temperature. Cancer can't grow when the body is warm.

So, what emotions don't you send the cancer cell when you are working on it? You don't send it fear or hate, because you will feed it. It will continue to grow, because that's its job: to collect toxic feelings. But if you send it love, what will happen? It can get confused, but it will also start to change back into a harmless form.

Because I have had lymphoma, I am not afraid of cancer and I do not have a problem with it. Cancer is simply what it is. Some people say that it has evolved from bacteria to virus, to fungus and then to cancer. I think that in some cases of breast cancer, this is the case. Nevertheless, I think that leukaemia gets a bad rap and so does lymphoma. I think lymphoma is like a cancer, but I do not think that leukaemia is a cancer at all.

In the body, cancerous tumours or polyps usually appear black or brown. Lymphoma and Hodgkin's grow big nodules on people. Don't buy into fear when you see these, just go up and ask the Creator to change them.

Intuitive Remedies

Of the many different diseases known to man, cancer seems to be one of the most receptive to energy healing.

Make the command that all cancer be gone from the person. Say, 'Creator, take care of this and create a healthy body.' Witness the changes made in the body.

For cancer that has been caused by radiation, command that built-up radiation to be released from the body. Command the tumour to shrink and go to the Creator's light and witness it done.

Ask if there has been heavy-metal poisoning. If there has been, the person should do an appropriate cleanse.

If a toxin is poisoning the body and you remove this from the cells, it will change the cancer to normal cells. There are supplements that can help pull toxins out too.

It is suggested that a person with cancer has an alkaline diet, does a parasite cleanse, takes a good calcium supplement and follows their progress. You may witness the Creator heal the person, but if all the other factors that are creating the cancer are not put into balance, the cancer may return.

Of the different cancers that we have worked on, we have found brain cancer and melanoma to be the most receptive to healing. These seem to be quite easy to shrink, disintegrate and make leave the body.

The most important aspect in healing cancer is to ensure that the person has a 7.2 balanced alkaline body. If they have created a cancer from negative programmes such as 'I hate this person' or 'I will die' or 'The doctor thinks I'm going to die', you need to do belief work as well.

Belief Work

When you start working on people with cancer, you're going to encounter many different emotions and beliefs. Beliefs that are typical of most cancers are 'I should suffer', 'I should die' and 'I hate this person'. See if the person can accept unconditional love and make sure they can accept healing. Instill 'I am worthy of God's love' and 'I am worthy of a healing'.

People with bladder cancer have an enormous amount of anger and will suddenly attempt to blame you for anything and everything. Please understand this is not the person, this is the cancer. Go in and pull the programmes of anger and make sure the belief 'I am healthy and strong' is instilled.

Also, ask the person what the cancer is doing to serve them. Many people will give you an actual reason, or something the cancer has done to change their life. Listen to them carefully.

If the cancer is caused by an emotional component and that component is removed, the cancer can be healed in an instant.

Test the person and see if you can find repressed anger, despair, loneliness or rejection.

To uncover negative programmes, start from their childhood and work up to the present. Pull any subconscious beliefs that are blocking their healings. Some people will die because the doctor expects them to die. Make sure you pull 'I have to die because the doctor says so'.

Another programme that clients with cancer have is 'I believe everything that the doctor says'. Just telling a person that they have cancer gives them the ability to create a slow and methodical death for themselves.

Acceptance and knowledge that the cancer is healed and they are healthy and strong will tell the subconscious to correct the problem.

Healing the Broken Soul

When you are working with someone who has cancer, ask the Creator of All That Is if their soul has been broken. (Do not use energy testing to find out if they have had this happen to them, as it will not be accurate on this particular challenge.)

Remember, when someone dies, the Creator repairs all the grief and sorrow from their life. The 'Healing the Broken Soul' exercise is a way of healing the soul while we are living. The Creator always gives us alternatives.

The Process for Healing the Broken Soul

Look into the person's eyes, because the eyes are the windows to the soul. You have taken these eyes with you in every lifetime. Even in the spirit world your eyes have been the same.

1   Centre yourself.

2   Begin by sending your consciousness down into the centre of Mother Earth, which is a part of All That Is.

3   Bring the energy up through your feet, into your body and up through all your chakras.

4   Go up through your crown chakra in a beautiful ball of light, out past the stars to the universe.

5   Go beyond the universe, past the white lights, past the dark light, past the white light, past the jelly-like substance that is the Laws, into a pearly iridescent white light, into the Seventh Plane of Existence.

6   Gather unconditional love and make the command: *'Creator of All That Is, it is commanded that* [name the person]*'s broken soul be healed and made whole once again at this time. Thank you! It is done. It is done. It is done.'*

7   Move your conscious into the person's crown chakra and go up and witness the healing. You may see a ball of light, or an orb, with cracks or tears in it. Watch as the Creator causes the ball to spin counter-clockwise, then slow down to a full stop. Then watch as the sphere begins to spin clockwise and the cracks and tears become whole. Occasionally, you may just be out in the universe, but wait until the ball appears. Never question what you witness; that's not your job. Your job is just to witness. Some people may take longer than others. If the person you're working on appears despondent, go back and ask the Creator if their process has finished. Avoid cancelling the technique in the middle. As with all healing, wait until it seems finished and ask, 'Creator, is it finished?' Then wait for the answer.

8   When it is finished, connect back to the energy of All That Is, take a deep breath in and make an energy break if you so choose.

Be aware that when people become mentally, physically or spiritually sick through being broken in their soul, they will become apathetic. When their soul is healed, their energy will come back. Joy will stimulate the adrenals and the spirit.

Once the soul has been repaired, the body's illnesses will begin to clear.

Sending Love to the Baby in the Womb

This exercise is beneficial in the treatment of many diseases and can have a positive effect on cancer. It is an amazing healing process.

You can do this exercise on yourself, on your children and parents. As a man or a woman, you have the right to give love to your child when it is in the womb. With your own parents, of course, you must realize that they have free agency as to whether they accept it or not. With clients, you must have their verbal consent to do this exercise.

The Process for Sending Love to Baby in the Womb

1 Centre yourself in your heart and visualize going down into Mother Earth, which is a part of All That Is.

2 Visualize bringing up energy through your feet, opening each chakra to the crown chakra. In a beautiful ball of light, go out to the universe.

3 Go beyond the universe, past the white lights, past the dark light, past the white light, past the jelly-like substance that is the Laws, into a pearly iridescent white light, into the Seventh Plane of Existence.

4 Make the command: *'Creator of All That Is, it is commanded that love be sent to this person as a baby in the womb. Thank you! It is done. It is done. It is done.'*

5 Now go up and witness the Creator's unconditional love surrounding the baby, whether that baby is you, your own child or your parents. Witness love filling the womb and enveloping the fetus, simply eliminating all poisons, toxins and negative emotions.

6 As soon as the process is finished, rinse yourself off and put yourself back into your space. Go into the Earth, pull Earth energy up through all your chakras to your crown chakra and make an energy break.

Supplements and Other Nutritional Recommendations

It is important for the person who is using supplements for cancer to understand that some herbs and minerals work well with others and some do not. It is the same with conventional medicine. Some herbs will not work well with certain conventional pharmaceutical drugs; in fact, there may be a negative effect as opposed to a positive one.

Second, if a person is undergoing chemotherapy, they cannot take many vitamins, because the vitamins will inhibit the chemotherapy. In many instances, you will have clients who want to take vitamins because they think that they know what is best for them. Until they have finished chemotherapy, only use healings with them. Then suggest that they take the vitamins and herbs applicable to the situation.

All the following supplements are good for cancer, but you have to give yourself a break from all herbs now and then. So take them for a while and then discontinue use for a while.

- a body cleanse and zinc supplement
- antioxidants
- alpha-lipoic acid
- CoQ10
- Echinacea (but not if the person is on chemotherapy or has leukaemia)
- Essiac tea
- a vegetable juice blend consisting of one carrot, half a beetroot, one stick of celery, a pinch of ginger and a pinch of garlic
- one cup of cottage cheese and 2T flaxseed oil
- molybdenum
- multivitamins
- noni (but not in conjunction with chemotherapy)
- pau d'arco
- Tahhebo tea
- vitamin C

Other useful remedies:

- Change to the alkaline diet.
- Do a fungus cleanse.
- Do not use wheat, processed sugar or Nutra-sweet and other artificial sugars.
- Liver cleanses (see the Liver).
- Make sure the person has enough copper, selenium and zinc.
- Nutritionally, a person with cancer should consider eating almonds, avocados and cucumbers.
- Use the lemon cleanse.

Bladder Cancer

Bladder cancer typically begins in the lining of the bladder, which is the balloon-shaped organ in the pelvic area that stores urine. Some bladder cancers remain confined to the lining, while others invade other areas.

Bladder cancer is the fourth most common cancer in males and the eighth most common in females. It's rated fifth in types of cancer that cause death. Most people who develop bladder cancer are older adults – more than 90 percent of cases occur in people older than 55, and 50 percent of cases occur in people older than 73.

Smoking is the greatest single risk factor for bladder cancer. Exposure to certain toxic chemicals and drugs also makes it more likely you will develop bladder cancer. Saudi/Gulf War syndrome can lead to bladder cancer.

One of the first signs of bladder cancer is blood in the urine and difficulty urinating. It is usually detected and diagnosed by a viewing scope and testing the urine.

Healing

Many bladder cancers are healed instantly. This is because toxins and heavy metals are the cause, not beliefs.

Belief Work

Where there are beliefs involved in bladder cancer, they revolve around resistance to change, resentment, anger, guilt and grudges.

Supplements

- a good vitamin and mineral complex
- all the green foods
- noni
- nutritional therapy
- pau d'arco

Bone Cancer

Bone cancer can be caused by a tumour isolating heavy metals inside the bones. Make sure it is not interfering with the bone. If the bone appears black and grey, this means there is a lack of calcium. This is usually caused by lead. If after a healing the tumour shrinks and grows again, there is still heavy-metal poisoning.

Intuitive Remedies

Command a healing and say, *'Creator, show me.'* Ask for the relief of all pain.

Belief Work

Check for:

God issues – work on issues of being supported by God.

Supplements

- selenium
- zinc (to pull the lead out; 50–100 mg a day)

Brain Cancer

Types

There are two types of brain tumour: primary brain tumours that originate in the brain and metastatic (secondary) brain tumours that originate from cancer cells that have migrated from other parts of the body.

Primary brain cancer rarely spreads beyond the central nervous system. Metastatic brain cancer indicates advanced disease and has a poor prognosis.

Primary brain tumours can be cancerous or non-cancerous. Both types take up space in the brain and may cause serious symptoms (e.g., vision or hearing loss) and complications (e.g., stroke). All cancerous (malignant) brain tumours are life-threatening because they have an aggressive and invasive nature. A non-cancerous primary brain tumour is life-threatening when it compromises vital structures such as arteries.

Causes

Vinyl chloride and genetic mutations are prevalent causes of brain cancer.

Clearing Radiation

This technique came from witnessing what the Creator did when brain tumours were released that were caused by too much radiation. It is a good example of a ThetaHealing technique that can be used upon yourself or others. I have used it to release the day-to-day radiation of cell phones, computers, fluorescent lights and other electrical equipment.

The Process for Clearing Radiation

1   Centre yourself in your heart and visualize going down into Mother Earth, which is a part of All That Is.

2   Visualize bringing up energy through your feet, opening each chakra to the crown chakra. In a beautiful ball of light, go out to the universe.

3   Go beyond the universe, past the white lights, past the dark light, past the white light, past the jelly-like substance that is the Laws, into a pearly iridescent white light, into the Seventh Plane of Existence.

4   Make the command: *'Creator of All That Is, it is commanded that all radiation that does not serve* [person's name] *be pulled, changed and sent to God's light. Thank you! It is done. It is done. It is done.'*

5   Witness the radiation being pulled and sent to God's light.

6   As soon as the process is finished, rinse yourself off and put yourself back into your space. Go into the Earth and pull the Earth energy up through all your chakras to your crown chakra and make an energy break.

Since radiation is not a substance that should be in the body, it is not necessary to replace it with anything.

Breast Cancer

I once had a client named Lucy who had breast cancer. She had been fighting it for about 15 years before she came to see me. Now the cancer was all through her bones, in her lungs, even in her brain. She was married to a man who was taking care of her faithfully.

To me, Lucy was the kindest, sweetest person you could ever see. We worked on amazing issues in our sessions together. Nevertheless, I always felt that she was avoiding something and I couldn't put my finger on what it was.

One day I asked her, 'What is the best thing that's happened to you since this cancer came into your life?'

She became very serious and told me, 'My husband cheated on me 17 years ago, and by God, if it's the last thing I do, I'm going to make his life miserable. Now that I'm sick he has to take care of me. He's never going to get out of this. I'm going to make sure he takes care of me morning, noon and night, so that every second he will know what his relationship with that other woman did to me. I want him to be tortured for the rest of his life.'

Stunned by this response, I said, 'My gosh, Lucy, would you like to pull that?!'

Without any hesitation she replied, 'No. I'm perfectly happy making his life miserable.'

Breast cancer is interesting. They say that one in eight women will develop it. In one woman it can take off and destroy the entire breast and in another woman it will take years to do the same thing.

Lucy's cancer seemed stable, then all of a sudden it was worse. Upon questioning her as to what she had been doing differently, I found out that she had been flying over to Hawaii to get oestrogen treatments. Apparently, there was a person in Hawaii who believed that if breast cancer clients got enough oestrogen, it would heal all their cancer. This could not be more wrong, since oestrogen makes most breast cancers grow – which is exactly what it did to Lucy. When she stopped using the oestrogen therapy, her condition began to improve once again. She would come in for sessions and show great improvement. Over the three years that I worked with her, she never did get better, but neither did she get any worse. All her doctors thought she was a miracle. She was the most resilient person they had ever seen. Nevertheless, the truth was that deep down in her heart, she harboured the most unbelievable anger and hatred for her husband. This kept her alive.

This is not true for everyone with breast cancer, as many are divorced and out of their poor relationships. However, many do still harbour hatred towards their former partner and anger that they ever let someone hurt and abuse them as they did.

With some women, massaging the breast can work as a preventive measure; however, periodic self-examination is one of the best preventatives for breast cancer.

Types

There are several types of breast cancer:

- *Ductal carcinoma in situ* is considered to be breast cancer in its early stage.
- *Infiltrating ductal carcinoma:* This is a cancer that arises in the lining of the milk ducts and invades the surrounding breast tissue.
- *Inflammatory carcinoma:* In this type of cancer the tumour arises in the lining of the milk ducts. As it grows, it plugs lymphatic and blood vessels in the breast.
- *Introductory carcinoma in situ:* This is a localized type of cancer in which cancer cells grow within the ducts.

- *Lobular carcinoma:* This is a breast cancer that arises in the lobes of the body.
- *Paget's disease of the nipple:* This cancer occurs when the cells from an underlying cancerous tumour migrate to the nipple.

Intuitive Insights

The conventional treatment for breast cancer is generally removal of the tumour, chemotherapy and radiation, along with backup from pharmaceutical drugs.

In the present day, doctors are leery about doing too many surgeries on breast-cancer patients because they have found that this can spread the cancer. However, when a person comes to you for a healing and they tell you that the oncologist wants to operate on the breast, you should ask them what they want to do. Do not go against the doctor's wishes, or the patient will be likely to turn against you. The view that a medical doctor is an all-powerful, all-knowing, omnipotent being is still very strong in Western society.

If the client is seeing a doctor when they come to you, do not discourage them. In fact, encourage them to continue because this will provide validation to them that the healings are working.

Many people with breast cancer that have issues with past relationships have a tendency to try to give you the responsibility and the decisions pertaining to the disease. This is why it is important to give responsibility back to the client and teach them to heal themselves. It may also be the cancer talking to you, not the person.

I have worked with a great many breast-cancer clients over my career. Early on, the best I could do was to stop the cancer's growth. These early clients did not actually heal until I began working on the cancer as a fungus-like essence in the body. Fungus grows in deep, dark places, so women should not wear tight bras. There seems to be a correlation (at least in some women) between the amount of time a woman has used a bra and breast cancer.

When men get breast cancer, it is also linked to fungus. Breast cancer often recurs within five years, so perhaps it spores out. It is important for the practitioner to understand that viruses, fungi and bacteria are interchangeable and that they can shift back and forth from one form to another in the body.

The right breast is where toxins are held and will work well with intuitive healing. If it is the right breast that is affected, the cause is usually environmental. A good example of this was where three women who worked together developed breast cancer at the same time.

The left breast holds emotional issues generally caused by the mother, father, husband or brother. This issue will fight the healing.

Some psychics think that breast cancer is a female entity, but there are many forms of it and they do not follow the same criteria, so I do not agree with this theory.

By the time the cancer has reached a certain size, it is almost as if it has become the person's friend. By the time it has grown twice its original size, it has become a whole way of life. I have watched people get locked into their diagnosis and their sickness. They can even claim they have the disease well after it has healed – even if the doctor has told them it is gone. Everything about them screams that they are healed and still they walk into my office and say, 'I have breast cancer.' I do a healing and then tell them to go to the doctor. I fully expect them to be completely healed, without any doubts.

Intuitive Remedies

When a client first comes to me with breast cancer, I ask the Creator if it is an irregular cell or if it is cancer. At this point, I will hear a 'yes' or 'no'. However, you should never tell a person that they have cancer, but rather suggest that they get tested for it.

When breast cancer is small, all you have to do is to go up to Theta and command a healing and in most instances, it is simply gone. However, if a person has a large protruding lump of any kind, I still tell them to go to the doctor and have it removed. It has happened that the cancer has gone by the time they have gotten to the doctor. If the cancer is pea- or marble-sized, it responds very well to healing. Unfortunately, many people do not come to me until the cancer is full-blown and in its later stages.

If the cancer breaks the skin and the person constantly views the lump, it can be harder to heal, because they see it every day and their anxiety and fear feed it. So, cover the cancer up before, during and after the healing. Instruct the client to keep the breast covered for two days and not look at it. In this way, once they do take the covering off they will see that there has been improvement in the breast. The reason we do this is that the eyes are the first witness to reality. If the person goes to a mirror after you have done the healing and does not see instant results, this may encourage the growth of the tumour and discourage the healing.

Pronounced breast cancer seems to take the same route. It starts in the breast, then moves to the lymphatic system, to the bones, onward to the lungs and then to the other breast. Once it goes into the bones, it can travel into the brain. Don't let this make you nervous. When you do healings on pronounced breast cancer you can literally watch people heal in their bones, their brain and their lungs. However, they can still have the same original tumour in the breast. Unless you treat it as if it is fungus, it's going to settle in and set up house.

With breast cancer, it is imperative to change the environment in all aspects – where the person lives, their diet, their relationships and so on.

Some deodorants should not be used on the lymph nodes, as this may be an environmental cause of the disease.

Belief Work

As soon as I began to release resentment and anger programmes in clients, I had better results with breast cancer. Now I know you can do healings on breast cancer with instant results if the person knows what it feels like to be loved, knows how to receive and accept a healing, thinks they deserve it and believes it can happen. Ask the client, 'What is the best thing you have learned from breast cancer?'

Breast cancer is almost always connected to poor relationships. These can be relationships with siblings, mates or parents. Look for:

Feelings and programmes of being taken advantage of and being abused.

Unreasonable, unresolved fears, resentments, regrets, anger and hatred.

Feelings of hopelessness, helplessness, hatred, being overburdened, being unable to change what you are feeling and wanting to get even.

'If I have breast cancer, it will make my family come together.'

'If I have breast cancer, I can live without any relationship.'

'No man will want me again if I have breast cancer.'

Be gentle and let the person talk so you can understand their issues. Men healers have to be extra gentle when they are searching for programmes in a belief work session. Some women immediately begin to think a male healer will take the side of whatever male is in their life now or was there in the past.

Even though the person may have been divorced for several years, it is best to go back to the point where resentments began and release them. It takes three to four years for problems from a miserable and hateful relationship or conflict in the family to accumulate as negative emotions in the body. Then the breast cancer will show up.

Beliefs pertaining to breast cancer are not usually things like 'I hate myself' or 'I hate this person', but rather there is a great deal of self-loathing, usually for not making changes in life.

Healers and sensitive women who get breast cancer have the tendency to get the disease so that they can bring their family back together. This seems to be the unconscious motivation behind it. This kind of self-sacrifice may seem noble, but it is ridiculous to waste your life in this way.

Ask the client, 'What is the worst thing that could happen if you were completely well?' You may find they have an absolute fear of letting anyone in to love them.

Use the following belief downloads for the digging work:

'I know how to live without resentment.'

'I know how to forgive.'

'I know how to have compassion for myself.'

Download:

'It is safe to be loved.'

'It is possible to create a life for myself.'

'It is possible that the breast cancer will go away completely.'

'The Creator of All That Is can heal anything.'

'I understand how to move forward in life.'

'I understand what it feels like to plan for the future.'

'I know the Creator's definition of and perspective on what it feels like to be intimate.'

'I know the Creator's definition of and perspective on what it feels like to be nurtured.'

'I know the Creator's definition of and perspective on what it feels like to be listened to completely.'

'I know the Creator's definition of and perspective on what it feels like to listen to your mate completely.'

'I know the Creator's definition of what intimacy is.'

'I know what it feels like to live my daily life without being victimized.'

Check to see if a divorced person feels free of any commitments to a prior mate. Test for:

'I am still in my previous marriage.'

Replace with:

'I have the Creator's definition of what it feels like to receive and accept love from a mate.'

'It's OK to feel sexual, sensual and sexy and still have good discernment.'

'I have the Creator's definition of what it feels like to enjoy sex with my mate.'

Check for beliefs involving molestation and receiving and accepting sexual love:

'I am married to God.' (Ask God for the correct programme to replace this.)

'It is my duty to have sex.'

'I have to be a sacrifice.'

'Sex is dirty.'

'I am afraid of sex in the dark or in any other environment.'

'I am embarrassed about sex.'

'I have to have sex all the time.'

'I am a sexual sacrifice.'

Replace with:

'It's OK to be sexy.'

'It's OK to have sex and be spiritual.'

'I know and understand my partner completely.'

'It's OK to enjoy sex.'

'It's OK to show sexual emotion.'

'It's OK to be sensual.'

'I respect my body.'

'It's OK to be in my body.'

'It's OK to be a girl or a boy.'

'It's OK to show emotions during sex.'

Check for being present in a relationship and issues around guilt. Download the programmes with the appropriate replacement, also:

'I know what it feels like to live without people taking advantage of me.'

'I know how to live without taking advantage of others.'

'I know how to live without having to receive pity.'

'I know what it feels like to accept love from my family without pity.'

'I know what it feels like to live without having to be a burden.'

'I know what it feels like to feel worthy of being taken care of.'

'I know it's safe to be nurtured.'

'I know it's safe to be innocent.'

'I know what it feels like to live without anger and regret.'

'I know what it feels like to live without the rejection of those I love.'

'I know what it feels like to be an important being of light.'

'I deserve to be loved.'

'I know what it feels like to live without driving other people crazy.'

'I know what it feels like to listen to other people's problems.'

'I know what it feels like to accept everything that breast cancer has to teach me and let it go.'

'I know what it feels like to have a plan for the future.'

'I know what it feels like to look at my life without regret.'

'I know what it feels like to take one day at a time and know I am doing well.'

'I know what it feels like to have a miraculous healing.'

'I know how to draw friends to me that are beneficial.'

Once I have done belief work on a client with breast cancer, I train them to work on themselves using energy healing and other alternative avenues. When they leave my office, they are empowered to heal themselves using ThetaHealing.

Supplements and Other Nutritional Recommendations

When a person gets breast cancer, they must put something out to the universe, because once they know that they have it, everyone else knows they have it as well. And everyone and their dog will send miracle cures for breast cancer. This is where people make a mistake: they take all of these different cures at once. There are some things that are good for cancer, breast cancer included, but they should be used alone, without other supplements.

Oestrogen therapy, for example, is OK for some cancers, but breast and ovarian cancer have a tendency to live off the oestrogen. In fact any hormone-related cancer is going to be triggered by an abundance of oestrogen. So never suggest any herb that has oestrogen in it. This means no black cohosh, no Damiana, no liquorice root, no maca and no suma!

Catnip tea is good for the liver and it can help breast cancer.

Cervical Cancer

Cervical cancer accounts for 11 percent of cancers. The cervix is the lower part of the uterus, the place where a baby grows during pregnancy. Cervical cancer is caused by several types of a virus called human papillomaviruses (HPV), which is spread through sexual contact.

Most women's bodies are able to fight HPV infection, but sometimes the virus leads to cancer. You're at higher risk if you smoke, have many children, use birth control pills for a long time or have HIV infection. It is suspected that the bleach used in tampons is carrying the papilloma virus and this may be one cause. A vaccine for girls and young women protects against the four types of HPV that cause most cervical cancer.

Cervical cancer may not cause any symptoms at first, but later you may have pelvic pain or bleeding from the vagina. It usually takes several years for normal cells in the cervix to turn into cancer cells. Your healthcare provider can find abnormal cells by doing a cervical smear test – examining cells from the cervix under a microscope. By getting regular smear tests, you can find and treat changing cells before they turn into cancer.

A woman once came to me because she had been diagnosed with cervical cancer and she was pregnant and the doctors wanted her to abort the baby. Apparently, they felt that in order to control the spread of the cancer, the child would have to go. You see, when a woman is pregnant, an incredible amount of growth hormone is released into the system. This could make the cancer spread at an exponential rate – at least this is what the doctors feared. But the woman wanted so badly to keep her baby! I believe that it was this desire, this unquenchable hope, that opened her to the healing. She certainly had enough motivation to dispel fear, doubt and disbelief. There was no belief work to be done; I simply witnessed the Creator come in and heal her. Afterwards, I told her to go to the doctor to be checked. It seems that she was suddenly cancer-free. She had the baby, healthy and strong.

Intuitive Remedies

Command a healing. Watch the Creator scrape the cancer out and hear the tone that will be sent to erase it. Cervical Cancer responds almost immediately to intuitive healings.

Belief Work

Check for guilt, self-esteem and worthiness issues. People with HPV virus have the same issues as those associated with herpes:

> 'It is wrong to have sex.'
>
> 'I am evil.'
>
> 'I am bad.'
>
> 'I have to be punished.'

Ask the client, 'What is the best thing you have learned from cervical cancer?'

Supplements

- folic acid
- foods high in protein
- selenium
- vitamin B complex
- vitamin C
- vitamin E
- zinc

Do not use black Damiana, maca, oestrogen, soy, suma or hormones, as these may accelerate the disease.

Colon Cancer

The human colon is a muscular tube-shaped organ measuring about four feet long. It extends from the end of your small bowel to your anus, twisting and turning through your abdomen. The three functions of the colon are to digest and absorb nutrients from food, to concentrate faecal material by absorbing fluids from it and to store and control evacuation of faecal material. The right side of the colon plays a major role in absorbing water and electrolytes, while the left side is responsible for the storage and evacuation of stools.

Colon cancer is detected through the use of a scope. It is second only to lung cancer as a cause of death.

Causes

Colon cancer tends to be genetic. Other causes can be a diet that is high in animal fat, build-up of toxins in the colon, continued problems with diarrhoea and constipation, inflammatory bowel disease, smoking and sometimes diabetes.

People who have had inflammatory bowel disease are at higher risk. A high-fibre vegetable diet is very good for these kinds of people.

Symptoms

Symptoms include:

- bleeding in the stools
- bloating
- colitis
- constipation
- weight loss

Belief Work

Beliefs will berelated to relationship problems, the inability to absorb love, the inability to express yourself, verbal, sexual and physical abuse (both childhood and adult abuse), regrets and the inability to let go of the past.

It is imperative that the bottom belief is found with colon cancer because this will have the quickest effect.

Larynx Cancer

See Oesophageal and Larynx Cancer.

Leukaemia

Leukaemia is considered a type of cancer. In my opinion, however, it is not really a cancer. Even though it is classified as such, I have found that if you deal with it in the same way as most cancers, you do not have the same results as if you deal with it as you would an infection.

Conventional medicine has no cure for leukaemia. Treatment involves chemotherapy, blood transfusions and bone-marrow transplants. These treatments can extend the life of the patient. In recent years, stem-cell research seems to be promising.

Types

The types of leukaemia are grouped by how quickly the disease develops – it is either chronic (gets worse slowly) or acute (gets worse quickly) – and by the type of white blood cell that is affected. Leukaemia can arise in lymphoid cells or myeloid cells. Leukaemia that affects lymphoid cells is called lymphocytic leukaemia. Leukaemia that affects myeloid cells is called myeloid leukaemia or myelogenous leukaemia.

Dependent on the type of leukaemia, the white blood cells attack some of the red cells.

In one type of leukaemia, the lymph system produces so many white blood cells that it does not know what to do with them. White blood cells attack irregular red blood cells, but in some cases of leukaemia the body is releasing too many red blood cells before they are adults and the white blood cells are trying to get rid of them, and so you have a high white blood cell count and a low red one. The blood cells have become dysfunctional.

Symptoms

Symptoms of leukaemia include:

- cuts that are slow to heal
- enlarged lymph nodes
- extreme weight loss
- fears
- nosebleeds
- paleness
- shortness of breath

Leukaemia is detected by a blood test.

Intuitive Insights

In order to see leukaemia in the body, you need to go into the bone marrow and the bloodstream.

I suspect that living near big electrical wires is a risk factor for leukaemia and little children are particularly vulnerable. The family needs to move away from these wires.

Intuitive Remedies

I have found that viruses have caused leukaemia, but one thing I usually find in blood diseases is mercury poisoning, so make sure you pull the mercury out of the body. Leukaemia can be healed, but if you do not take the mercury out of the body, the leukaemia may come back.

Love is the key when working on leukaemia. Go in and tell the body to produce the right red blood cells. Then go to the blood and make sure the red blood cells are at a healthy level and that the white blood cells accept them. Witness it as done. Command that the damaged cells be pulled from the blood and sent to the light of the Creator. Command the white blood cell count to lower and the red blood cell count to rise. Of course, ask the Creator for guidance.

Belief Work

Any time I work on someone who has leukaemia or non-Hodgkin's lymphoma, I make sure they know that they are loved and we work on resentment issues. These people do have a lot of old resentments! Teach them how to feel nurtured and loved.

Babies are prone to leukaemia if they do not have enough nurturing and love, but some of them are little warriors who have come into this world to teach their parents how to love each other. These babies are easy to heal. Just go up and ask the Creator.

It is important to work with the parents, too, because you can make babies go into remission, but they will not stay in remission until they know they are loved.

With adults as well, if you do not work on their resentments and teach them how to feel loved, you will not be able to hold the results. Once they feel loved, though, the results are likely to be good. Download:

'I know what it feels like to be loved.'

'I know how to absorb love.'

'I know what it feels like to be cherished.'

'I know what it feels like to be adored.'

'I know what it feels like to be important.'

'I know what it feels like to be appreciated.'

'I know how to be appreciated.'

'I know it's possible to be appreciated.'

'I know what it feels like to communicate my thoughts easily and effortlessly.'

'I know what it feels like to have hope.'

'I know what it feels like for all the organs of my body to communicate in unison.'

'I know what it feels like to appreciate and love my body.'

'I know what it feels like to be surrounded by love.'

'I know what it feels like to know that this Earth is not a bad place.'

'I know what it feels like to know that this Earth is safe.'

'I know what it feels like to know I am safe.'

'I know what it feels like to know that it is safe to be well.'

'I know what it feels like to live without being too tired.'

'I know what it feels like for my body to grow stronger every day.'

'I know that it is possible for the people around me to co-operate.'

'I know what it feels like to know I am important.'

'I know what it feels like to live with hope for myself and others.'

'I know how to be contagious with this hope.'

'I know what it feels like to live with my self-esteem getting better all the time.'

'I know what it feels like for people to love me.'

'I know what it feels like to utilize every moment in the highest and best way.'

Supplements

- It is suggested that all amalgam fillings are pulled when dealing with leukaemia.

- Liver flushes and selenium are excellent aids for leukaemia.
- Pull mercury out of the body by suggesting ALA.
- Use stinging nettle as a supplement.

***

- Do not suggest Echinacea, goldenseal or melatonin – they will make leukaemia worse.

Lung Cancer

Lung cancer forms in the tissues of the lungs, usually in the cells lining the air passages. It is the leading cause of death by cancer among both men and women. The age of diagnosis is generally 60 years old. Doctors detect it by image screening, biopsy and blood tests.

Smoking accounts for almost 80 percent of lung cancer cases. Other instances are caused by alcohol abuse and exposure to asbestos, herbicides, nickel, pesticides, pollution and radon.

Treatment options include chemotherapy, immunotherapy, radiation therapy, surgery and vaccine therapy.

Types

The two main types are small cell lung cancer and non-small cell lung cancer. These types are diagnosed based on how the cells look under a microscope.

Symptoms

Signs and symptoms of lung cancer include:

- fatigue
- loss of appetite
- recurring pneumonia
- shortness of breath
- weight loss

Intuitive Remedies

Witness the cancer being gently scraped from the lungs and send to the Creator's light. This is an obedient cancer to healings. Permit the Creator to show you what to do.

Belief Work

If there is not an instant healing, belief work will be necessary.

This disease can be caused by sorrow and resentment. The practitioner should consider using 'The Heart Song' exercise (*see Cardiovascular Disease*).

Ask the client what was going on in their lives when they first got sick. Ask the client what would happen if they were completely healed.

Download:

'I know what it feels like to breathe clearly.'

'I know what it feels like to make quick and decisive decisions.'

'I know what it feels like to accept the breath of life.'

'I know what it feels like to forgive myself.'

'I know what it feels like to clean my body.'

'I know what it feels like to eat good food.'

'I know what it feels like to live without tobacco.'

'I know what it feels like to live my day-to-day life feeling important.'

'I know what it feels like to be completely healed.'

'I know that it's possible to be completely healed.'

'I know what it feels like to be able to express my emotions.'

'I know what it feels like to live without being angry all the time.'

Supplements

- noni
- Sibu berry drink
- slippery elm
- vitamin C
- vitamin E

Lymphatic Cancer/Lymphoma

Lymphoma is a type of cancer involving cells of the immune system, called lymphocytes, which fight infection. Just as cancer represents many different diseases, lymphoma represents many different cancers of lymphocytes – about 35 different sub-types.

Lymph nodes are found in the abdomen, chest and under the arms. Other parts of the lymph system include the adenoids, bone marrow, thymus gland and tonsils.

Types

Cancer that develops in the lymph system is classified as Hodgkin's or non-Hodgkin's lymphoma.

In non-Hodgkin's, the body's ability to fight off infection is significantly decreased, because it has fewer normal white blood cells. Older adults are at higher risk.

Causes

The causes of lymphoma are linked to viruses. Risk factors include AIDS, black hair dye, mercury, exposure to herbicides and pesticides, heredity, immune system dysfunction, immuno-suppressant therapies and receiving an organ transplantation.

Lead or mercury poisoning can also cause lymphatic cancer. It will pull bone marrow out of the bone and attach itself to the bone. The spleen will swell. There is the need to clean out the heavy metals so the body will heal.

Symptoms

Symptoms of lymphoma include:

- a feeling that something is stuck in the throat
- chronic disorders of the mouth, tongue or throat that do not heal
- difficulty swallowing
- discoloured patches in the mouth or throat area
- loss of feeling in the mouth

A biopsy should be done if lymphoma is suspected.

Intuitive Insights

People with lymphoma have a need to please others and have issues with lack of love. They are generally having problems with one of their parents and cannot express their feelings about the relationship.

Running away is a symptom of non-Hodgkin's on all levels – physically, mentally and spiritually.

Usually, the parent that brings a child with lymphoma to you will tell you that they are having problems with the other parent. There is undoubtedly abuse in these families, but sometimes these children are so sensitive that the abuse could be something as simple as the parents screaming at one another. Overall, the parents will not go out of their way to make the abusive situation any better and will expect the child to deal with it.

Intuitive Remedies

Witness the lymphoma being pulled and sent to the Creator's light.

Since toxins cause Hodgkin's and non-Hodgkin's lymphoma, healings have great results, but you always have to follow up on non-Hodgkin's with belief work.

Alcohol should be completely avoided for those who have lymphoma.

Belief Work

Work on the person being able to express themselves, defend themselves and move forward. Download:

'I am allowed to stick up for myself.'

'I know how to express myself.'

'I am allowed to defend myself.'

'I am allowed to move forward.'

These are only a guideline; you still have to do the digging work to find out with whom the person is having issues. Giving them back their identity is very important.

Download:

'I know the Creator's definition of love.'

'I know the Creator's definition of how to shine.'

'I know the Creator's definition of what a home feels like.'

'I know how to make a home on this Earth.'

'I know the Creator's definition of what the breath of life feels like.'

'I am worthy of communicating with the Creator.'

'I am worthy of living without the fear of being alone.'

'I know what it feels like to understand what the person next to me is feeling.'

'I know what it feels like to care about another person.'

'I know how to live without permitting negative thoughts in.'

'I can live without another person taking advantage of me.'

'I know what it feels like to live my life in true harmony with God.'

'I know what it feels like to hear truth.'

'I know what it feels like to be able to hold my pride.'

'I know how to live without permitting others to make me sad.'

'I know what it feels like to live without having to be needy.'

'I know how to give back to the world.'

'I know what it feels like to live my life without resenting everyone who helps me.'

'I know what it feels like to live without resenting anyone.'

'I know what it feels like to appreciate those who are there to help me.'

'I know how to release people from obligations of making me angry.'

'I know what it feels like to live without being angry at the world.'

'I know what it feels like to live without the fear of moving forward.'

'I know what it feels like to move forward.'

'I know that it's possible to move forward.'

Oesophageal and Larynx Cancer

Oesophageal cancer forms in tissues lining the oesophagus, the muscular tube through which food passes from the throat to the stomach.

This cancer is more prevalent in women than men.

Types

Two types of oesophageal cancer are squamous cell carcinoma (cancer that begins in flat cells lining the oesophagus) and adenocarcinoma (cancer that begins in cells that make and release mucus and other fluids).

Causes

The causes of oesophageal cancer are not clearly understood by medical science, but risk factors include coeliac disease, heredity, obesity, radiation therapy, reflux disease and smoking.

Symptoms

Symptoms include:

- difficulty in swallowing
- excess mucus
- hoarseness
- vomiting blood
- weight loss

Belief Systems

Emotions connected to oesophageal and larynx cancer include the inability to express feelings and then guilt from the over-expression of feelings. Beliefs pertain to guilt, taking on the burden of another person's feelings and problems, and attachment to the past.

Supplements

- a diet high in green leafy vegetables
- vitamin A, not to exceed 25,000 units
- vitamin C

Oral Cancer

Oral cancer includes cancer of the cheeks, floor of the mouth, gum, hard palate, lips, minor salivary glands and tongue. It usually occurs in people over the age of 45, but can develop at any age.

Symptoms

The following are the most common symptoms:

- a lump on the lip or in the mouth
- a lump on the neck

- a sore on the lip or in the mouth that does not heal
- a white or red patch on the gums, tongue or lining of the mouth
- bad breath
- difficulty opening the jaw
- difficulty or pain with chewing or swallowing
- loose teeth
- oral pain that does not go away or a feeling that something is caught in the throat
- sensory loss of the feelings in the face
- swelling of the jaw that causes dentures to fit poorly or become uncomfortable
- unusual bleeding, pain or numbness in the mouth

Intuitive Remedies

I have only worked on this particular kind of cancer five or six times, but in every instance it has healed instantly.

Belief Work

I recommend following up with the belief work and instilling the programmes of being able to express yourself and not worrying about what other people think of you. When you are compulsively worrying about what everyone thinks of you, you cannot express yourself. Download:

'I know how to express myself.'

'I know how to feel good about myself in spite of what others think.'

Supplements and Other Nutritional Recommendations

- fresh fruits and vegetables
- omega 3 fatty acids
- rinsing with Melaleuca oil (Be careful, this is strong stuff!)

Ovarian Cancer

Ovarian cancer is a disease produced by the rapid growth and division of cells within one or both ovaries, the reproductive glands in which the ova, or eggs, and the female sex hormones are made. The ovaries contain cells that, under normal circumstances, reproduce to maintain tissue health. When growth control is lost, the cells divide out of control and a cellular mass or tumour is formed.

If the tumour is confined to a few cell layers, such as the surface cells, it does not invade surrounding tissues or organs, so is considered benign. If it spreads to surrounding tissues or organs, it is considered malignant, or cancerous.

If ovarian cancer is treated early, the survival rate is quite high. Unfortunately, it is known as the silent disease, as there are very few symptoms until it is quite advanced. Ovarian cancer moves very quickly in the body. If it metastasizes to the bone, then there is a problem. Chemotherapy can, however, work well.

Causes

The causes of ovarian cancer are unknown; however, radiation exposure and other toxins are suspected.

Risk factors are a diet high in animal fat, a history of other cancers, HPV virus and obesity. However, the use of birth control pills seems to lower the risk of ovarian cancer by 50 to 60 percent.

Symptoms

Symptoms include:

- a malnourished or wasted appearance
- abdominal/pelvic discomfort or pressure
- back or leg pain
- bloating
- changes in bowel function or urinary frequency
- fatigue
- gastrointestinal symptoms (e.g., gas, long-term stomach pain, indigestion)
- nausea or loss of appetite
- unusual vaginal bleeding

Intuitive Insights

Because ovarian cancer is a fast-moving cancer, a thorough and complete healing must be done and the client should get scanned and tested by a doctor. Ovarian cancer can come back and be all over the body within a few weeks. So if someone comes to you with ovarian cancer, make sure they go to their doctor immediately, before you start doing healings with them.

People do not come to me with ovarian cancer very often. Usually, by the time they do, the cancer has spread all through their organs and they are convinced that they are going to die. I have only one session to work with them.

When you start dealing with people with fast-moving cancers like ovarian cancer, make sure that they understand that they have purpose in life so they can finish living. If they do not have a purpose, sometimes they do not want to do anything but die.

Intuitive Remedies

This disease is responsive to healing.

Go to the person's space to find out if toxins caused the cancer. If so, a simple healing is in order. These toxins could be asbestos, mercury or lead. They will inhibit the person's ability to express themselves in relationships.

Use the 'Sending Love to the Baby in the Womb' exercise and 'The Heart Song' exercise to clear the person of toxins.

Always send them to their doctor for validation after a healing.

Belief Work

People with ovarian cancer have a tendency to be very defensive, so it is best to make it very clear that this cancer is likely to be caused by genetic beliefs or toxins.

Ovarian cancer always comes with programmes connected to relationship issues. There seems to be the pervading belief that the person must die to redeem themselves.

These are also issues around trust and blame. People with ovarian cancer may try to place the blame for the disease on their husband or the healer: 'You cheated on me in the past and that is why I am sick.' Or: 'You did a healing on me and it didn't work, so it's all your fault.'

Start with relationship issues: husband, mother and father issues.

Then look at issues of inadequacy in relationships.

Download:

'I know how to live my day-to-day life feeling important.'

'I know what it feels like to know that I am important in my relationship.'

'I know what it feels like to make decisions in my relationship that are important to me.'

'I know what it feels like to live my life without being abused.'

'I know I have the strength to move forward and go on.'

'I know what it feels like to make good decisions based on my heart.'

'I know it's wrong to stay where I am unhappy.'

'I know what it feels like to be happy, joyful and strong.'

'I know it's possible to be in a good relationship and be full of joy.'

'I know it's possible to live my life knowing I am completely healed.'

'I know it's possible to live my life without being angry at anyone that helps me.'

'I know what it feels like to live my life without despair, anger and disappointment.'

'I know what it feels like to have a purpose.'

Supplements

Only use these supplements if the person has chosen not to have chemotherapy or if they have finished with it:

- ALA
- CoQ10
- glutathione
- noni
- omega 3s

Pancreatic Cancer

Pancreatic cancer is one of the most serious of cancers. It develops when cancerous cells form in the tissues of the pancreas, a large organ that lies horizontally behind the lower part of the stomach. The pancreas secretes enzymes that aid digestion and hormones that help regulate the metabolism of carbohydrates.

Pancreatic cancer spreads rapidly and is seldom detected in its early stages, which is a major reason why it's a leading cause of cancer death. Signs and symptoms may not appear until the disease is quite advanced. By that time, the cancer is likely to have spread to other parts of the body and surgical removal is no longer possible.

For years, little was known about pancreatic cancer. But researchers are beginning to understand the genetic basis of the disease. This knowledge may eventually lead to new and better treatments. Just as important, you may be able to reduce the risk of pancreatic cancer with some lifestyle changes.

Intuitive Insights

Pancreatic cancer looks black and brown in the pancreas in the body and is fast-growing.

Intuitive Remedies

Pancreatic cancer is the second fastest cancer to respond to intuitive healings, the fastest being brain cancer. Make the command and witness the Creator dissolve the tumour.

Prostate Cancer

I first met Ipu Brown in Australia when she came to one of my classes. She walked up to me during break time and offered to give me a therapeutic massage. She came highly recommended by my seminar co-ordinator, so I said OK. Ipu was a beautiful woman of Maori descent. During the massage, we found we liked one another and I invited her to another of my classes. From the start, I could sense something in Ipu, a fierce goodness that pervaded her. She was a traditional Polynesian dancer, massage therapist and healer. She still had many connections with traditional Maori people in New Zealand.

After I had met her, the Creator told me that I was going to go to New Zealand to bring ThetaHealing to the Maori people and it was through Ipu that I was going to accomplish this.

In time, Ipu became one of my ThetaHealing teachers (and one of my finest friends) and took the work to the Maori. We staged an 'Intuitive Anatomy' class in Rotorua, right in the heart of the Maori culture.

What you need to understand about the Maori culture is that they believe. They heal easily because they do not have so many subconscious beliefs blocking them from healings.

During the 'Intuitive Anatomy' class, we invited outside people to come and participate in healing circles, so the students could practise their new-found skills on them. One of these participants was an elder, a Maori man with advanced prostate cancer. He had been told that he only had a few days to live. As I worked with him, I witnessed the Creator come into his space and give him an instant healing. The cancer was gone and he was healed.

The Prostate Gland

The prostate is a gland found only in men. It is situated just below the bladder and in front of the rectum. It is about the size of a walnut. The tube that carries urine (the urethra) runs through it and it contains cells that make some of the semen that protects and nourishes the sperm.

Prostate cancer is the second leading cause of cancer death in men. (Lung cancer is the first.) However, while one man in six will get prostate cancer during his lifetime, only one man in 35 will die of this disease. It is prevalent in men over 50.

A client of mine told me about his father, who died within a week of the diagnosis. Apparently, he was so afraid that he was going to die that he just gave up. The prostate cancer probably would not have killed him for 30 years, and the doctor had told him that, but he was quite literally scared to death.

This shows you how important it is with prostate cancer to work with the psychological issues. You may have to pull programmes such as 'Cancer is a death sentence'.

The PSA Test

By the time men get to the age of 50, doctors will run a test called the PSA (prostate-specific antigen) test. This measures the possibility of cancer in the system. It is not an accurate test. The man who developed it says it isn't accurate because men over 50 will normally have elevated PSAs. However, other tests accompany the PSA test that tell a doctor if a man has prostate cancer.

Just because you have a high PSA doesn't mean you have cancer.

And remember that it is normal for a few small cancer cells to be in the prostate.

Be aware that if you are going to get your PSA checked and are doing any kind of liver cleanse using something such as milk thistle, your PSA levels will be abnormally high. In addition, anytime you have a swollen organ, your PSA test will be high. Therefore, if you are having problems with your kidneys when you are tested, your results will probably be higher than normal. If you are using any herbs or supplements, make sure to discontinue use of them for three days before a PSA test for a more accurate reading.

Intuitive Remedies

Most prostate cancer can be instantaneously healed. I have seen prostate cancer that has metastasized to the bone go in one healing. If prostate cancer is healed instantly, it is generally caused by toxins in the body.

Prostate cancer can usually be changed with cleanses and dietary changes.

Belief Work

One of my clients was diagnosed with prostate cancer and came for a healing. During the reading, I scanned his body and told him, 'It looks as though you're in a very difficult relationship.'

He replied, 'I am married to the meanest woman you ever saw.'

I asked him, 'Why do you stay married? Why don't you change this situation?'

He said, 'I would rather die than go through a divorce.'

And that's what he did: he died instead of going through a divorce.

You see, healing toxic feelings is like healing toxic substances. You can give the person a healing that will clear the problem, but if the toxin is reintroduced into the system, the disease re-establishes itself.

Men have a tendency to 'make a relationship work' no matter what, because if they divorce, their wife is going to get 50 percent of all the couple has accumulated. You may not think that this is a big deal, but it is a big deal with many men. I know men who have been in relationships with abusive and miserable women for years, yet they would rather die than face the emotional and financial upheaval the break-up would cause. Unfortunately, it is likely that the relationship created the prostate cancer in the first place, because prostate cancer is usually associated with problems in relationships. The cancer attaches itself to the weakened area of the body, the area under distress, the area with the emotion that is out of control and out of order.

Advanced prostate cancer makes a person very tired. Sometimes it takes energy to fight it. So simply telling your client that they need to fight for who they are or change things in their life or work on their feelings so they can love everyone may not work. These issues are too deep to begin with. Instead begin with:

'I know how to have energy.'

'I know how to get better.'

Then continue with the relationship issues.

When it comes to prostate cancer, you have to work on how to have love in a spiritual sense. You have to teach the person that it is OK to have opinions and it is OK to have emotions, too. How many men are allowed to cry when they are children and adults? Men are told to be strong, to be in control and not to show emotion! Holding emotions inside is a likely reason why some men are susceptible to prostate cancer.

The person has to know what it feels like to be completely loved and how to change their life. Otherwise they will stagnate and not have the emotional component necessary to follow through. However, this is easily done, because they will not struggle to keep the beliefs.

Ask them, 'How has this cancer benefited you? What is the best thing that has happened to you because of this cancer?'

Listen to what they say. Many of the answers will surprise you, such as, 'If I have this cancer, I will get love from my wife' or 'If I have this cancer, I can finally rest.' The answer to this dilemma is to get the client to understand that they can have these things without the cancer.

Download:

'I know how to express myself in relationships.'

'I know how to feel good about myself.'

Supplements and Other Nutritional Recommendations

To keep the prostate in good shape, use:

- CoQ10
- lipids
- liver cleanses (see the Liver)
- plenty of fluids
- regular ejaculation
- saw palmetto
- vitamin A
- vitamin B complex
- vitamin C
- vitamin E
- zinc

***

- Avoid tobacco, tobacco smoke, noxious chemicals and food additives.
- Cut back on red meat.
- Drink freshly made vegetable and fruit juices daily.
- Eat grapefruit, tomatoes and watermelon.
- Eat foods high in omega-3 fatty acids such as herring, salmon and sardines.
- Eliminate alcoholic beverages, coffee and teas.
- Include in your diet foods that are high in zinc, such as mushrooms, pumpkin seeds, spinach, sunflower seeds and wholegrains.

- It has been found that the hormone DHEA blocks an enzyme that promotes the growth of cancer cells.
- Maintain a wholefood diet with plenty of fresh fruit and vegetables, including blueberries, Brazil nuts, cantaloupe melon, cherries, grapes, legumes, strawberries and walnuts.
- Oregano oil kills parasites in the prostate.

Skin Cancer

Skin cancer is the abnormal growth of skin cells. It most often develops on skin exposed to the sun. However, this common form of cancer can also occur on areas of the skin not ordinarily exposed to sunlight, such as the palms, spaces between the toes and the genital area. Skin cancer affects people of all skin tones, including those with darker complexions.

Most skin cancers can be prevented by limiting or avoiding exposure to ultraviolet (UV) radiation. If skin cancer is found early enough, it can be successfully treated with conventional methods.

Not all skin changes are cancerous. The only way to know for sure is to have your skin examined by a doctor or dermatologist.

Skin cancer begins in the skin's top layer, the epidermis. This is as thin as a pencil line and provides a protective layer of skin cells that the body continually sheds.

The epidermis contains three types of cells:

- *Squamous cells* lie just below the outer surface.
- *Basal cells*, which produce new skin cells, sit beneath the squamous cells.
- *Melanocytes*, which produce melanin, the pigment that gives skin its normal colour, are located in the lower part of the epidermis. Melanocytes produce more melanin when you are in the sun to help protect the deeper layers of your skin. Extra melanin produces the darker colour of tanned skin.

Normally, skin cells within the epidermis develop in a controlled way. In general, healthy new cells push older cells toward the skin's surface, where they die and eventually are sloughed off. This process is controlled by the DNA; skin cancer occurs when this process malfunctions. When the DNA is damaged, changes occur in the instructions, which can cause new cells to grow out of control and form a mass of cancer cells.

Types

There are three major types of skin cancer:

- basal cell carcinoma
- squamous cell carcinoma
- melanoma

Basal cell carcinomas and most squamous cell carcinomas are slow growing and highly treatable, especially if found early. However, squamous cell carcinoma also can spread internally. Melanoma affects deeper layers of the skin and has the greatest potential to spread to other tissues in the body.

All three types of skin cancer are on the rise.

Basal Cell Carcinoma

This is the most common skin cancer and the most easily treated. It is the least likely to spread. It usually appears as one of the following:

- a pearly or waxy bump on the face, ears or neck
- a flat flesh-coloured or brown scar-like lesion on the chest or back

Squamous Cell Carcinoma

Squamous cell carcinoma is easily treated if detected early, but it is somewhat more likely to spread than basal cell carcinoma. It usually appears as one of the following:

- a firm, red nodule on your face, lips, ears, neck, hands or arms
- a flat lesion with a scaly, crusted surface on your face, ears, neck, hands or arms

Melanoma

Melanoma is the most serious form of skin cancer and is responsible for most skin-cancer deaths. It can develop in otherwise normal skin or in an existing mole that turns malignant. Although it can occur anywhere on the body, it appears most often on the upper back or face in both men and women.

Warning signs of melanoma include:

- a large brownish spot with darker speckles located anywhere on the body

- a simple mole located anywhere on the body that changes in colour or size or bleeds
- a small lesion with an irregular border with red, white, blue or blue-black spots on the trunk or limbs
- dark lesions on the palms, soles, fingertips and toes, or on mucous membranes lining the mouth, nose, vagina and anus
- shiny, firm, dome-shaped bumps located anywhere on the body

If not treated and released, melanoma can be life-threatening. However, if the disease is treated early, chances of recovery are good.

There are four types of melanoma, each with slightly different characteristics:

Acral lentiginous melanoma is the most common type among people of African and Asian descent. The lesions have flat dark brown areas with bumpy portions that are brown to black or blue to black in colour. They most likely appear on the palms, soles of the feet and in the nail beds of the fingers and toes.

Lentigo maligna melanoma is more common in women than in men. The lesions generally occur on the face, neck and ears or other areas that have been heavily exposed to the sun. This type of melanoma rarely occurs before the age of 50 and is usually preceded by a pre-cancerous stage called *lentigo maligna*.

Nodular melanoma is a type of disease that attacks the underlying tissue without first spreading across the surface of the skin. It is more common in men than in women; the lesions may resemble blood blisters and coloration can be from pearly white to blue-black. Modular melanoma tends to metastasize sooner than other types of melanoma.

Superficial spreading melanoma is the most common type. It occurs primarily in Caucasians and more often in women than in men. It begins as a flat mole, most often in the lower legs or upper back that develops an irregular surface.

Less Common Skin Cancers

Less common types of skin cancer include:

Aposi Sarcoma

This rare form of skin cancer develops in the skin's blood vessels and causes red or purple patches on the skin or mucous membranes. Like melanoma, it is a serious form of skin cancer. It is mainly seen in people with weakened immune systems.

Merkel Cell Carcinoma

In this rare cancer, firm, shiny nodules occur on or just beneath the skin and in hair follicles. They may be red, pink or blue and can vary in size from a quarter of an inch to more than two inches. Merkel cell carcinoma is usually found on sun-exposed areas on the head, neck, arms and legs. It grows rapidly and often spreads to other parts of the body.

Sebaceous Gland Carcinoma

This uncommon and aggressive cancer originates in the oil glands in the skin. It usually appears as hard, painless nodules. These can develop anywhere, but most occur on the eyelid, where they are often mistaken for benign conditions.

Pre-cancerous skin lesions, such as an actinic keratosis, also can develop into squamous cell skin cancer.

Actinic keratoses appear as rough, scaly, brown or dark-pink patches. They're most commonly found on the face, ears, lower arms and hands of fair-skinned people whose skin has been damaged by the sun.

Causes

UV Light

Much of the damage to the DNA in skin cells results from ultraviolet (UV) radiation found in sunlight and in commercial tanning lamps and tanning beds. UV light is divided into three wavelength bands:

> ultraviolet A (UVA)
>
> ultraviolet B (UVB)
>
> ultraviolet C (UVC)

Only UVA and UVB rays reach the Earth. UVC radiation is absorbed by atmospheric ozone.

At one time, scientists believed that only UVB rays played a role in the formation of skin cancer. UVB light does cause harmful changes in skin cell DNA, including the development of oncogenes, which are a type of gene that can turn a normal cell into a malignant one. UVB rays are responsible for sunburn and for many basal cell and squamous cell cancers.

UVA also contributes to skin cancer. It penetrates the skin more deeply than UVB does and weakens the skin's immune system to increase the risk of cancer, especially melanoma. Tanning beds deliver high doses of UVA, which makes them especially dangerous.

Other Factors

Sun exposure does not explain melanomas or other skin cancers that develop on skin not ordinarily exposed to sunlight. Genetics may play a role. Skin cancer can also develop from exposure to toxic chemicals or because of radiation treatments. Bear in mind the following risk factors:

- A *family history of skin cancer:* If one of your parents or a sibling has had skin cancer, you may be at increased risk of the disease. Some families are affected by a condition called familial atypical mole-malignant melanoma (FAMMM) syndrome.

- A *history of sunburn:* After sunburn, your body works to repair the damage. Having a lot of blistering sunburn as a child or teenager increases your risk of developing skin cancer as an adult. Sunburn in adulthood is also a risk factor.

- A *personal history of skin cancer:* If you have developed skin cancer once, you're at risk of developing it again. Even basal cell and squamous cell carcinomas that have been successfully removed can recur in the same spot, often within two to three years.

- A *weakened immune system:* People with weakened immune systems are at greater risk of developing skin cancer. This includes people living with HIV/AIDS or leukaemia and those taking immunosuppressant drugs after an organ transplant.

- *Age:* The risk of developing skin cancer increases with age, primarily because many skin cancers develop slowly. The damage that occurs during childhood or adolescence may not become apparent until middle age.

- *Excessive sun exposure:* Anyone who spends considerable time in the sun may develop skin cancer, especially if the skin is not protected by sunscreen or clothing. Tanning is a risk. A tan is your skin's injury response to excessive UV radiation.

- *Exposure to environmental hazards:* Exposure to environmental chemicals, including some herbicides, increases the risk of skin cancer.

- *Fair skin:* If you have blond or red hair, light-coloured eyes and you freckle or sunburn easily, you are much more likely to develop skin cancer than if you have darker features.

- *Fragile skin:* Skin that has been burned, injured or weakened by treatments for other skin conditions is more susceptible to sun damage and skin cancer. Certain psoriasis treatments and eczema creams might increase your risk of skin cancer.

- *Medication:* Certain types of medication can cause the skin to be more susceptible to the sun. These include acne medicine, antibiotics, antidepressants, antihistamines, birth control pills, diuretics and oestrogen.

- *Moles:* People who have many moles or abnormal moles, called dysplastic nevi, are at increased risk of skin cancer. If you have a history of abnormal moles, check them regularly for changes.

- *Pre-cancerous skin lesions:* Having skin lesions known as actinic keratoses can increase your risk of developing skin cancer. These pre-cancerous skin growths typically appear as rough, scaly patches that range in colour from brown to dark pink.

- *Sunny or high-altitude climates:* People who live in warm climates are exposed to more sunlight than people who live in colder climates. Living at higher elevations, where the sunlight is strongest, also exposes you to more radiation.

If you notice any suspicious change in your skin, consult your doctor immediately. As with all cancers, early detection increases the chances of successful treatment. Do not wait for the suspected area to start hurting, because skin cancer seldom causes pain. Remember, this is your skin, the largest organ in the body. It is connected to all the nerve endings, blood cells and the lymphatic system.

Intuitive Insights

A great deal of fear surrounds melanoma, and it is true that it is very dangerous. If it grows to a certain point, it will spread all through the skin and to the rest of the body very quickly. One of my clients named Sally, who told her story in *ThetaHealing*, was healed of eight melanoma lesions in her brain. If you had been Sally's doctor, you would have told her that she had only a few months to live. This is exactly what she had been told by the doctors. When she came in for a healing, she had nothing to lose, so she was open to anything.

In my opinion, the reason that melanoma is so responsive to healing is because it is generally caused by some kind of toxin or radiation.

Seen on the skin, not all melanoma has a rough-edged appearance.

Sometimes it is just a little spot on the body that looks odd. Sometimes melanomas can look like little scabs. I have also seen melanoma that looks like different colours in the skin pigment. Therefore, if you have a spot on your body that you are not sure of, you might want to get it checked.

If a client comes to you with a spot and you ask the Creator if it's cancer, you might get a 'yes' or 'no' answer, but when it comes to melanoma, make sure that they get it checked by their doctor to make sure it's not in the bloodstream. The reason I'm saying this is not because I don't trust your ability to listen to the Creator. I'm saying this so that you don't set yourself up for somebody to blame you because of a melanoma that developed two weeks after they left your office.

If you see odd-looking liver spots with a funny shape, this could be melanoma or basal cell cancer. Basal cell cancer is recognized by rough edges. This is conventionally treated by being burned off.

Intuitive Remedies

I think that melanoma is one of the most responsive cancers to healing. This is, however, no reason to become arrogant and direct the person away from receiving that extra validation from their doctor. I think that people should go to a doctor, then a healer, then back to the doctor for validation.

One thing that works on melanoma is commanding all excess radiation to leave the body. You also have to teach people to pick their doctor. You do not have to go to a doctor that you do not like.

Belief Work

Since the skin is the first line of defence, most of the belief programmes will be associated with the things that it does for us. Replace with:

'I am protected.'

'I am secure.'

'I believe that melanoma can be healed.'

Melanoma is very responsive to belief work.

If you do not like some of your moles, check to see whether you are carrying the belief that it is wrong to have moles. Many women were killed in the times of the witch-hunts because they had a mole in a certain place, particularly from the neck up, where people could see it. Some women were also considered witches if they had birthmarks.

Supplements

For basal cell cancer:

- Put ALA and selenium directly on the cancer and it will dissolve.
- You can also use a herbal salve called black salve.

For melanoma, use:

- a multivitamin and mineral combination
- black salve
- burdock root
- CoQ10
- essential fatty acids
- glutathione and ALA, 600 mg
- noni
- selenium
- vitamin A
- vitamin B complex
- vitamin C

Stomach Cancer

The most common form of cancer that affects the stomach is adenocarcinoma, which arises in the glands of the innermost layer of the stomach. This tumour tends to spread through the wall of the stomach and from there into the adjoining organs (pancreas and spleen) and lymph nodes. It can then spread through the bloodstream and lymph system to distant organs. This disease is more common in men than in women. The age group is generally past 40. The risk factors are:

- A chronic infection of *Helicobacter pylori*, which is a common cause of chronic gastritis and peptic ulcer disease.
- A family history of stomach cancer.
- A prior diagnosis of pernicious anaemia (a chronic progressive disease caused by the failure of the body to absorb vitamin B12).
- A diet deficient in fresh fruits and vegetables and rich in salted or smoked fish or meats and poorly preserved foods.
- Blood type A.
- Tobacco and alcohol abuse.

Treating benign stomach or duodenal ulcer disease is performed by removing part of your stomach and is associated with an increased risk of cancer developing in the remaining stomach, especially 15 years or more after the surgery.

Symptoms

Symptoms include:

- acid indigestion
- anaemia
- black and tarry stools
- blood in the faeces
- fatigue
- pain in the stomach after eating
- vomiting after eating
- weight loss

Intuitive Insights

When you go to the stomach, the cancer will have made the lining look as though it is turning grey instead of being the beautiful pink colour it is supposed to be.

Healings are effective with stomach cancer.

Belief Work

When you meet people with stomach cancer, they can be a little grouchy. It is likely that their belief systems will pertain to how they can absorb love.

I have seen these programmes attached to stomach cancer:

'Everything is against me.'

'What's the use? I might as well be dead.'

'I've given up.'

Supplements

- ALA
- *Aloe vera* juice

- antioxidants
- green vegetables and less meat
- noni
- omega 3s
- selenium
- vitamin C
- vitamin E

Testicular Cancer

Testicular cancer occurs in the testicles (testes), which are located inside the scrotum, a loose bag of skin underneath the penis. The testicles produce male sex hormones and sperm for reproduction. Compared with other types of cancer, testicular cancer is rare. However, it is the most common cancer in American males between the ages of 15 and 34.

Testicular cancer is highly treatable, even when the cancer has spread beyond the testicle. Depending on the type and stage, you may receive one of several treatments or a combination. Testicular cancer does respond to chemotherapy and radiation.

Regular testicular self-examinations can help identify growths early, when the chances of successful treatment of testicular cancer are highest. However, cysts may be misdiagnosed as cancer.

Intuitive Remedies

Testicular cancer seems to be caused by heavy metals in the body. It may metastasize to the bone, but responds very well to healings.

Belief Work

Belief work is generally necessary. This cancer is connected to relationship and sexual issues – how one feels about sex, how one feels about women, and so on.

Supplements

As well as eating tomatoes, watermelon and wholegrains, take:

- ALA
- omega 3s
- vitamin E

CANDIDA

Many people suffer from an overgrowth of the micro-organism *Candida albicans*, a condition called Candidiasis.

Symptoms

There is a wide variety of symptoms, which may vary greatly and includes:

- *Allergies to foods and/or airborne chemicals:* The number of offending substances keeps increasing until many people become 'universal reactors' of *Candida*.

- *Fatigue: Candida* can cause continual fatigue that is more noticeable after eating.

- *Gastrointestinal problems: Candida* can cause bloating, constipation, diarrhoea, heartburn, poor digestion, stomach cramps and wind.

- *Genito-urinary problems:* Candida can cause impotence, infertility, menstrual problems, prostatitis, rectal itch, urinary infections and vaginal infections.

- *Neurological problems: Candida* can cause anxiety, depression, dizziness, a 'fogged in' feeling, headaches, irritability, migraine, mood swings, poor concentration and sugar cravings.

- *Respiratory problems: Candida* can cause asthma, bronchitis, congestion, earaches, post-nasal drip, sore throats and a suppressed immune system.

Intuitive Remedies

Candida is always present in the body, so you cannot command all of it to leave. It is only when there is an imbalance that it becomes a problem. This can be caused by taking too many antibiotics and can spread between partners.

A *Candida* cleanse can work well.

It is important to move the dosage up slowly because during and after the cleanse, the person will feel a little ill. This is because as the *Candida* dies off in the body, it leaves behind a toxic substance called acetlyaldehyde. This can cause allergies, aching joints and memory impairment and can be difficult to flush from the body. In order to clear it, try a molybdenum supplement, because molybdenum attaches to acetlyaldehyde and creates uric acid, and uric acid is more easily flushed from the body than acetlyaldehyde. A suggested regimen is to start with 100 micrograms of molybdenum a day, move up to 300 micrograms a day the second week and then gradually move up to 500 micrograms a day.

One of the primary feelings associated with *Candida* is resentment. The beliefs of resentment are the same as those in fungus.

Supplements and Other Nutritional Recommendations

To heal someone with *Candida,* you need to make sure they give up all their white bread and gluten.

Use one of the following:

- *Aloe vera* juice
- comfrey tea
- fungi cleanse
- grapeseed extract
- noni
- olive-leaf extract (an excellent herb for *Candida*)
- oregano oil
- pau d'arco
- platinum trace mineral
- Tahhebo tea
- the alkaline diet

Add these supplements to the diet:

- ALA: 300 mg
- acidophilus
- CoQ10
- MSM (for four months)

CARDIOVASCULAR DISEASE

Cardiovascular disease is a broad term used to describe a range of diseases that affect the heart or blood vessels. They include coronary artery disease, heart attack, heart failure, high blood pressure and stroke. The term 'cardiovascular disease' is used interchangeably with 'heart disease' because both terms refer to diseases of the heart, arteries and blood vessels. By whatever name, it's clear that this is a serious problem. Cardiovascular disease is the number one worldwide killer of men and women.

'Cardiovascular disease' is used most often to describe damage caused to the heart or blood vessels by atherosclerosis. This disease affects the arteries. These are blood vessels that carry oxygen and nutrients from your heart to the rest of the body. Healthy arteries are flexible, strong and elastic. Over time, however, too much pressure in the arteries can make the walls thick and stiff. This sometimes restricts blood flow to the organs and tissues. This process is called arteriosclerosis, or hardening of the arteries. The major risk factors for developing atherosclerosis, and in turn, cardiovascular disease, are an unhealthy diet (saturated fats), lack of exercise, being overweight and smoking.

Some forms of cardiovascular disease are not caused by atherosclerosis. These include cardiomyopathy (disease of the heart muscle), congenital heart disease, heart infections and heart valve disorders.

Medical Terminology

Aneurysm: A section in a blood vessel where the wall becomes thin and bulges outward.

Angina pectoris: Pain or heavy pressure in the chest that is caused by insufficient supply of oxygen to the heart.

Angiogram: A diagnostic picture produced by injecting a dye that is visible on X-ray into the heart and/or blood vessels.

Angioplasty: A procedure in which a small balloon is inserted into a blocked or partially blocked artery to compress the plaque on the blood vessel wall to widen the artery to allow blood to flow through it.

Aorta: The main channel for heart arterial circulation; the large artery into which oxygenated blood is pumped by the heart.

Aortic stenosis: A condition in which the aortic valve is narrowed, restricting blood flow to the heart into the aorta.

Arrhythmia: Disturbance in the normal rhythm of the heartbeat. There are different kinds of arrhythmia; some are quite dangerous, even life-threatening, while others are merely annoying and pose no particular danger.

Cardiac arrest: This occurs when the heart stops beating. When this happens, the blood supply to the brain is cut off and the person loses consciousness.

Cardiomegaly: The medical term for enlargement of the heart.

Cardiomyopathy: Any group of diseases of the heart muscle that results in impaired heart function and ultimately heart failure.

Cardioversion: A procedure used to correct arrhythmia in which electrical current is applied to the heart to restore normal rhythm.

Carditis: Inflammation of the heart muscle.

Carotid artery: The major artery to the brain.

Catheterization: A procedure used to diagnose the condition of the heart and/or circulatory system. A hollow tube called a catheter is inserted through the blood vessel to detect artery blockage or discover malformations of the heart.

Claudication: Clamp-like pains in the legs that are the result of poor circulation in the legs.

Congenital heart defect: A heart defect that is present at birth, though not necessarily inherited.

Congestive heart failure: Chronic heart disease that results in fluid accumulation in the lungs.

Coronary arteries: The arteries that supply blood to the heart.

Coronary artery disease: Arteriosclerosis of the coronary arteries.

Echocardiogram: A diagnostic procedure that uses ultrasound technology to form an image of the heart.

Electrocardiogram: A diagnostic test that tracks electrical impulses in the heart.

Embolism: A circulatory condition in which a foreign object such as air, gas, tissue or a piece of a tumour is transported around the body and becomes trapped in a blood vessel, obstructing the flow of blood.

Fibrillation: An irregular heartbeat characterized by a slow or fast beating of the heart. It is often a complication of a heart attack.

Heart attack: The medical term is 'myocardial infarction'. In a heart attack, the heart is cut off from oxygen. Depending on the size and location of the area(s) affected, the attack may be described as mild or severe.

Heart murmur: Sound made by the heart that may or may not be a heart condition.

Mitral valve prolapse: A condition where the mitral valve, which controls blood flow from the left atrium to the left ventricle (the heart's main pumping chamber), protrudes too far into the left atrium while it is pumping. In many cases, this causes no symptoms at all, although some people experience occasional dizziness, fatigue and palpitations.

Stroke: An interruption of blood flow to the brain.

Thrombosis: The formation of a clot in a blood vessel.

Valvular disease: A disorder that impairs the functioning of one or more of the heart valves. It may be caused by a congenital defect or an illness such as rheumatic fever or endocarditis, which is an infection of the heart muscle.

Conventional Treatment

There is a variety of conventional treatments for cardiovascular disease:

- ACE inhibitors inhibit the formation of the hormone angiotensin, which narrows the blood vessels.

- Anti-coagulants are commonly prescribed for people in particular danger of developing blood clots.

- Beta blockers induce the heart to beat more slowly and with less force.

- Calcium channel blockers relax blood vessel muscles.

- Central adrenergic inhibitors prevent the nervous system from increasing the heart rate and narrowing blood vessels.

- Diuretics, or water pills, help the kidneys get rid of sodium and water, reducing the volume of blood in the body and therefore the strain on the heart.

- Helidac is a treatment for *E. pylori*, which is now seen as a culprit in heart disease. It contains three different drugs: bismuth subsalicyle, metronidazole and tetracycline.

- Studies have shown that people who take a supplement of coenzyme Q10 following a heart attack are less likely to have a second attack within five years.

- For those who have had a heart attack, it is best to avoid high levels of salt, sugar and white flour and, of course, alcohol and tobacco abuse.

Intuitive Insights

Scientists have discovered that some species of bird are the longest-lived creatures, based on the way their heart beats. This is an indication of how special the actions of the heart are for us.

The heart receives constant hormonal messages that create an electrical pulse. It has its own internal pacemaker that monitors itself and several backup systems.

If there are problems in the heart, it will be very loud in a reading. It will call to you to help it. You will try to move to scan the other parts of the body, but you will constantly get pulled back to the heart until you ask the person if they have challenges with their heart.

A long time ago, I worked with a man who had heart problems. Deep into the trance-like state of Theta, I watched an angel come into his body and take one heart valve out and plug it into another spot. Many years later he went in for heart surgery. They found out that he had a valve that had rejoined itself to another part of the heart.

One of the most important things you can do for your heart is keep good company. This is because you are affected by the thoughts of the people around you. So the person you are with should have a vibration that matches your own. Communication with this person is important. You might be with your soul mate and not know it, because you do not communicate with them. Work with the blood and heart to learn how to communicate. If you dwell on negative thoughts, it will drain your body and create what you dwell on, such as a heart attack.

You can keep your heart in perfect order by keeping your liver in perfect order. The cleaner your liver, the better your heart is going to work. Your liver processes the food for the heart and through the heart to the brain.

Anytime someone has a heart operation of any kind they are going to get abrasive and easily annoyed. If someone has had bypass surgery, it is typical for them to be short-tempered. Many men will have associated problems with the prostate. Sometimes you will discern problems in the prostate when you scan the body before you pick up the heart problems.

Belief Work

Love and joy are prevalent emotions in the heart, so people who have heart problems may not know how to give or receive joy or love. My theory is as follows: if it is the arteries that have the problem, they do not know how to give love; if it is veins, they do not know how to receive love.

Heart problems always have something to do with love, or fear of life. If a person has major heart problems, I know there is probably a reason why. I also know that they are going to have a lot of old anger coming up, so I have to be careful in my wording or they might have a need for confrontation!

Sometimes when people have many affairs, the heart chakra suffers because they don't know how to love someone completely and wholly.

I find that many people have heart problems because the person they are in love with has changed over time and they no longer really want to be with them.

Other people think that in a relationship they have to become what the other person wants, so that is what they do. After three or four years of doing this, however, they get really tired of it and become resentful.

This works with family relationships as well. Sometimes you try so hard to be what the family entity wants you to be and find it's a hard thing to maintain, so you begin to resent all of them for it. It's the same with individual family members – sometimes you are trying so hard to be what your mother or father want you to be, or perhaps what they don't want you to be, that this can bring up resentments and lead on to heart problems.

When a client has a hurt or broken heart, they will be complaining about chest pain. You will need to teach them how to accept love easily.

If, after seeking the Creator's wisdom, you feel that it is a physical problem with the heart, intuitively witness the Creator cleaning out all the valves in the heart area. Keep an eye on them. Be prepared to work on their heart when it needs to be worked on. Suggest medical advice. Check whether they know how to love someone completely and wholly and accept them for who they are and still be themselves. Also energy test for:

'I have to give up who I am in order to be in a relationship.'

'I have to give up my identity in order to be in a relationship.'

Download:

'I know the Creator's definition of what it feels like to respect myself.'

'I know what it feels like to respect my family and others.'

'I know what it feels like to respect Theta work.'

'I know the Creator's definition of what it feels like to be sweet.'

'I understand what it feels like to be loved.'

'I know what a mother's love feels like.'

'I know what a father's love feels like.'

'I know what a child's love feels like.'

'I know what it feels like to live my day-to-day life without despair and sorrow.'

'I understand what it feels like to communicate with others.'

'I know what it feels like to be important enough to communicate my thoughts easily and effortlessly with others.'

'I know how and when to communicate.'

'I know that it's possible to communicate.'

'I know that it's possible to live my life without being selfish and self-centred.'

'I know what it feels like to live my life caring about others.'

'I know what it feels like to still care about myself while caring for others.'

'I know what it feels like to take in the breath of life.'

'I know how to deal with confrontation.'

'I know how to interact with others.'

'I know how to live without fighting for my right to be.'

'I know how to say no.'

'I know how to live without people taking advantage of me.'

'I know how to honour my boundaries and those of others.'

'I know what it feels like to learn easily and effortlessly.'

'I know how to confront someone in the highest and best way.'

'I know how to be aware of other people's feelings.'

'I know how to be assertive.'

'It's easy for me to be respected.'

Intuitive Remedies

For problems in the heart, use the 'Healing the Broken Soul' (*see Cancer*) and especially 'The Heart Song' exercises.

The Heart Song

'The Heart Song' exercise, which is designed to release sorrow and anger via a tone that comes from the heart, has already been outlined in *Advanced ThetaHealing*, but is given here for reference, as it is invaluable for healing the heart.

Only the voice of the client is able to release the sorrow and pain from the heart. The practitioner cannot release it for them and can only assist the client by encouraging them to create the tone.

Many of the people who do this exercise will connect to the universal tone that releases anger, hatred and sorrow on a world level.

There are three molecules that are connected to the soul and go with it everywhere it goes. These molecules are distributed to three places in the body when we enter into this life:

- One is in the pineal gland and releases emotions and physical programmes.
- One is in the heart and releases old sorrow and anger.
- One is at the base of the spine and activates the molecule in the heart to release sorrow.

The practitioner should guide the client through the process in the following way:

The Process for the Heart Song

1   Centre yourself in your heart and visualize going down into Mother Earth, which is part of All That Is.

2   Visualize bringing up the energy through your feet, opening each chakra to the crown chakra. In a beautiful ball of light, go out to the universe.

3   Go beyond the universe, past the white lights, past the dark light, past the white light, past the jelly-like substance that is the Laws, into a pearly iridescent white light, into the Seventh Plane of Existence.

4   Make the command: *'Creator of All That Is, I command that sorrow be released from the song of the heart through a tone of my voice. Thank you. It is done. It is done. It is done.'*

5   Imagine going to the Law of Music and asking for the tone that will release the sorrow and anger from the heart. Imagine that you are going down deep into your heart. Listen to the sad song your heart sings. Let it come out in your voice, in the tone that you sing.

6   As you listen to the sound that the heart sings, listen to all the resentments, all the frustrations with war, famine, hatred and anger that are locked in the heart. Let the sound that is locked in the heart come out of your mouth and be released. Then do the same for all the organs in the body.

7   When you have finished, connect back to the energy of All That Is, take a deep breath in and make an energy break if you so choose.

The way to tell that the process has finished is that the client feels finished. They will feel as though they have released all the built-up sorrow and anger from the heart.

This process can be done more than once if the client needs to release layers of sorrow and anger from the heart.

The client may not be completely happy releasing all their stored sorrow with another person. If so, tell them that they can use the process when they are alone, perhaps as they relax in a hot tub of water. This process is capable of creating amazing healing properties for the body.

Also, download the feeling and the knowing of:

'Everything I have experienced matters.'

'I can wake others up to their divine selves.'

'This time I can wake them up.'

Supplements

*   Magnesium is necessary in order to make the heart work properly. It can clear up issues of the heart.

Heart Attacks

Symptoms

Symptoms include:

*   anxiety
*   chest pain

- difficulty swallowing
- dizziness
- fainting
- loss of speech
- nausea
- shortness of breath
- sudden ringing in the ears
- sweating
- vomiting

The severity of chest pain will vary from one person to another. Some people have intense pain, while others feel only mild discomfort. Many mistake the signs of a heart attack for simple indigestion. Some have no symptoms at all, a situation referred to as a 'silent' heart attack.

Many illnesses mimic heart attacks, such as fibromyalgia, a gall bladder attack and reflux disease. Regardless, if you have chest pain it is best to see a doctor.

Intuitive Insights

Your heart cells live an entire lifetime and, according to conventional medicine, never regenerate themselves. In the instance of a heart attack, half of the heart can be affected, and doctors will tell you that it is impossible for the heart to be as it was before. They believe that the damage can never be made good, but I do not believe this to be true.

A woman once came to me saying her doctor had said she had only 17 percent of her heart function left. She could barely walk into my office. I did some work with her and she ended up getting a divorce. After her divorce, she was tested and her heart was up to about 60 percent of its normal functioning. The doctors were stunned by this inexplicable event. They could not figure out why her heart cells had regenerated.

You have to realize that your body produces stem cells, and these can become anything the body needs. I think that we all have the ability to regenerate ourselves, but this ability has been forgotten. There are many scientific instances where children who are unaware that they cannot grow back a hand or finger will grow one back.

I had a man come to my class who had accidentally cut the tip of his finger off. He stuck his finger in a jar of honey so it would heal slowly, the idea being that the skin and bone would grow back. He grew his whole finger back, including the nail.

Little children can have a stroke that destroys part of their brain and body, but still have the fetal memories of regeneration and so be able to repair the damage.

Your body is in fact constantly repairing itself. It is a miracle! It is continually working to bring the cells oxygen and food. It constantly sends messages back and forth to ensure that there is enough sugar in the bloodstream, enough oxygen in the bloodstream, and so on. These autonomic responses are going on every second throughout our lifetime.

I believe ThetaHealing can trigger the forgotten ability of regeneration so that the body heals itself.

Intuitive Remedies

Call for an ambulance! Use CPR if you know how to do it.

Also, do a healing. Command the veins and arteries to clear and blood flow to resume. Command the heart to beat until the right rhythm is restored and give it energy from the Creator. Use stem cells to rebuild the heart.

Belief Work

Heart attacks always relate to not receiving love.

After a heart attack, the person is supposed to live with less of the heart's pumping capacity. This can cause people to create programmes relating to those around them. Download:

'I understand the Creator's definition of what it feels like to be nurtured.'

'I have the Creator's definition of how to nurture myself.'

'I understand how to be loved.'

'I understand how to accept love.'

'I understand how to have joy.'

'I understand what joy feels like.'

'I know what it feels like to live without giving up who I am in order to be in a relationship.'

'I know what it feels like to live without having to give up my identity in order to be in a relationship.'

'I know how to love someone completely and wholly.'

'I know how to give love.'

'I know how to deal with confrontation in the highest and best way.'

'I live without fearing life.'

Supplements

Lack of copper and magnesium can cause a heart attack. Useful supplements are:

- ALA
- CoQ10
- grapeseed extract
- hawthorn (as a preventive measure)
- Lecithin
- magnesium
- potassium (if the person's medication allows)
- selenium

High Cholesterol

Cholesterol is a fat-like substance that your body needs to function normally. It is naturally present in cell walls or membranes everywhere in the body, including the brain, heart, intestines, liver, muscles, nerves and skin.

The body uses cholesterol to aid in the production of hormones, vitamin D and the bile acids that help to digest fat. It takes only a small amount to meet these needs. If you have too much cholesterol in your bloodstream, the excess may become deposited in arteries, including the coronary (heart) arteries, where it contributes to the narrowing and blockages that cause heart disease.

Coronary heart disease is caused by cholesterol and fat being deposited in the walls of the arteries that feed nutrients and oxygen to your heart. Like any muscle, the heart needs a constant supply of oxygen and nutrients, which are carried to it by the blood. Fixed narrowing in the arteries that is often calcified (hardened) can cause angina. Less severe narrowing may contain unstable blockages called fatty plaque. Unstable atherosclerotic plaque can rupture, resulting in clot formation, no blood flow and possibly a heart attack.

If the blood supply to a portion of the heart is completely cut off by total obstruction of a coronary artery, the result is a heart attack. This is usually due to a sudden closure of the artery from a blood clot forming on top of unstable plaque.

A simple blood test is used for high cholesterol. Knowing your total cholesterol level is not enough. A complete lipid profile measures your LDL (low-density lipoprotein, the bad cholesterol), total cholesterol, HDL-high density lipoprotein (the good cholesterol) and triglycerides, another fatty substance in the blood.

A desirable total cholesterol level is 200 mg/dL or lower. A desirable LDL is 100 mg/dL, 130–159 is borderline high, 160 is high, 190 is very high. HDL, the 'good cholesterol', should be around 40 mg/dL or greater. With HDL, the higher the number, the better, and 60 mg/dL is protective against heart disease.

Too many people have high levels of total cholesterol and LDL (the bad cholesterol). A diet high in saturated fat (a type of fat found mostly in foods that come from animals and certain oils) raises LDL levels more than anything else. You also eat cholesterol directly in your diet, although the effect of saturated fat in the diet is greater than the effect of dietary cholesterol. Trans-fatty acids (seen in processed foods and many 'fast foods') can also increase LDL levels. Dietary cholesterol is found only in foods from animal products. Genetic factors combined with eating too much saturated fat and cholesterol are the main reasons for the high levels of cholesterol that lead to heart attacks. Reducing the amount of saturated fat and cholesterol you eat is an important step in reducing your blood cholesterol levels.

There is a heightened incidence of high cholesterol in people from northern regions. With people from the equator, it tends to be lower.

Intuitive Remedies

Balance the hormones of the heart in the brain. Have the Creator show you. Make sure the person knows how to receive and accept love and how to give love.

Supplements

- ALA
- fibre and oat bran
- Lecithin
- omega 3
- selenium

***

- Getting proper sunlight seems to lower cholesterol levels.
- Most vegetarians do not usually eat the good fats in their diet – they should eat avocados and evening primrose. If you do not have the

right lipids when you are a vegetarian, your cholesterol may be high. You may even gain weight and get depressed.

- Using virgin olive oil in your diet seems to lower cholesterol.
- Vitamin C is helpful for high cholesterol, but you should not use more than 3,000 to 5,000 mg, sporadically during the day at no more than 1,000 mg at a time.

Hypertension/High Blood Pressure

Hypertension can be a precursor to heart problems. It is a common form of cardiovascular disease. It usually results from a decrease in the elasticity in the interior diameter of the arteries. This may be caused by arteriosclerosis, defects in sodium metabolism, enzyme and electrolyte imbalances, nutritional deficiencies and stress. By the time it becomes advanced enough to cause symptoms such as dizziness, rapid pulse, shortness of breath and sweating, it is much harder to treat. Many people do not even know that they have hypertension until it is too late. This is why it is called the 'silent killer'. Women are as likely to suffer from this condition as men are.

If blood pressure is high, it doesn't relax when the body and heart are relaxed, and the pressure on the veins can become too much. It will find a weak spot in the veins and the person can develop a heart attack, kidney failure or a stroke. (When I refer to a stroke, I am referring to an aneurism where the blood vessel wall becomes thin, bulges and bursts, causing a stroke.) Any time there is a blockage in the carotid arteries, there will be symptoms of hypertension.

If your blood pressure is high, your body may not be breaking down salts the way it needs to. Your lipids are not being maintained in the body and this can cause a problem.

People with hypertension have a tendency towards sleep apnoea. This is a dangerous condition in which the person stops breathing for short periods while they sleep.

Types

Blood pressure is usually divided into two categories, primary and secondary. Primary hypertension is high blood pressure that is not due to an underlying disease. The precise cause is unknown, but the risk factors include cigarette smoking, drug abuse, excessive use of stimulants such as coffee or tea, high sodium intake, obesity and stress.

When elevated blood pressure is the result of an underlying health problem, this is called secondary hypertension. The causes of secondary hypertension may be arteriosclerosis, poor kidney function or sometimes liver problems.

Blood Pressure Measurements

Blood pressure is measured as the blood is pumping through the veins and the body and the heart are relaxed.

The systolic (higher) measurement is the highest pressure that the blood pumps out of the heart. The diastolic (lower) measurement is when the system is between beats, known as the resting pressure. This should be 60–80, while the systolic measurement should be 120–140, though 120 is better.

If there is too much range between the systolic and the diastolic numbers, there is cause for concern. If the lower number is too high, there is too much standing pressure in the system. If the systolic measurement is high, the person is more liable to have a stroke.

When either number is too high, the pressure can blow out your kidneys and this could blow out the top of your heart.

The heart itself should pump at between 50 and 100 beats per minute and the pulse should be between 50 to 70 beats a minute.

Intuitive Remedies

Witness the balancing of the hormones of the heart that are sent from the brain. Have the Creator show you.

Suggest that the person do a liver cleanse (*see the Liver*).

Belief Work

Beliefs of blood pressure are centred around stress.

'No matter what I do it is not enough.'

'I must always do more.'

'There is no time for rest.'

Supplements and Other Nutritional Recommendations

- amino acids, apart from phenylalanine and tyrosine
- apple pectin (from apple juice)
- CoQ10
- garlic
- Lecithin

- magnesium
- selenium
- vitamin B
- vitamin C
- vitamin E
- zinc

***

- Avoid alcohol, tobacco and excessive caffeine.
- Be cautious in the use of gingko biloba, as there is the risk of stroke.
- Cucumber is amazing for regulating blood pressure.
- Do not use antihistamines.
- Lower the sodium intake.
- Note that some acupuncture procedures and some chiropractic back adjustments will affect blood pressure.
- Omega 3s will help prevent cholesterol build-up in the veins.
- Start a diet high in fibre.
- Start moderate exercise.

Hypotension/Low Blood Pressure

In some instances, pharmaceutical medication for high blood pressure can cause low blood pressure, which is called hypotension. The symptoms of hypotension are fainting, fatigue, nausea, sweating and even loss of consciousness.

If someone is very agitated and has low blood pressure, it is possible that something is wrong.

CARPAL TUNNEL SYNDROME

Carpal tunnel syndrome is associated with a lack of vitamin B6.

Intuitive Healing

After giving the person vitamin B6, go to the Seventh Plane and witness the tendons slowly going back to where they should be. Command the nerves to grow back to as they were before they became injured.

By commanding relief, you should have drastically improved the carpal tunnel syndrome, if you have not alleviated it altogether. Remember the command that is made is always: *'Creator, change this. Thank you, it is done, it is done it is done.'*

Downloads

'I know when to rest.'

'My determination is rewarded.'

'I can love myself.'

Supplements and Other Nutritional Recommendations

- vitamin B6 for two weeks, then B complex
- zinc, 100 mg to 150 for a month on a full stomach, then lowering it to 50 mg

CATARACTS

See the Eyes.

CEREBRAL PALSY

Cerebral palsy is caused by oxygen being cut off from the brain at birth. When the brain lacks oxygen, parts of it burn out and die.

Intuitive Remedies

Cerebral palsy responds well to healing. Ask that the dead tissue be removed and the brain be 'rebooted'. The cells have a fetal code, and you can go in and rebuild what needs to be done using this code. Ask the Creator what to do and witness it being done.

Belief Work

Children with cerebral palsy respond quickly to healings, but the belief systems of the parents can get in the way. The father is often so hurt over the situation that it takes time for him to accept it. The mother often wants to immediately fix it.

First work on the mother, in case she is holding the baby to its defect, since she can become co-dependent on the situation. Then work with the father to convince him that the child can be healed.

It only takes the belief of one parent to change to make it possible for the child to heal. If possible, show the parents how to do the healings themselves.

The child itself rarely needs digging work and only needs downloads and healings. The parents are the ones in need of deep digging work.

Downloads for the child:

'I can grow and become normal.'

'Normal is good.'

'I am special.'

'I am surrounded by love.'

'I bring positive energy to everyone around me.'

'I am cherished.'

'I am important.'

'It is easy for people to love me.'

'It is easy for me to love myself.'

'I am patient with myself.'

'I become stronger every day.'

'It's safe to be strong.'

'Life is full of opportunity.'

'I believe my body can and will heal.'

'I know what it feels like to know I am special.'

When doing digging work with the parents, check for:

'My life will never be normal.'

'No one will ever love me with a child like this.'

'It is impossible for me to share my child's love with anyone.'

'My child's condition is my fault.'

Replace with:

'I know what it feels like to still have a life.'

'I know how to let other people in to love me.'

CHEMICAL POISONING

Chemical and environmental poisoning can be a severe problem, especially for those who are sensitive or immune-compromised.

Types

One of the most prevalent chemical pollutants is formaldehyde. This is an industrial chemical manufactured from methanol, natural gas and some of the lower petroleum hydrocarbons and found widely in the urea formaldehyde foam insulation used in homes and mobile homes.

Another group of environmental poisons is herbicides and pesticides. One form that was used in the past was DDT.

One of the most dangerous toxic substances is asbestos. Once it gets into the lungs, it opens up like barbed wire and hooks to the sides of the lungs. This is what it looks like in the body.

There are other many forms of pollution, including:

Environmental Pollution
- acid rain
- carbon monoxide
- mycotoxins – cryptosporidium
- plastics
- refinery emissions
- soil treatment sprays – herbicides, fungicides, pesticides
- solvents
- waste treatment plant emissions

Electromagnetic Pollution
- communication frequencies
- electrical appliances
- mobile phones
- power lines
- transformers

Magnetic Fields: Direct Impact
- aircraft
- bed frames
- belt buckles

- cars
- dental work
- hair grips
- jewellery
- spectacles
- steel buildings and structural beams
- underwired bras

Toxic Substance Radiation
- carpets and upholstery
- foam rubber
- household cleaners
- pesticides
- plastics
- polyurethane
- synthetic fabrics

Toxic Ingestion
- *drinks:* artificial sweeteners, refined sugar
- *drugs:* alcohol derivatives, phenol, synthetic carrying agents
- *food:* harmful chemicals, enhancers, preservatives

Magnetic Fields and Toxic Substance Radiation
In the home:

- appliances
- carpets
- curtains
- electricity in the walls and floors
- fabrics
- foam padding
- kitchen cleaners
- lights
- mattresses
- upholstery

- walls

In the workplace:

- carpets
- lighting
- machinery
- office equipment
- panelling
- power tools
- steel buildings
- telephones

Belief Work

Test for:

> 'I fight with the environment.'
>
> 'I have to fight for everything I have.'
>
> 'The world is trying to kill me.'

Downloads

> 'It is safe to be on this planet.'
>
> 'I know how to live in my environment in peace and harmony.'
>
> 'My body is always healthy and strong.'
>
> 'I know how to live without absorbing toxic substances.'
>
> 'I know how to live without fearing my environment.'
>
> 'I am impervious to the toxins in my world.'

For more beliefs and downloads, see Heavy Metals (Prologue), Lead Poisoning and Mercury Poisoning.

Supplements and Other Nutritional Recommendations

For pesticides and herbicides:

- ALA
- blue-green algae
- calcium
- zinc

For asbestos:

- chlorella
- spirulina

CHLAMYDIA

This sexually transmitted disease is caused by the bacteria *Chlamydia trachomatis*. Men and women can get it through vaginal, anal or oral sex. The more sexual partners a person has, the greater risk there is of infection. Because there are often no symptoms, people may unknowingly pass the disease on.

An infected mother can also pass *Chlamydia* to her baby during childbirth. These babies can have weakened immune systems. They can get conjunctivitis or develop pneumonia.

Chlamydia has very little effect on the man that contracts it, but if left undetected for a long time in a woman it can create pelvic inflammatory disease, which can result in so much scar tissue in the Fallopian tubes that the woman may not be able to have children. As well as scarring the female organs, it will start in on the intestinal tract, causing scars and inflammation. It is terribly painful. I have seen women in such intense pain from their Fallopian tubes that they cannot work.

Antibiotics are used to treat and cure *Chlamydia*. There are antibiotics that are safe to use during pregnancy. Women are often at risk of reinfection, however, if their sexual partners are not treated, and reinfection places them at higher risk of serious reproductive health complications.

Symptoms

Chlamydia is known as a 'quiet' disease, because 75 percent of infected women and at least half of infected men have no symptoms at all. Most people do not know they have it, at least in its initial stages. If symptoms do occur, they usually appear within one to three weeks of contact.

Symptoms in women, if any, include a burning sensation when urinating, itching, painful intercourse and an abnormal vaginal discharge that resembles cottage cheese. However, even if the infection spreads from the cervix to the uterus and Fallopian tubes, some women may still have no symptoms.

Symptoms in men include a burning sensation when urinating and a clear watery discharge from the penis. Men might also have burning and itching around the opening of the penis or pain and swelling in the testicles, or both.

The bacteria also can infect the throat from oral sexual contact with an infected partner.

Intuitive Remedies

Pelvic inflammatory disease responds well to the basic healing. Go up to the Creator of All That Is and command that the reproductive organs are restored to perfect health. Witness the scar tissue changed into healthy tissue.

Belief Work

The programmes that are associated with Chlamydia and pelvic inflammatory disease cycle around issues of mental and sexual abuse, worthiness, the inability to stand up for yourself and the inability to receive love. Download:

'I know what it feels like to be assertive and self-confident.'

'I know how to be assertive and self-confident without overcorrection.'

'I know when to be assertive and self-confident.'

'I know what it feels like to know I am worthy of God's love.'

'I know it's possible to be with someone who loves me.'

'I know what it feels like to live without pain.'

'I know what it feels like to live without abuse.'

'I know what it feels like to live without being taken advantage of.'

'I know how to live a stress-free life.'

CHRONIC FATIGUE SYNDROME

The interesting thing about chronic fatigue syndrome is that before the disease was 'accepted' by the conventional medical industry, thousands of people would go to the doctor with it and either be told that they were hypochondriacs or be misdiagnosed. The alternative medical industry accepted CFS as a viable disease long before conventional medicine did.

CFS can affect people of all ages, ethnic backgrounds and socio-economic classes. More women than men are diagnosed with it. It can be hard to diagnose, because there is no lab test for it and many of its symptoms are also signs of other illnesses or medical treatments.

Symptoms

A person with CFS generally feels completely worn out. This extreme tiredness makes it hard to do daily tasks such as bathing, dressing or eating. Sleep or rest does not make the fatigue go away. People who contract CFS suddenly feel fine one day and then feel extremely tired the next. Many people say it started after an infection, a cold or a stomach bug. It also can follow an attack of infectious mononucleosis (mono), the 'kissing disease' that depletes your energy, or a time of great stress, such as a death in the family or major surgery.

There may be muscle pain, trouble focusing or insomnia. The extreme tiredness may come and go.

Supposedly, CFS is not life-threatening, but I have seen people in such pain that my contention would be that it can be life-threatening.

Intuitive Insights

I believe that CFS is most likely caused by contracting a virus, such as the Epstein-Barr virus. A high percentage of the population of the United States carry this virus.

Heavy-metal poisoning can also be a cause of CFS.

Intuitive Remedies

When a person comes to you and tells you they have CFS, go out of your space and see if they have the Epstein-Barr virus. You should look for this in the bloodstream. It is of the herpes virus variety and can be overcome by using belief work to change it into a form that is harmless to the body. See Epstein-Barr Virus.

From a nutritional standpoint, CFS can be overcome with proper nutrients and a healthy diet.

Supplements

- acidophilus
- calcium

- chromium
- CoQ10
- Lecithin
- magnesium
- vitamin C
- vitamin E

CIRRHOSIS

There are few organs in the body that can compare with the liver in terms of what it does for us. As with the heart, all the roads of the body lead to the liver.

One of the most important of the liver's functions is the secretion of bile for digestion. Bile is integral in the absorption of vitamins and nutrients. Once these vital nutrients have been processed in the digestive system, they are sent to the liver for the extraction of iron, vitamin A and B12 for future use.

The liver also synthesizes fatty acids, amino acids and sugars and creates a substance called glucose tolerance factor, which balances blood sugars in the body.

The liver filters pesticides, drugs and innumerable other toxins from the rest of the body.

It is responsible for regulating thyroid function by converting thyroxine (which is a thyroid hormone) into its more active form, tridothyronine. Inadequate conversion of these thyroid hormones may lead to hyperthyroidism.

The liver also breaks down hormones such as adrenaline, aldosterone, insulin and oestrogen after they have performed their necessary functions.

Cirrhosis causes healthy liver tissue to be replaced with scar tissue. This eventually blocks the flow of blood through the liver and slows the processing of drugs, hormones, nutrients and toxins and the production of proteins and other substances made by the liver.

According to experts, cirrhosis is the seventh leading cause of death by disease.

Causes

Hepatitis A, a fatty liver and alcohol abuse are the most common causes of cirrhosis in the USA, but anything that damages the liver can be responsible, including:

- alpha 1 antitrypsin deficiency, the absence of a specific enzyme in the liver
- blockage of the bile duct, from the liver to the intestines
- cystic fibrosis
- diabetes
- glycogen storage diseases
- haemochromatosis, a condition in which excessive iron is absorbed and deposited into the liver and other organs
- hepatitis B, C and D
- obesity
- repeated bouts of heart failure with fluid backing up into the liver
- Wilson's disease, caused by the abnormal storage of copper in the liver

Symptoms

The symptoms of cirrhosis vary with the stage of the illness and include:

- a brownish or orange tint to the urine
- blood in the stool
- bruises
- confusion, disorientation, personality changes
- fever
- fluid retention (oedema) and swelling in the ankles, legs and abdomen
- itchy skin
- lack of energy
- light-coloured stools
- loss of appetite
- weight loss or sudden weight gain
- yellowing of the skin (jaundice)

Conventional Treatment

- Diet and drug therapies can help improve the altered mental function that cirrhosis can cause.
- Diuretics are used to remove excess fluid and to prevent oedema from recurring.

- For cirrhosis caused by alcohol abuse, the person must stop drinking alcohol to halt the progression of the disease.
- If a person has hepatitis, the doctor may prescribe steroids or antiviral drugs to reduce liver-cell injury.
- Laxatives such as lactulose may be given to help absorb toxins and speed their removal from the intestines.
- Oedema and ascites (fluid in the abdomen) are treated by reducing salt in the diet.

Intuitive Remedies

Seen intuitively in the body, cirrhosis of the liver should not be confused with cancer of the liver, which looks very different. Liver cancer is denser in structure, darker and has a different structure from the scar tissue of cirrhosis. Cirrhosis has a grey colour.

If the cirrhosis has been caused by alcoholism, the person may not want to change. Simply telling someone that they should stop drinking does not mean that they will. It is best that they have stopped drinking by the time that they get to you, so that you can put them on a decent regime and they will accept the healing in a much more conducive way.

The anger needs to be pulled from the liver to enable it to function properly. Go up to the Creator of All That Is and ask that the liver be cleansed.

Witness the Creator cleanse the liver at least twice. You should never witness the toxins being pushed out into the body but rather changed into something different.

Some of the ThetaHealing processes that can be used are the 'Sending Love to the Baby in the Womb' exercise (*see Cancer*), the 'Heart Song' exercise (*see Cardiovascular Disease*) and 'The Broken Soul' exercise (*see Cancer*).

Belief Work

Cirrhosis of the liver causes people to be bitter and angry. They are generally bitter about the past and angry about the future.

They also have a tendency to overstep their boundaries with other people. They may take money that is not theirs and push themselves onto other people. They should be taught what it feels like to know their boundaries. Download:

'I know what it feels like to live without overstepping the boundaries of others.'

'I know what it feels like to respect the boundaries of others.'

'I know what it feels like to have my boundaries respected.'

'I know what it feels like to live without others taking advantage of me.'

'I know what it feels like to live without taking advantage of others.'

'I know what it feels like to live without pain.'

'I know what it feels like to live in a perfectly healthy body.'

'I know what it feels like to be happy.'

'I know what it feels like to feel strong.'

'I know what it feels like to take charge of my own life.'

'I know what it feels like to see the good side of things.'

'I know what it feels like to allow others to love me.'

'I know what it feels like to live without resentment.'

'I know what it feels like to live without anger.'

'I know how to live without fear.'

'I know how to live without feeling guilty.'

'I know how to live without regret.'

'I know how to live without feeling regret about the past.'

'I know what it feels like to forgive myself.'

'I know what it feels like to go forward.'

'I know how to forgive old abuse in the highest and best way.'

'I know what it feels like to accept and receive love.'

'I know it is possible to become stronger and healthier every day.'

'I know what it feels like to know my body can recover.'

'I know it is possible that my body can recover.'

'I know what it feels like to treat my body with respect.'

Supplements and Other Nutritional Recommendations

- ALA will help the liver, 300 mg to 600 mg.
- Do not use liver cleanses for cirrhosis of the liver, as they might be

too severe. The only liver cleanse I recommend in this case would be milk thistle, because it detoxifies the liver with ease, and only for two weeks at a time.

- Drink fresh vegetable juices such as a mixture of beetroot, carrot, garlic, a little ginger and a stick of celery.
- Eat plenty of foods high in vitamin K. Persons with cirrhosis of the liver are often deficient in vitamin K. Good sources of vitamin K include sprouts and green leafy vegetables.
- Echinacea will help to stimulate the liver.
- It is recommended to have a diet of 75 percent raw foods, consisting of fresh vegetables.
- Lidtke Technologies has a product called 'Cleanse and Build' that is wonderful for the liver.
- Olive-leaf extract is helpful for cirrhosis of the liver.
- Omega 3s, 6s and 9s are useful.
- Red clover will stimulate and cleanse the blood.

COELIAC DISEASE

Coeliac disease is a digestive condition triggered by eating the protein gluten, which is found in biscuits, bread, pasta, pizza crust and many other foods containing wheat. Barley, rye and even oats may also contain gluten.

When a person with coeliac disease eats gluten, an immune reaction occurs in the small intestine resulting in damage to its surface. Normally, the small intestine is lined with tiny hair-like projections called villi. Resembling the deep pile of a plush carpet on a microscopic scale, these work to absorb vitamins, minerals and other nutrients from food. Coeliac disease results in damage to the villi, and without them, the inner surface of the small intestine is unable to absorb the nutrients and instead they are eliminated with the stool.

The decreased absorption of nutrients can cause vitamin deficiencies that can lead to other illnesses. These can be especially serious in children, who need proper nutrition to develop and grow. However, coeliac disease can be managed through changing the diet.

Some experts conjecture that coeliac disease has been around since humankind switched from a foraging diet of meat and nuts to a cultivated diet using wheat.

Causes

Coeliac disease is often inherited. It can occur at any age, although problems do not appear until gluten is introduced into the diet.

The disease can emerge after some form of trauma, such as an infection, a physical injury, the stress of pregnancy and severe stress or surgery.

Symptoms

The symptoms of coeliac disease can mimic other conditions such as a nervous condition, anaemia, Crohn's disease, gastric ulcers, irritable bowel syndrome, parasite infections and skin disorders. Most people with the disease have complaints such as intermittent abdominal pain, bloating and diarrhoea, but some have no gastrointestinal symptoms at all.

The disease can present itself in less obvious ways that include depression, irritability, joint pain, mouth sores, muscle cramps, neuropathy, osteoporosis, skin rashes and stomach upsets.

Indications of the malabsorption that may result from coeliac disease include:

- abdominal cramps, gas and bloating
- diarrhoea
- fatigue and weakness
- foul-smelling or greyish stools
- osteoporosis
- pronounced weight loss
- stunted growth in children

Intuitive Remedies

Witness the gene work and the healing.

Belief Work

With coeliac disease, the belief systems are of being a victim and perfectionist, never being good enough and not being able to absorb love. Download:

'I know how to receive and accept love.'

'I receive love.'

'I have good discernment about people.'

'I can live without being a victim.'

'I know how to live without being ill.'

Supplements

The following will all help the damage to the intestine:

- *Aloe vera*
- chlorophyll
- Jerusalem artichoke
- olive-leaf extract
- spirulina

See also Irritable Bowel Syndrome.

COLON DISORDERS

Most colon disorders are associated with the fact that the elimination system of the body is holding digested faecal matter for too long.

Intuitive Remedies

Make sure that the ileocecal valve is opening as it should.

Another method of healing for the colon is coloured light therapy. This seems to be extremely productive.

Belief Work

Use belief work to release hatred and resentment.

The emotions that are held in the colon are:

- anger
- fear
- guilt
- old abuse
- resentment
- the inability to accept love

Download:

'I know what it feels like to live without fear.'

'I know how to live without fear.'

'I know how to live without resentment.'

'I know the Creator's definition of what it feels like to be safe.'

'I know the Creator's definition of what it feels like to be protected.'

'I know the Creator's definition of what it feels like to be secure.'

Supplements and Other Nutritional Recommendations

- Aloe is a good laxative and strengthens the colon.
- Chelated calcium and magnesium are beneficial.
- Make sure the person's body is alkaline.
- Suggest that the person removes wheat and gluten from their diet.

See also Irritable Bowel Syndrome.

COMA

One day a man walked into my office with a dilemma. His nephew was in a coma in hospital and he was wondering if I would intuitively talk to the boy to see if I could wake him up. I asked him where the boy was, asked his name and told the man that I would go and talk to him the first chance I had.

That night I went out of my space and searched for the boy. When I found him, his spirit was out of his body. I began to talk to him and told him that he needed to return to his body. He told me he was afraid to enter his body because it would hurt. I told him that he needed to make the decision whether to leave to go to the Creator or to go back and reconnect with his body. I encouraged him to go back into his body and told him that it would be alright. I told him to wake up slowly, and only when he was ready, and then left him.

The next day, I received a jubilant call from the uncle, thanking me for waking the boy up.

It seems that after the boy woke up he began to talk about the 'angel lady' who had come to him in the coma, encouraging him to return to his body. He told his parents that she had long brown hair and green eyes, and gave a good description of me.

I have also brought myself out of a coma to return to my loved ones.

Intuitive Insights

When a person is in a coma, the spirit may have left the body and become lost or disoriented. Quite often it has actually been knocked out of the body by a traumatic experience such as an accident. It knows the pain it may encounter if it returns to the body, so it avoids returning.

Even though the spirit has left the body, or cannot find the body to return to, there is an umbilical cord running between spirit and body. You can use this to locate the spirit and return it to the body.

Intuitive Remedies

You can wake the person by the following process:

The Process for Waking a Person from Coma

1. Centre yourself in your heart and visualize yourself going down into Mother Earth, which is a part of All That Is.

2. Visualize bringing up the Earth energy through your feet, opening up all of your chakras as you go. Continue going up out of your crown chakra in a beautiful ball of light, out to the universe.

3. Go beyond the universe, past the white lights, past the dark light, past the white light, past the jelly-like substance that is the Laws, into a pearly iridescent white light, into the Seventh Plane of Existence.

4. Make the command, 'Creator of All That Is, it is commanded that I find [name the person]'s spirit and return it to their body in the highest and best way. Thank you! It is done. It is done. It is done.'

5. Move your consciousness over to the person's space. Go over into their body through their crown chakra and witness the spirit return to the body.

When dealing with children whose spirits have left the body, it is vital that you remember that a child's soul is afraid of pain and it may not be easy to bring it back. You must be persistent with children and coax them to return to life.

Belief Work

For those who come out of a coma, download:

'I know how to go on without the fear of relapse.'

'I know how to overcome the fear of never being normal.'

'I know what it feels like to go back to being normal.'

'I know how to receive love.'

'I know how to live without pushing myself too hard.'

'I know what it feels like to permit my body to heal.'

'I know what it feels like to live without fearing others.'

'I know what it feels like to live without the fear of dying.'

'I know what it feels like to live without the fear of a coma happening again.'

'I know what it feels like to be grateful to be alive.'

'I know how to cherish every moment.'

'I know what it feels like to cherish every moment.'

'It is safe to cherish every moment.'

'It is safe to live again.'

'It is safe to dream again.'

CROHN'S DISEASE

Crohn's disease is a type of inflammatory bowel disease that may be caused by bacteria. Researchers are also finding that heavy-metal poisoning may be one of the causes.

In Crohn's disease the lining of the digestive tract becomes inflamed, causing severe diarrhoea and abdominal pain. The inflammation often spreads deep into the layers of the tissues of the bowel and food just runs right through the intestinal tract without any of the nutrients being extracted from it. The current medical treatment is steroids to slow the digestive system.

Like ulcerative colitis, Crohn's disease can be both painful and debilitating. It can eventually cause death if the person does not get some kind of treatment for it. There is no known medical cure. However, treatment can greatly reduce the symptoms and many people afflicted with Crohn's disease are able to function normally in everyday life.

Symptoms

- abdominal pain and cramping
- arthritis
- blood in the stool
- diarrhoea
- eye inflammation
- fatigue
- fever
- fistula or abscess
- inflammation of the liver or bile ducts
- reduced appetite and weight loss
- skin disorders
- ulcers

Intuitive Remedies

I believe Crohn's disease is caused by bacteria and also by unbalanced cortisone levels. Unbalanced cortisone levels cause the body to produce too much histamine. When you have too much histamine, it will begin to attack the inner colon.

Belief Work

People with Crohn's disease tend to be Type A personalities, with a perfectionist nature. They never stop. They feel that they can never do enough. They have a tendency to have poor communication skills. They feel that they have not been given a fair chance in life. They may be attempting to escape from their situation.

Download:

'I know how to live my life seeing perfection in everything.'

'I know what God's definition of perfection is.'

'I know how to live without the world irritating me.'

'I know what it feels like to make decisive decisions.'

'I know what it feels like to live without intentionally hurting other people's feelings.'

'I know what it feels like to live without having to fight all the time.'

'I know what it feels like to live without feeling that I'm under attack.'

'I know what it feels like to choose friends who uplift me.'

'I know what it feels like to live without pain.'

'I know what it feels like to permit other people to be kind to me.'

'I draw to me people who are kind and loving.'

'I know what it feels like to live without having to fight for everything I have.'

'I know what it feels like to live without feeling overwhelmed.'

'I know what it feels like to live my life without overcorrecting.'

'I know what it feels like to live my life without becoming aggressive.'

'I know what it feels like to be understood.'

'I know what it feels like to have compassion.'

'I know what it feels like to live without resentment of past abuse.'

'I know what it feels like to move forward in a good way.'

'I know it's safe to ask questions.'

'I know how to live without having to defend the world.'

'I know what it feels like to rest.'

'I know what it feels like to live without thinking things are never done.'

'I know what it feels like to have reasonable expectations of myself.'

'I know what it feels like to live without pain.'

'I know what it feels like to eat without pain.'

'I know what it feels like to communicate easily.'

'I know what it feels like to live without feeling that life cheats me.'

'I know what it feels like to feel happy about my life.'

'I know what it feels like to live without wishing I was in someone else's body.'

'I know what it feels like to accept and love my own body.'

'I know what it feels like to know it is possible to be well.'

'Through God, everything is possible.'

'I know it's possible to live without regret.'

'I know how to live without taking advantage of others.'

Supplements and Other Nutritional Recommendations

Aloe vera is very helpful and omega 3s are very important. The alkaline diet is helpful. Other useful supplements:

- acidophilus
- calcium–magnesium
- Jerusalem artichoke
- slippery elm
- vitamin C

The person with Crohn's should avoid alcohol, caffeine, tobacco and wheat products.

CUSHING'S SYNDROME

See Adrenal Disorders.

CYSTIC FIBROSIS

Cystic fibrosis (CF) is an inherited illness that is the result of a defect in chromosome 7. This chromosome is responsible for the instructions for a protein that regulates the passage of salt in and out of the cells of the body's exocrine glands. Even this one tiny protein defect in the DNA can result in a disease of the mucus and sweat glands. It affects the intestines, liver, lungs, pancreas, sex organs and sinuses, causing the mucus to be thick and glutinous. The mucus then clogs the lungs, causing breathing problems and making it easy for bacteria to grow. This can lead to problems such as repeated lung infections and lung damage.

The symptoms and severity of CF vary widely. Some people have serious problems from birth. Others have a milder version of the disease that does not show up until they are teenagers or young adults.

Although there is no known medical cure for CF, treatment has improved greatly in recent years. Many of the symptoms are treated with drugs or nutritional supplements. Attention to and prompt treatment of respiratory and digestive complications have dramatically increased the expected lifespan of a person with CF. While several decades ago most died before the age of two, today about half of all people with CF live past the age of 31.

Belief Work

Children with cystic fibrosis can benefit from using the gene work. Most of them are wonderful beings who want to live. Often it is their parents who are preparing them to die. So the parents usually need belief work so that they do not give up hope. They must believe that recovery is possible. In many instances, the parents' guilt holds the child back from a healing.

Downloads for the parents:

'It is possible that my child can be healed.'

'I know what it feels like to expect a healing from the Creator.'

'I know it's possible that DNA can be changed.'

'I know it's possible to expect good things from the Creator.'

'I know what it feels like for my child to accept a healing.'

'I know what it feels like to live without the fear of getting my hopes up.'

'I know it's possible to be happy.'

'I know how to let my child be happy.'

DEAFNESS

See Hearing Impairment.

DEPRESSION

There is a vast difference between feeling depressed and suffering from clinical depression. The hopelessness of clinical depression is unrelenting and overwhelming. Some people describe it as 'living in a black hole' or having a feeling of impending doom. They can't escape their unhappiness and desolation. However, some people with depression don't feel sad at all. Instead, they feel lifeless and empty. In this apathetic state, they are unable to experience pleasure. Even when participating in activities they used to enjoy, they feel as if they're just going through the motions. The signs and symptoms vary from person to person, and they may wax and wane in severity over time.

Women with depression may not have enough oestrogen, or be low in serotonin. During menopause, some women will become depressed because their hormones are off-balance. There is a need to clean out the liver. If a woman's mother or another relative is also depressed, there are likely to be programmes to pull.

Intuitive Remedies

If a person is depressed, a good mineral and vitamin supplement may be needed. A good mineral supplement may also be needed to pull heavy metals out of the body. Mercury is one of the most toxic of substances and can make a person very depressed.

You can then command the noradrenaline and serotonin levels to be balanced. When in balance, noradrenaline and serotonin enable people to react to events in reasonable ways, whereas an imbalance of these key brain chemicals can either increase aggression or lower it.

The Process for Normalizing Brain Chemicals

1   Centre yourself in your heart and visualize going down into Mother Earth, which is a part of All That Is.

2   Visualize bringing up the energy through your feet, opening each chakra to the crown chakra. In a beautiful ball of light, go out to the universe.

3   Go beyond the universe, past the white lights, through the gold light, past the dark light, past the white light, past the jelly-like substance that is the Laws, into a pearly iridescent white light, into the Seventh Plane of Existence.

4   Make the command, 'Creator of All That Is, it is commanded that [name the person]'s noradrenaline, serotonin and hormone levels be balanced in the highest and best way as is appropriate at this time. Thank you! It is done. It is done. It is done.'

5   Move your consciousness over to the person's space. Go into their brain and witness the noradrenaline, serotonin and hormone levels being balanced as is proper for the person.

6   As soon as the process is finished, rinse yourself off and put yourself back into your space. Go into the Earth and pull the Earth energy up through all your chakras to your crown chakra and make an energy break.

Belief Work

Check for fear of failure and success. Download:

'I know how to live my day-to-day life without being depressed.'

'I know the Creator's definition of joy.'

'I know what it feels like to live without having to create depression.'

'I know what it feels like to live without being stuck inside myself.'

'I know what it feels like to help others.'

'I know what it feels like to see life from a higher perspective.'

'I know what it feels like to live without feeling hopeless.'

'I know what it feels like to create wonderful things in my life.'

'I know how to create wonderful thoughts.'

'I know how to live without donating large parts of my day to depression.'

'I know what it feels like to know that I can find joy.'

'I know what it feels like to be able to deal with any situation.'

'I know what it feels like to draw the breath of life.'

'I know what it feels like to live without the "poor me" attitude.'

'I know what it feels like to be cherished by God.'

'I know what it feels like to have hope and understanding.'

'I know what it feels like to cherish myself.'

'I know it's possible to cherish myself.'

'I know the Creator's definition of cherishing myself.'

'I know the difference between my feelings and those of another.'

'I know how to live without taking on other people's sorrow and sadness.'

'The sadness of others is automatically changed to love.'

'I know what it feels like to live without the whole world resting on my shoulders.'

'I know what foods are best for me.'

'I know it's safe to be awake and alive.'

'I know it's safe to be intuitive.'

'I know it's safe to be myself.'

'Every day in every way I feel stronger.'

'Every day in every way I feel happier.'

'Every day in every way I find solutions.'

'Every day in every way I see the possibilities in life.'

Supplements and Other Nutritional Recommendations

In many instances depression and nervousness are caused by a lack of vitamins and minerals. Try the following:

- alpha-lipoic acid to remove heavy metals (which may be the cause)
- calcium–magnesium
- 5 HTP
- omega 3s
- Royal Camu
- the alkaline diet
- vitamin B complex

- D phenylalanine-EndorphiGens from Lidtke Technologies are good, but you cannot use D phenylalanine and depression medication at the same time.
- St John's Wort can be used for depression and nervousness, although not if you have hypoglycaemia.
- There may be the need for more tryptophan, which is found in chocolate, eggs, pasta, popcorn and turkey.

DIABETES

Diabetes is a disease in which the body does not create or properly use insulin. Insulin is a hormone that 'unlocks' the cells of the body, allowing glucose to enter and fuel them with the energy needed for daily life.

Types

Pre-diabetes
This is a condition that occurs when a person's blood glucose levels are higher than normal, but not high enough for a diagnosis of Type 2 diabetes. There are 54 million Americans who have pre-diabetes, in addition to the 20.8 million with diabetes.

Gestational Diabetes
This affects about 4 percent of all pregnant women.

Type 1 Diabetes
Often called 'childhood diabetes', Type 1 results from the body's failure to produce insulin.

Type 2 Diabetes
This results from insulin resistance (a condition in which the body fails to

use insulin properly), combined with relative insulin deficiency. Most people who are diagnosed with diabetes have Type 2 diabetes.

'Insulin resistance' is a term used for the body's inability to use its own insulin. When we eat, our body changes all our carbohydrates into glucose, which enters into the bloodstream. The blood sugar rises and the body releases insulin, which attaches to the cells like a gatekeeper, allowing glucose to enter and energy to be stored. In the event that the insulin is unable to reach the cells, it stays in the bloodstream. The blood sugar is high and the pancreas continues to release insulin. The pancreas is therefore overworked and begins to wear out and then the blood sugar begins to rise.

Basically, there are three things needed to overcome insulin resistance:

1. An exercise regime.

2. Weight loss.

3. Proper medication.

Causes

The cause of diabetes continues to be unknown, although both genetics and environmental factors such as diet, lack of exercise and obesity appear to play roles.

Ongoing studies of those with diabetes have uncovered new information that is shedding light upon the development and causes of the disorder:

- One indication of diabetes is when the eyebrows stay dark while the rest of the hair turns grey.

- According to a study, if a woman is a size D bra or larger at the age of 20, she may be up to five times more likely to develop diabetes.

- New research suggests that the month in which you are born could play a role in the development of Type 1 diabetes. Spring babies seem to be more at risk.

- Previously overlooked, hearing loss has now been linked to diabetes as a complication.

- If you have periodontal disease or tooth loss you are at increased risk of diabetes.

- People who are exposed to high levels of pesticides and herbicides have been found to be at increased risk of diabetes.

- In some people, diabetes has been traced to fetal development.

Conventional Treatment

Insulin is necessary when treating Type 1 diabetes. As Type 1 diabetes occurs when the pancreas stops making insulin, people with this type need to inject insulin to keep their blood glucose from soaring out of control.

Type 2 is managed with pharmaceutical drugs, though insulin is also used if oral medication is not enough to keep blood glucose levels within a normal range.

Proper nutrition is all-important in managing any form of diabetes, and information on this is readily available.

Testing and Monitoring

As a means of testing for diabetes, people use an electronic device with a strip to give a numerical readout of the glucose level. You simply prick your finger with a spring-loaded needle and apply a drop of your blood to a test strip. This gives you an immediate blood sugar result.

What is a normal blood sugar glucose level? If you're fasting, when you first wake up in the morning, it should be 4.0 to 5.6 mmol/l. From 6.0 to 7.0 mmol/l can show impaired glucose tolerance and is considered to be borderline; 7.0 mmol/l and over for a two- or three-day period is likely to indicate diabetes.

If you are not fasting, your blood sugar levels should be 7.8 mmol/l or less, two hours after you've eaten. If your levels are higher than this in either of these scenarios, there may be cause for concern.

A haemoglobin A1 C (HbA1c) test can be taken to find out your average sugar levels for the past three months.

A regular eye test is important as well.

The Challenges of Diabetes

Hypoglycaemia/Low Blood Glucose

One of the challenges of diabetes is that of low blood glucose, or hypoglycaemia.

Low blood glucose is caused by not enough of the right kind of food, too much exercise without fuel for the body and too much medication at any one time. The warning signs are blurred vision, cold sweats, confusion, headache, hunger, irritability, lightheadedness, rapid heart rate and shakiness. A glass of cold milk or orange juice will raise the blood glucose levels.

Emergency foods are three to four commercial glucose tablets, one glass of orange juice, one glass of skimmed milk, one teaspoon of honey or four to six Lifesavers. Rest for 15 minutes and then test glucose levels. If the blood glucose is still low, have another 15 g of carbohydrates. Continue these steps as needed until the blood sugar returns to normal.

Hyperglycaemia/High Blood Glucose

If the blood glucose levels are high, it is called hyperglycaemia.

High blood glucose is caused by not enough or too much of the wrong kind of food (carbohydrates), not enough exercise, too much stress and any unrelated illness. The warning signs are blurred vision, dry itchy skin, fatigue, frequent urination, hunger and increased thirst.

A diabetic should always test for high blood glucose with a blood glucose monitor. They should not rely upon how they feel, because there may be no symptoms at all.

Diabetic Ketoacidosis

Ketoacidosis is glucose that stays in the blood instead of entering the cells. When your blood sugar is high, it means that your blood cells are unable to use the glucose as they should, so it stays in the blood. When the cells are starved of glucose, the body breaks down fat for energy. The cells cannot use fat completely, however, and ketones are left. These enter the bloodstream and make the blood acidic. Ketoacidosis is more likely to occur in those who are insulin dependent.

Diabetics should test for ketones when they feel ill. The warning signs are alcohol-smelling breath, blood sugar over 13.0 mmol/l, difficulty breathing, nausea, stomach pain, vomiting and weakness.

Diabetes and Illness

When there is an illness that is unrelated to diabetes it is possible that there will be an increase in hormones in the body that can make the blood glucose levels higher. So, if you have diabetes, it is especially important to take care of yourself during an illness. The blood sugar should be checked every two to four hours and recorded. Ketones should also be checked every four hours. You should continue taking your medication as directed and take the amount of insulin prescribed by your doctor. Follow your diet plan as closely as possible. Drink plenty of water and stay in contact with your doctor until you are better.

Non-prescription Medication

A person with diabetes should be aware that non-prescription medicine may contain ingredients that can affect the blood sugar. Some recommendations:

- Avoid aspirin in large doses.
- Avoid products containing sugar. (Use sugar-free cough syrups or cough drops.)

- Be careful of decongestants.
- Choose products containing little or no alcohol, because alcohol contains glucose and is high in calories.
- Use tablets or capsules rather than liquid medicine because they contain no alcohol and no sugar.

Stress

When we are under stress, our body releases substances called stress hormones. These cause the release of stored glucose into the bloodstream and also interfere with the way insulin works, creating insulin resistance.

People with diabetes should consider taking up relaxation techniques such as yoga, ThetaHealing and learning to laugh, as well as getting the proper amount of sleep, having a healthy diet and identifying what is stressing them.

Depression

Clinical depression is much more common among people with diabetes than the general population. Why this is so is not fully understood. It may be that the extra demands of diabetes management itself – blood testing, diet restrictions – are difficult and can result in depression. Diabetes opens feelings of anger, guilt, sadness and not being in control. Those with clinical depression tend to have poorer blood sugar control and less compliance with their treatment.

Symptoms that are common to depression are:

- apathy and social withdrawal
- excessive emotional sensitivity
- ideas of suicide
- irritability
- moodiness and despair
- low self-esteem
- pessimistic thinking
- the inability to experience joy or happiness

The Kidneys

Diabetes is the leading cause of kidney failure in the USA. This is because high blood glucose levels have a tendency to damage the kidneys over time, causing a condition called diabetic neuropathy. As the damage increases, the kidneys lose their ability to remove waste products from the body.

There are five stages of neuropathy:

1. The flow of blood increases, causing hyper-filtration and increased urine output. The kidneys become enlarged.

2. The rate of filtration remains elevated and the filtering units begin to show damage.

3. Increased amounts of protein are lost in the urine and can be detected in routine urine tests. High blood pressure can develop.

4. Advanced clinical neuropathy: the filtration rate decreases and large amounts of protein are passed into the urine. High blood pressure is a result.

5. End-stage renal disease: the attrition rate drops severely and the symptoms of kidney failure occur.

In order to prevent kidney disease, a person with diabetes should:

- control blood pressure
- drink plenty of water
- get a yearly check at the doctor's
- keep the blood glucose levels normal
- prevent kidney infection
- restrict protein intake
- watch for symptoms:
  back pain just below the rib cage
  blood in the urine
  chills and fever
  cloudy urine
  feeling weak and tired
  high blood pressure
  increased amounts of urine
  ketones in the urine
  pain or burning during urination

Kidney disease is treated with:

- a low-protein diet
- a low-sodium diet

- antibiotics
- controlling blood pressure through ACE inhibitors
- keeping blood glucose under control

The Cardiovascular System

Diabetics are more prone to heart disease than any other condition. Because of the circulatory problems that are associated with high blood sugar, high levels of insulin, insulin resistance and lipid abnormalities, the heart can be very vulnerable to disease. This is why self-management is so important with diabetes as it pertains to the heart and arteries.

The Feet

Those with diabetes have a higher risk of developing problems with the feet. Decreased circulation and the accompanying high blood sugar can cause cell damage and make it difficult to heal an infection or injury. An unhealthy foot cannot handle the pressure of the body's weight because of the damage from diabetes. The problems that can occur (especially with chronic high blood sugar levels) can include:

- a greater chance of developing hammer toe and arch collapse
- a greater chance of skin breakdown and infection that results in gangrene and amputation
- an increased risk of athlete's foot or toenail fungus
- increased development of calluses or corns
- numbness or tingling that make it difficult to sense an injury or sore

This is why foot care is so important for those with diabetes. The feet should be washed every day, well dried, a moisturizing lotion applied and medicated powder used. The feet should be inspected daily, checking between the toes for blisters, cuts, scratches and colour changes. Calluses and corns should be properly removed. Tight stockings should not be used and a diabetic should not go barefoot.

Educate yourself. The more you know about diabetes, the better you will be able to get it under control.

Diet and Exercise

They say that an apple a day will keep the doctor away. But an apple-shaped figure will increase the likelihood of heart disease and diabetes. High levels of triglycerides and fatty acids cause insulin resistance. These acids tend to collect in the abdomen, hence those with an apple figure are twice as likely to develop insulin resistance.

What you eat is important here. Choose foods that do not have saturated fat in them. Animal fats should be kept to a minimum. However, be sure to consume adequate protein and to drink enough water to remain hydrated. Many foods that are low in carbohydrates will in turn keep the blood sugar to reasonable levels.

In many instances, diabetes can be improved with exercise and a diet low in carbohydrates. Eating 30 carbohydrates a meal and 15 to 20 in two snacks a day will reduce body weight and lower the blood glucose levels. Reading labels pertaining to carbohydrates is the key to a proper diet for those with diabetes. Increasing fibre will help as well.

An exercise plan that fits your lifestyle is also incredibly important, even if it is only for 10 minutes a day.

One suggestion might be to use weight training. Weight resistance builds muscles and lowers glucose even when you are at rest. It helps insulin to be used correctly in the body and prevents injuries to the body by building strong muscles and bones. Alternating between the upper body and lower body is a good regime. To begin with, use very light weights. Start with five to eight repetitions, gradually working up to 15 to 20 repetitions.

Intuitive Remedies

Diabetes is hard to detect intuitively since the medication the person is taking will fool you into believing that the body is balanced.

Find out what kind of diabetes the person has. If the Creator takes you to the pancreas, there is an imbalance in the blood sugar. Command it to be healed. Command that the pancreas balances the production and release of insulin. Ask the Creator to show you.

Healing the liver is generally where the Creator begins to heal a person with diabetes.

Go in and command that the chromosomes change so that they produce the right amount of insulin and the right number of neurons and receptors needed to take the messages to create the proper amounts of insulin.

Command the insulin level to return to the level that it was before the diabetes took hold of the body.

If the Creator tells you that there is a weakness in a gene that is causing the diabetes, use the gene work to pull and replace the gene that is shown to you. With all genetic defects, where one defect is found, another one exists. The Creator will show you the other defect and repair this also.

In some instances, you may find that the diabetes seems to have been caused by an interaction with a mild virus over the outside of the cells, which blocks them from hearing each other correctly. Go in and witness the virus being changed to a harmless form.

Belief Work

One of the first things I will do for diabetes Type 2 is to give the person a diet that is low in carbohydrates.

Then I will work on their feelings of being defeated. On some level, especially on the genetic level, they will feel as though they have lost the battle. Ask about their ancestors. In many instances you will see that their grandfather lost a farm, or their father lost everything, or their parents have made them feel defeated.

Always start with issues of defeat and boredom with life. I have had instant healings just by working with these issues.

This works particularly well with diabetes Type 2. The beliefs and feelings are of sorrow and emotional shock; the joy is gone in life, and the person is judgemental and angry.

People with diabetes are independent and also have over-controlling issues such as 'I have to control everything and everyone'. Download 'I know how to be healthy', allow the person to visualize themselves as healthy and ask them what it would feel like if they were completely healthy. This will lead you to a bottom belief. They might say, for example, 'If I were completely healthy, I would go back to my old ways. I would leave my wife and my world would fall apart.' This person thinks that diabetes is keeping them reliable and responsible, so they have no reason to heal it. This belief should be changed to 'I can be reliable and responsible without diabetes'. Diabetes makes people take care of themselves. Many people who have a fear of getting better suffer from it.

Download:

'I know what it feels like to live without defeat.'

'I know what it feels like to live without this disease defeating me.'

'I can achieve without diabetes.'

'I know what it feels like to live without diabetes.'

'I can achieve abundance without diabetes.'

'I can maintain control without diabetes.'

'I can care for my body without diabetes.'

'I can care for my family without diabetes.'

'I can be a mature person without diabetes.'

'I can permit someone to love me without the fear of dying.'

'I can be close to the Creator without diabetes.'

'My family will still love me without diabetes.'

'Diabetes is an inconvenience that I know how to live without.'

'I know how to take care of my body without diabetes.'

'I know what it feels like to live without resenting everyone and everything around me.'

'I know what it feels like knowing that I have the freedom to choose.'

'I know what it feels like to be allowed to be happy.'

'I know how to motivate myself.'

'I know what it feels like to know I am safe.'

'I know what it feels like to live without resenting the past.'

'I know what it feels like to be completely strong and healthy.'

'I know it's possible to be completely strong and healthy.'

'I know how to live without being bored.'

Supplements and Other Nutritional Recommendations

- calcium–magnesium
- chromium
- cinnamon
- CoQ10
- dandelion
- DHEA
- goji juice
- noni
- omega 3s, 6s and 9s

***

- Alpha-lipoic acid helps to normalize blood sugar levels but, as with all supplements, should be used with caution.
- Do a liver cleanse (*see the Liver*)! Suggest 'Cleanse and Build' by Lidtke Technologies.
- Do not use wormwood or oregano.
- Glucophage is a pharmaceutical aid.

THE DIGESTIVE SYSTEM

Mouth Enzymes

The enzymes of the mouth are the beginning of the digestive system. They help to digest starch, as well as destroying powerful bacteria as they enter the body. These enzymes are swallowed with the food and travel down the oesophagus to aid in digestion.

The Stomach

The stomach is located on the left side of the body. It thinks it is always busy and extremely important. If people do not know what it feels like to be loved and accepted, the stomach is affected and the food does not get digested properly. If you become angry because you have eaten something that perhaps you truly should not have, there is the possibility that the food will not be digested correctly because of your emotion. This is how sensitive the stomach is and how the intuitive person can permit their emotions to affect their health.

The Intestinal Tract

The food is carried by villi through the intestines, and small openings allow food and nutrients to go through them. Minerals have to be ionized in order to be small enough to be absorbed in this way. Colloidal minerals can be absorbed by plants, but are too big to be absorbed by the human digestive system.

Due to an improper diet and perhaps other factors, some people have sluggish bowel movements. You are supposed to have a bowel movement about half an hour after eating. You will have regular bowel movements if you eat the right foods and are alkaline enough to process them correctly. The more belief and feeling work you do, the more balanced your pH becomes. Belief work alone can help a sluggish bowel.

The Digestive System and Abuse

The digestive system is where emotions of abuse are often stored. 'Abuse' is quantified as 'experiencing physical, emotional, verbal, spiritual and sexual abuse as a child'.

What registers in the mind of one person as abuse might not seem like abuse to another. Abuse can be the medical treatment given to a child on whom the doctors are running tests. It can be an enema given to a child. Or when an adult says to a child, 'You are ugly,' or when children tease each other with derogatory statements. The body can collect all these memories and place them in patterns inside the organs. If a person witnesses another person being abused, the body can also store this as abuse. When we go through the intestinal tract we can identify and release these old emotions and programmes.

Repetitive abuse or 'ritual abuse' is any kind of abuse that happens over and over again, constantly, like a ritual. It does not have to be satanic ritual abuse.

The lower right side of the abdomen holds sexual abuse, while the lower left side of the body holds emotional abuse.

The solar plexus holds shame.

The liver holds anger.

The spleen area holds fear and guilt.

With the permission of the client, the practitioner can gently touch these areas to bring up these issues or have the client put their hand on their own abdomen when doing abuse work.

Go up to the Creator and command the trauma to leave the body in the highest and best way, then begin using the belief work to find the bottom beliefs.

When you are working with abuse, download the following:

'I understand what the Creator's definition of love is.'

'I understand what it feels like to be loved.'

'I understand what it feels like to be cherished by the Creator.'

'I understand the Creator's definition of what it is to love and cherish myself.'

'I understand what it feels like to really love someone.'

'I understand what it is to be loved by the Creator of All That Is.'

'I understand the Creator's definition of acceptance.'

'I understand the Creator's definition of what it is to be safe, protected and completely loved.'

'I know how to live without allowing others to abuse me.'

'I know how to live without abusing myself or others.'

Also, for the digestive system, download:

'I know what it feels like to live without fear.'

'I know how to live without fear.'

'I know how to live without resentment.'

'I know the Creator's definition of what it feels like to be safe.'

'I know the Creator's definition of what it feels like to be protected.'

'I know the Creator's definition of what it feels like to be secure.'

DOWN'S SYNDROME

Down's syndrome (DS) is a condition in which additional genetic material causes delays in the way a child develops and often leads to mental retardation. It affects one in every 800 babies born. It can be detected before a child is born.

Causes

Normally, at conception a baby inherits genetic information from its parents in the form of 46 chromosomes: 23 from the father and 23 from the mother. In most cases of Down's syndrome, however, the child gets an extra chromosome. It's this extra genetic material that causes the physical and cognitive delays associated with DS.

In Down's syndrome, 95 percent of all cases are caused by one egg cell having a duplicate of the twenty-first chromosome. So, the resulting fertilized egg has three twenty-first chromosomes, making a total of 47 chromosomes instead of 46. The scientific name for this is trisomy 21. Recent research has shown that in these cases, approximately 90 percent of the abnormal cells are the eggs. The cause of the non-disjunction error isn't known, but there is definitely a connection with maternal age of the eggs. Research is currently aimed at trying to determine the cause and timing of the non-disjunction event.

Symptoms

The symptoms of Down's syndrome can vary widely. While some children with DS need a lot of medical attention, others lead very healthy and independent lives. The health problems that can go along with DS can be treated and there are many resources within communities to help kids and their families who are living with the condition.

Intuitive Remedies

Ask the Creator what needs to be done.

In some cases, the child will have a compromised immune system.

In rare instances, the child has chosen this existence and the practitioner is instructed by the child's higher self not to work on it.

Witness the Creator realign and balance the brain and use the gene work.

DRUG ABUSE

Entity Energy in Drug Abuse

All the drug-addicted people that I have experienced psychically have had strange entities attached to them. Each drug seems to have an entity that is peculiar to it and intuitively looks the same from person to person. These are some of the forms that addictive energies take when seen intuitively:

- A heroin spirit looks like a shrivelled old man with hollow eyes.
- A marijuana spirit looks like an emaciated brown-haired woman with glowing green eyes.
- A cocaine spirit looks like an emaciated white-blonde woman with skin the colour of snow and electric blue eyes. Her energy will be flowing around the addicted person.
- A crystal methamphetamine spirit looks like an emaciated white-blonde woman with blank holes for eyes.
- Each type of alcohol has a different spiritual energy attached to it. Why do you think they call it spirits?

Waywards may also be present, as drug addiction and alcoholism can cause a spiritual energy drain that opens the person to parasitic energy, and waywards are then able to intrude into their weakened 'space' or aura.

Intuitive Remedies

To help the person, alter their serotonin level as the Creator directs, and go into their space to see if anything needs to be detached and sent to the Creator's light. If they are on drugs, the relevant entity will be attached to them, whispering the words that keep them addicted to the substance. This entity must be sent to the Creator's light to ease the suffering of the addicted person and give them a chance for recovery.

Warning! The abuse of methamphetamine creates raw dopamine in the brain. This actually eats the feeling parts of the brain. This is why feelings for parents and loved ones seem non-existent with a methamphetamine addict. Depending on the severity of the addiction, it can take a year for these feelings to return to normal, if ever. Command the feeling centres of the brain to be as they were before the addiction.

Also command any waywards to go to the Creator's light.

Belief Work

Look at issues of worthiness. Download:

'I know what it feels like to live my day-to-day life without feeling dependent upon a drug.'

'Every day in every way I get healthier and stronger.'

'Life is beautiful.'

'I can enjoy life without the use of drugs or alcohol.'

'I know what it feels like to live without having to feel sad.'

'I know what it feels like to get high on life.'

'I no longer feel happy with alcohol.'

'I no longer feel happy with drugs.'

'I no longer feel happy with tobacco.'

'I can feel the breath of life without alcohol and drugs.'

'Alcohol is a waste of time.'

'Drugs are a waste of time.'

'I feel clean.'

'I breathe the air.'

'I feel joy.'

'Life is full of possibilities.'

'There is magic in all things.'

'I can feel magic without the use of drugs and alcohol.'

'I am connected to God.'

'I am full of energy and change.'

Supplements and Other Nutritional Recommendations

- Echinacea cleans drugs out of the blood.
- Niacin cleans drugs out of the body.

The following can also be beneficial:

- a sauna cleanse
- folic acid
- glutathione IVs from a certified practitioner
- goji juice
- liver cleanses (*see the Liver*)
- molybdenum, 300 mg
- omega 3s
- the alkaline diet
- vitamin B complex

See also Alcoholism.

DYSLEXIA

Do not change it, ever! If a person has dyslexia, then there is also a genius gene present! Some of the most intelligent people in the world have dyslexia. You can, however, ask for the dyslexia to be toned down. Ask the Creator to show you what needs to be done.

E. COLI

See Food Poisoning.

THE EARS

See Hearing Impairment.

EMPHYSEMA

Emphysema is a long-term progressive disease of the lungs that causes shortness of breath. It is included in a group of diseases called chronic obstructive pulmonary disease, or COPD. It is called an obstructive lung disease because the destruction of lung tissue around smaller airways, called bronchioles, makes them unable to hold their shape properly when you exhale.

Causes

Possible causes include:

- air pollution
- asthma
- cigarette smoking
- genetic defects

Intuitive Remedies

Witness the Creator holding the lungs up and breathing in love and life to recreate the cells. Witness the Creator changing the emphysema and witness the dark patches being sent to the Creator's light.

Downloads

'I am worthy of God's love.'

'I know what it feels like to have love for myself.'

'I have compassion for myself.'

See Asthma for other beliefs.

THE ENDOCRINE SYSTEM

There are three major components of the endocrine system:

- *Glands:* These are specialized cell clusters or organs.
- *Hormones:* These are chemical messengers secreted by the glands in response to stimulation. They transfer information and instructions from one set of cells to another.
- *Receptors:* These are gateways or doorways for the hormone to trigger cell responses.

The glands of the endocrine system and the hormones they release influence almost every cell, organ and function in the body. The endocrine system also regulates our emotions, which can contribute to our general health. If joy and love are experienced, the body will heal much faster than if anger or hatred are prevalent.

Intuitive Remedies

Make the command: *'Creator, balance the hormones and chemicals in this body in the highest and best way and show me. Thank you. It is done. It is done. It is done.'* Witness the process as done.

Feeling Work

Certain feelings can be taught to the endocrine system in order to balance the emotions and give the person the conscious choice to change. Download:

'I know how to live without anger.'

'I know how to live without depression.'

'I know how to live without fear.'

'I know how to live without regret.'

'I understand how to relax.'

'I understand what it feels like to rest.'

'I understand how to have fun.'

'I know how to make decisions easily.'

ENDOMETRIOSIS

Endometriosis is a common health problem in women. It gets its name from the endometrium, the tissue that lines the uterus. In women with this problem, tissue that looks and acts like the lining of the uterus grows outside the uterus, forming growths, tumours, implants, lesions or nodules.

Symptoms

Symptoms include:

- chronic pain in the lower back and pelvis
- fatigue
- heavy and/or long menstrual periods
- infertility
- intestinal pain
- pain during or after sex
- pain with periods that gets worse over time
- painful bowel movements or painful urination during menstrual periods
- spotting or bleeding between periods
- very painful menstrual cramps

Causes

Endometriosis can be genetic, caused by problems with the liver or created by beliefs.

Intuitive Remedies

Command that the endometriosis shrink to balance the body. The 'Free-floating Memories' exercise (see Alcoholism) can prove effective.

Belief Work

Check for:
'I feel taken advantage of.'

'I have to fight for all I have.'

'I am never allowed to rest.'

'I am not good enough.'

See Fibroids for other beliefs.

Supplements and Other Nutritional Recommendations

- alpha-lipoic acid
- calcium–magnesium
- liver cleanses (*see the Liver*)
- vitamin C

EPILEPSY

Epilepsy is a brain disorder that causes people to have recurring seizures. These happen when neurons in the brain send out the wrong signals. People with epilepsy may have odd sensations and emotions or behave strangely. They may have violent muscle spasms or lose consciousness. In a *grand mal* seizure, the heart actually stops.

Doctors use brain scans and other tests to diagnose epilepsy. It is important to start treatment right away. There are many medicines that can control seizures. When medicines are not working well, surgery or implanted devices such as vagus nerve stimulators may help. Special diets can help some children with epilepsy. Some children will grow out of the challenge. Good results have been obtained by treating people with male/female hormones.

Causes

Epilepsy has many possible causes, including abnormal brain development, brain injury and illness. Fetal stress due to the mother's stress can throw off neurotransmitters. In many cases, the cause is unknown.

There are many things that can trigger seizures, including alcohol, brain injuries, caffeine, flashing lights, hormones, medication, memories and traumatic events. They can also be learned behaviour. Some of the conventional medicine given for seizures can actually create them, because of overdoses.

Seizures are also triggered when the brain doesn't get enough oxygen, so the body tries to catch up and begins to shake. The shaking is not the seizure; it is the body attempting to recover.

Intuitive Insights

Epilepsy is intuitively seen as a short-circuit going through the back of the brain, or lesions in the front.

Intuitive Remedies

The best way to pull someone out of a *grand mal* seizure is to touch them, command the body to stop shaking and imagine energy moving up through the feet.

To heal epilepsy, connect to the Creator, make the command, '*Show me*,' and witness the changes. Witness the neurons reconnecting and clear any free-floating memories with the 'Free-floating Memories' exercise (*see Alcoholism*). Go in and change the foetal memory and tell the growing baby not to worry and that it is safe.

Supplements and Other Nutritional Recommendations

- alpha-lipoic acid
- blue light (avoid flashing red lights)
- hormone therapy administered by a doctor
- maca
- Panax ginseng
- the alkaline diet

THE EPSTEIN-BARR VIRUS

This is a herpes virus. It is a type of herpes that can make the spleen swell. A high percentage of the population carries it and it is likely to manifest when the carrier has a lowered immune system.

Symptoms

Symptoms include:

- aching muscles
- blood-pressure problems
- fatigue
- headaches
- memory loss

- nasal congestion
- sore throat

Belief Work

Beliefs are likely to involve victimization. Test for:

'I can't help myself.'

'People are picking on me.'

and replace with

'I know how to live without being miserable.'

'I know how to enjoy my day-to-day life with joy.'

Supplements and Other Nutritional Recommendations

- Suggest a fungi cleanse, such as cumin, myrtle or oregano.
- Multimineral and multivitamins are a must, especially vitamin B complex.

See also Chronic Fatigue Syndrome, Fibromyalgia, Herpes and Viruses (Prologue).

THE EXCRETORY SYSTEM

The excretory system is the system that rids the body of waste products. The word 'excretion' means 'removal of wastes from the body'. Without the excretory system, we would all be dead, because it cleans the blood and sends the wastes from the blood out in the urine. It also regulates the chemical composition of bodily fluids by removing metabolic wastes and retaining the proper amounts of water, salts and nutrients. Components of this system in vertebrates (mammals) include the kidneys, liver, lungs and skin.

The Bladder

The bladder is a place where uric acid is held so that it can leave the body. It harbours old resentment and old anger.

The Kidneys

The kidneys' job is to maintain hydration throughout the body as well as getting rid of excess uric acid. They hold anger, resentments and grudges. If people aren't healing, go 'through the back door' to the kidneys and do resentment work.

See also Kidney Disease.

THE EYES

The eyes consist of the cornea, lens, optic nerve and retina.

We all see slightly differently and use other senses to compensate. In my view, there is too much emphasis on what we call 'normal eyesight'. The accepted values for normal eyesight are 20/20–20/15, with 20/10 as better than normal sight. So when the last number goes down, the eyesight becomes better.

To focus at a distance, the lens relaxes over the eyes, the muscles relax and the lens slants and bends so the light rays go directly to the back of the eyes.

When muscles in the eye contract too much, the eye lens becomes more rounded. At the point where the image goes through the lens, the objects will become blurred, causing near-sighted vision. This occurs when the lens reaches its maximum curvature to create a proper image.

Diseases and Disorders of the Eye

- astigmatism
- cataracts
- glaucoma
- farsightedness
- kidney failure
- macular degeneration
- near-sightedness

Near-sightedness

Near-sightedness occurs when the eyeball is too long and pointed. Instead of focusing on the retina's surface, the image is focused in front of it. You need to readjust this part of the surface until you are able to make the focus correct.

Farsightedness

Farsightedness occurs when the eyeball is too short, causing the image to focus behind the retina instead of on the surface. You can correct this by changing the surface of the eye.

Unlike near-sightedness, farsightedness can come from the mother having taken birth-control pills at conception, or it may be caused by beliefs.

For Astigmatism, Cataracts and Glaucoma, see below.

Intuitive Insights

The eyes are the windows to the soul. They are a reflection of all our experiences. We are allowed to take one thing with us throughout all our lifetimes: the energy of our eyes. Sometimes the eyes are different colours from existence to existence, but the same energy of sight follows us and the memory of the past is held in the eyes.

Iridologists believe that if the eyes have a green tinge, then there is extra bile in the blood, which is a sign of liver congestion. I believe that eye colour is genetic. Green, red and blue are the only true colours in the spectrum and the rest are a mix of these. However, I have seen slight colour variations in the eyes with liver cleanses.

Intuitive Remedies

The eyes are a good indicator of a person's belief systems and of the truth. Working on them brings up a wealth of emotions. Let the person know that when you work with their eyes many emotions will come up each time programmes are released and replaced or physical healings are done.

When you work on the eyes, make sure the person's glasses and contacts are off. The reason for this is that otherwise the command to repair will not be accepted because the eyes are already 'seeing' close to 20/20 vision and so the brain and the soul will accept these facts as real.

All parts of the eyes heal quickly, including the retina. Ask the Creator for the best vision possible for the person.

If you ask for better sight, this will also increase the person's intuitive sense of 'sight'.

When you work on the eyes, go into the person's space, witness the changes with the Creator and get out fast to avoid fear, doubt or disbelief! If you see something with the physical eyes, in one sense it is witnessed in this reality as a manifestation. The eyes are one of the processors of intuitive energy and if information is sent through them to the brain, it is perceived as real in this plane of existence because of the connection to the nervous system.

You do not have to know the intricate structure of the eye to heal it. Imagine the light as it enters the eye hitting the back of the eye evenly and correctly. If the person is farsighted, have them look at an object in the distance that they can see clearly as the healing is done. If they are near-sighted, have them focus on something close at hand that they can see clearly as you correct how the light enters into their eye. Stay with this process and watch it until the light actually hits the back of their eye in the correct position. In many instances you will only witness a flash and the Creator is finished. If this happens, you may ask for a replay of the healing.

In many instances, the eyes need coaching to change eyesight. You may need to change it gradually, with more than one healing session. A gradual improvement is much easier for the person's system and the attached emotions.

Sometimes the eye refuses to correct completely. This means that there is too much emotion for the mind to deal with.

If you have done a healing on the eyes and there is little or no improvement, it may be that a good liver cleanse is in order (*see the Liver*). The liver directly affects the eyes, and a liver cleanse is a must in some situations with the eyes. You may have to do an additional liver cleanse to follow up.

Diabetes or pregnancy can cause challenges with the eyesight, so do not forget to look for physical explanations.

You can intuitively clean out a burst blood vessel in the eye. These are caused by lack of vitamins and minerals.

For chronically dry eyes, intuitively clear out the tear ducts and glands.

Belief Work

Follow up with belief work anytime you do healings on the eyes.

In finding programmes and beliefs associated with the eyes, you must find out if there is something the client does not want to see. They have to want to see the truth. If there is something that they don't want to see, their eyesight will not improve. We often have a tendency to push aside what we don't want to see in ourselves instead of learning from it and integrating it.

Also, go in to look for any history-level memories of why they can't see. Explore programmes that are associated with the time in their life that their eyesight began to fail them.

With some people it is necessary to use the gene work.

Also look for programmes about the person's ego. There is a Native American saying, 'If your ego isn't your amigo, you are in trouble.' A person's ego is important to them, and you should not attempt to command it to go away.

Your ego is what you are. Where is your own ego taking you? Ask yourself if your ego is balanced. Ego*tism* is what you want to avoid.

Also, look for any jealousy issues and the comparisons the person is making between themselves and others.

Test for blocks over the third eye from past, present and future times. What is blocking the person from seeing and achieving their dream? Make sure that they are unafraid of the future and are 'living in this moment, focused on the future'.

With near-sightedness, check for programmes concerned with not wanting to see the present as it is.

Download:

'It's OK to see.'

'I can see the truth.'

'I am allowed to see clearly.'

'I know what it feels like to live my day-to-day life without self-sabotaging.'

'I know the Creator's definition of my soul's true potential.'

'I have the Creator's definition of what it feels like to witness the highest truth.'

'I have the Creator's definition of how to see myself through the Creator's eyes.'

'I have the Creator's definition of how to see others through the Creator's eyes.'

'I know what it feels like to live my life without discouragement.'

'I know what it feels like to live my life without disappointment.'

'I know what the Creator's definition of hope is.'

'I know what it feels like to live my life without feeling hopeless.'

'I have the Creator's definition of what it feels like to have my dreams come true.'

'I know what it feels like to live my life without competing with my fellow ThetaHealers.'

'I have the Creator's definition of how to reach my highest potential.'

'I have the Creator's definition of what it feels like to have my boundaries respected by others.'

'I have the Creator's definition of what discernment is.'

'I have the Creator's definition of what true communication is.'

'I have the Creator's definition of what it feels like to have ethics.'

'I have the Creator's definition of what it feels like to have integrity.'

'I have the Creator's definition of what it feels like to be honest with myself and with others.'

'I have the Creator's definition of how to live without having to trade one of my senses for power.'

'I have the Creator's definition of what it feels like to have the ability to see all truth in the highest and best way.'

'I have the Creator's definition of what it feels like to have clarity.'

'I understand what it feels like to witness the highest truth.'

'I have the Creator's definition of what truth feels like.'

'I know how to live without thinking that the only time I have no demands from others is when I am not wearing my glasses.'

Supplements and Other Nutritional Recommendations

- Look for vitamin deficiencies when working with sight problems. Suggest a liver cleanse, as a congested liver can affect the eyes.
- Alpha-lipoic acid helps with some eye challenges.
- Using beta-carotene for a week will help night blindness.
- Vitamin A will clear allergies in the eyes.
- Zinc helps the eyes to focus.

Astigmatism

Astigmatism is an unequal curving of one or more of the refractive surfaces of the eye, usually the cornea. It prevents light rays lying in specific planes from coming into focus on the retina, thus producing blurred vision. Ask the Creator to readjust the curvature of the eye so that it is correct for 20/20 vision.

The eyes usually need coaching and will change gradually. So change contacts and glasses as you go and follow up with a liver cleanse. Belief work should always be done.

Cataracts

Belief Work

Cataracts are connected to programmes of seeing truth and being sheltered from reality.

Intuitive Remedies

To pull off a cataract, you need to go into the eye and imagine the cataract being gently removed from the eye. Ask the Creator to show you what should be done.

Supplements and Other Nutritional Recommendations

Rinse the eyes with comfrey to dissolve the cataracts: add two pinches of comfrey to a quart of water, seep for three to four minutes, cool and put a dropper's worth on the eye, once a day before bedtime until the cataract is gone.

Glaucoma

Glaucoma causes blindness due to increased pressure within the eye that leads to damage of the optic disk. This is caused by a blockage in the blood flow to the optic nerve. The result is the degeneration of nerve fibres. Those who are at greatest risk are people over 60, people with diabetes or high blood pressure, smokers, steroid users and those with severe myopathy or a family history of glaucoma.

Types

- The most common form of glaucoma is called *open angle glaucoma*. This has no symptoms until it is quite advanced and only half of the people with this disorder are aware that they have it. Open angle glaucoma has no visible blockage in the structure of the eye and it appears normal. The most pronounced symptom is a gradual loss or darkening of peripheral vision and a marked decrease in night vision. This leaves a person with tunnel vision, low-grade headaches and the need for frequent changes in glasses' prescription.

- A far less common but more serious form of glaucoma is *closed angle glaucoma*. This never manifests any symptoms until very late on. By this time the vision can be irreversibly damaged. Attacks of this type of glaucoma occur when the channels through which the eye fluids drain suddenly become constricted or obstructed. Early warning signs that a problem is developing include blurred vision, eye pain or discomfort, mainly in the morning, the inability of the pupils to adjust to a dark room and seeing halos around lights. Some symptoms can be accompanied by nausea and vomiting. Permanent visual damage can occur in as little as three to five days, making treatment within the first 24 to 48 hours imperative.

- *Normotensive glaucoma* manifests even though there is normal fluid pressure within the eye. With this condition, the optic nerve is damaged and vision is impaired in much the same way as with open angle glaucoma but without the increased fluid pressure. This has led researchers to shift their focus to the optic nerve itself. It is believed that mechanisms other than pressure may cause changes in the eye that can damage the optic nerve.

Causes

Scientists believe that glaucoma may be closely linked to stress, nutritional problems or disorders such as diabetes and high blood pressure. Another factor might be glutamate, an amino acid that might somehow be in excessive amounts in the body. Problems with collagen, the most abundant protein in the human body, have been linked to glaucoma. Collagen acts to increase the strength and elasticity of tissues in the body, especially those of the eye. Collagen and tissue abnormalities at the back of the eye contribute to the clogging of the tissues through which fluid normally drains.

For those at risk of glaucoma, a yearly eye test is necessary.

Belief Work

Most of the people with glaucoma that I have worked with have had the associated disease of diabetes, so many of the belief systems have been the same:

- allowing other people to treat you inadequately
- being blind to what is going on around you
- feeling inadequate
- feeling unable to accomplish your life's mission
- fear of how others perceive you
- fear of seeing the truth of a situation
- having to deal with the people in your life

Ask the person what was going on in their life when the first symptoms appeared. Make them think back to what their feelings were at that time and who in their life was making them not want to see something.

Healing

Go into the eye and witness the blood flow increase by opening the capillaries and then witness the Creator repairing any damage. This is the most successful way to work on glaucoma.

Suggestions

People with glaucoma should avoid prolonged eye stress such as reading, watching television and using a computer for long periods. Take focus breaks every 20 minutes and avoid alcohol, coffee and smoking.

Supplements/Recommendation

DHEA

* vitamin B complex
* vitamin C

***

* Avoid taking high doses of niacin.

FIBROCYSTIC BREASTS

Fibrocystic changes occur in about half of all women, mostly during childbearing years. The cause appears to be normal hormonal fluctuations. This is because the symptoms of fibrocystic breasts usually increase right before menstruation, subside after menstruation and usually stop after menopause. Fibrocystic breast changes were once referred to as a disease, but since the condition is so prevalent, it is no longer considered so.

Symptoms

The following symptoms usually peak right before menstruation:

- a feeling of fullness in the breasts
- breast pain and tenderness
- nipple discharge or sensation changes
- non-cancerous cysts
- thickened, lumpy areas in the breast tissue

Mammogram results for women with fibrocystic breasts may be difficult to read due to the breast tissue being denser than normal tissue. However, a definitive diagnosis can be made with a combination of mammography, an ultrasound and sometimes a minimally invasive needle biopsy.

Intuitive Remedies

Fibrocystic breasts are generally an inherited condition. However, if the person uses liver cleanses and keeps their liver clean, they will have good results in stopping the growth of these fibroids, as well as shrinking them.

The basic healing works well in shrinking fibroids.

A good-fitting bra with good support will also help.

Belief Work

Most of the issues around fibrocystic breasts cycle around sexuality.

Supplements and Other Nutritional Recommendations

Conventional medicine prescribes calcium and magnesium to shrink fibroids. Some of the following self-help measures may alleviate the symptoms:

- Eliminate caffeine from the diet.
- Restrict fat intake to 25 percent or less of daily calories.
- Use oral contraceptives – discuss this with a doctor

Try the following supplements:

- ALA
- amino-acid complexes
- burdock
- red clover
- vitamin A
- vitamin C

FIBROIDS

A uterine fibroid is the most common benign (non-cancerous) tumour in a woman's uterus. Fibroids start in the muscle tissues of the uterus. They can grow into the uterine cavity, into the thickness of the uterine wall or on the surface of the uterus into the abdominal cavity. Although these tumours are called fibroids, this term is misleading because they consist of muscle tissue, not fibrous tissue. They may grow as a single tumour or in clusters.

Uterine fibroids can cause excessive menstrual bleeding, pelvic pain and frequent urination. They occur in about 25 percent of all women and are the leading cause of hysterectomy (removal of the uterus) in the United States. Of every woman older than 35 years, one in five has a uterine fibroid. Medication and newer, less invasive surgery can control the growth of fibroids.

Intuitive Remedies

Go into the body and command that the fibroids go away. Make sure that you work on any unresolved hurts the person may have.

Supplements and Other Nutritional Recommendations

- Fibroid tumours can be shrunk easily by adding more calcium-magnesium to the diet and doing a liver cleanse (*see the Liver*).
- If the person is biting their fingernails, consider this another indication that their body might be needing calcium.
- Maca, a herb from South America, will shrink fibroids, also.
- Suggest alpha-lipoic acid, too.

FIBROMYALGIA

Fibromyalgia is a chronic condition typified by widespread pain in the muscles, ligaments and tendons, as well as overall fatigue. It is more common in women than in men and is characterized by pain in specific areas of the body when pressure is applied. The pain generally persists for months at a time and is often accompanied by stiffness.

People with fibromyalgia often wake up tired even though they seem to get plenty of sleep. Studies suggest that this is the result of a sleep disorder called alpha wave interrupted sleep pattern, a condition in which deep sleep is interrupted.

Irritable bowel syndrome is considered to be a complication of fibromyalgia. Symptoms include abdominal pain, bloating, constipation and diarrhoea. These are common in people with fibromyalgia. Many people who have fibromyalgia also have headaches and facial pain that may be related to tenderness or stiffness in their neck and shoulders. It is also common for people with fibromyalgia to report being sensitive to bright lights, noises, odours and touch.

Doctors do not know what causes fibromyalgia; however, information currently centres on a theory called 'central sensitization'. This states that people with fibromyalgia have a lower threshold for pain because of increased sensitivity in the brain to pain signals.

Intuitive Insights

Fibromyalgia is actually a symptom of a disease that gets in the muscles. It can sometimes be caused by the Epstein-Barr virus. It can develop when the person is under a great deal of stress and the immune system becomes fatigued.

People who are on the go all the time and never stop have a tendency to develop fibromyalgia. Sometimes I think that the body creates a mild disease in order to produce a desired effect. It's as if it says, 'Since you don't know how to rest, I'm going to make you.' It knows the person won't rest unless they have a good enough reason to rest and what better reason than illness?

So, if you have workaholic tendencies, you may want to download:

'My muscles know how to rest.'

'I know how to rest.'

'I know how to receive love.'

Supplements

- ALA
- calcium–magnesium
- cayenne pepper (to stimulate the immune system)
- Echinacea (to cleanse the blood)
- milk thistle (to cleanse the liver)
- raw fruit juice consisting of beetroot, carrots, celery, garlic and ginger (to relieve the pain)

FOOD POISONING

Food can cause gastrointestinal disorders in man and animals if it is contaminated by micro-organisms and their secondary metabolites. Generally, 'food poisoning' is a term applied to illness caused by common bacteria like *Staphylococcus* or *E. coli*. However, classic food poisoning, sometimes incorrectly called ptomaine poisoning, is caused by a variety of different bacteria. The most common are *Salmonella*, *Staphylococcus aureus*, *Escherichia coli* or other *E. coli* strains, *Shigella* and *Clostridium botulinum*. Each has a slightly different incubation period and duration, but all except *C. botulinum* cause inflammation of the intestines and diarrhoea.

The strains of bacteria that I work with most commonly are *E. coli*, *Salmonella* and *Giardia*. You will find *Salmonella* in uncooked chicken.

Intuitive Remedies

Go up to the Creator, command that a healing be done and witness the bacteria being flushed from the whole system. There have been times when I have done a healing and the person has vomited immediately afterwards. Get them to drink plenty of liquids, as there is a danger of dehydration.

If you have food poisoning yourself, it can be difficult to get into a deep enough Theta wave to witness a healing, so I suggest that you use a little thyme in the form of Listerine to flush out the bacteria. Two teaspoons for two days at a time is recommended.

Before you eat any food, be sure to go above your space and ask the Creator if the food is contaminated. You should be particularly careful at salad bars, because the more food sits out, the more prone it is to the rapid growth of bacteria. Always keep food such as mayonnaise and eggs refrigerated. Never use eggs if they are cracked. Be particularly wary of the possibility of meat contaminating other food. Clean cutting boards and utensils if they come into contact with poultry, and thaw all meat in the refrigerator.

E. coli

There are some *E. coli* that are naturally in the body, so do not command that they are all destroyed.

Intuitive Remedies

Command that the body is balanced.

Supplements and Other Nutritional Recommendations

- Two capsules of thyme for two days or charcoal to settle the stomach.

Giardia

Giardia is a bacterium that is contracted through contaminated water and food. It can cause violent vomiting and diarrhoea.

Supplements and Other Nutritional Recommendations

- *Giardia* listens and responds to the voice of healing.
- One teaspoon of Listerine works well in an emergency.
- If you are in an isolated area, a little charcoal from a campfire mixed with water can settle the stomach.

FUNGUS

See Prologue.

GALLSTONES

Gallstones are a solid formation of cholesterol and bile salts. However, research shows that approximately 80 to 90 percent of all gallstones are cholesterol gallstones, which form when the liver begins secreting bile that is abnormally saturated with cholesterol. The excess cholesterol crystallizes and then forms stones, which are stored in the gallbladder or the cystic duct. Gallstones can also form due to low levels of bile acids and bile Lecithin.

Risk factors that can lead to increased incidence of gallstones include the 'Four Fs' – fat, female, fertile and flatulent – as well as sickle-cell disease (bilirubin), cirrhosis, Crohn's disease, diabetes, hyperparathyroidism and pancreatic disease.

Intuitive Remedies

For small gallstones, consider using gallstone cleanses and liver cleanses (see the Liver). You can also go in and command the stones to break down into small pieces. As with any healing, it is best to ask the Creator what is best for the person.

Supplements and Other Nutritional Recommendations

- Drink one cup of milk with a touch of ginger and two tablespoons of castor oil.
- Watermelon, apple juice, lemon juice and magnesium all break down stones.

As with any disorder, always consult your doctor.

GANGRENE

Gangrene is dead and rotten tissue left after a bacterial infection. There is no blood flow to it (since it is dead), so it is now open to infection.

Intuitive Remedies

Gangrene responds well to the intuitive introduction of new tissue.

Make the command: *'Creator, show me.'* Clean up the gangrene and command the whole area to regenerate. See the old tissue pulled out and watch the new tissue come in.

GASTROESOPHAGEAL REFLUX DISEASE

See Heartburn.

GIARDIA

See Food Poisoning.

GLAUCOMA

See the Eyes.

GONORRHOEA

See Sexually Transmitted Diseases.

GOUT

Gout is a common type of arthritis that occurs when there is too much uric acid in the blood and muscle tissues.

Uric acid is the end product of the metabolism of the class of chemicals known as purines. In people with gout, the body does not produce enough of the digestive enzyme uricase, which oxidizes relatively insoluble uric acid into a highly soluble compound. As a result, uric acid accumulates in the blood and tissues, ultimately crystallizing. When it crystallizes, it takes on a shape like that of a needle and, like a needle, jabs its way into the joints. It usually affects the big toe, but can affect the knees, wrists and even the fingers.

Acute pain and joint inflammation are usually the first symptoms. The affected area can be sensitive to touch. Gout generally affects men between the ages of 40 and 50. It may be inherited or brought on by alcohol abuse, certain types of medication, injury to a joint, overeating, stress or surgery.

Intuitive Remedies

Witness a healing. You may watch the instructions to the DNA change in the way that the body breaks down uric acid.

Belief Work

The belief systems of gout are similar to those of arthritis: fear of moving forward, guilt, resentment and sorrow.

The pain of the gout will also make a person with it feel that they have to be stubborn and fight you over everything you're trying to tell them. They do not want to change. They feel they have to be right all the time. They feel they have to carry everyone.

How we do belief work on gout is dependent on where it is in the body. For instance, if it is in the knee, we will work on issues of moving forward.

Supplements and Other Nutritional Recommendations

- A deficiency in pantothenic acid (vitamin B5) produces excessive amounts of uric acid, so consider a B vitamin supplement.
- A person who develops gout should only eat raw fruit and vegetables for about two weeks. They should consider eliminating all meat and fried or rich foods from the diet for that time.
- Avoid white flour.
- Avoid the amino acid glysine. (Glysine can be converted into uric acid more rapidly in people who suffer from gout.)
- Cortisone is commonly prescribed for relief of acute attacks. However, this may put added strain on the adrenal glands.
- No alcohol should be consumed.
- Tart cherry juice breaks down uric acid.
- Treatment with honey bee venom has provided relief for some gout sufferers.
- Try supplementing the diet with:
  bilberry
  devil's claw
  yucca

GRAVES' DISEASE

Graves' disease is the most common form of hyperthyroidism. It occurs when your immune system mistakenly attacks your thyroid gland and causes it to overproduce the hormone thyroxine. This can greatly increase the body's metabolic rate, leading to a host of health problems, including affecting the tissue behind your eyes as well as parts of your skin. The disease can be recognized by bulging eyes, loss of weight and hair loss. The tissue around the eyes will have to be rebuilt. Graves' disease is, however, rarely life-threatening.

Although it may develop at any age and in either men or women, Graves' disease is more common in women and usually begins after the age of 20.

Scientists believe that there is no way to stop the immune system from attacking the thyroid gland. However, treatment can ease symptoms and decrease the production of thyroxine.

Intuitive Remedies

Ask the Creator how to repair the thyroid and witness it done. In many instances this can be an instant healing. In any event, Graves' seems to respond quickly to healings.

For beliefs, see the Thyroid.

GULF WAR SYNDROME

See Saudi Syndrome.

THE GUMS

See the Teeth.

HAEMOPHILIA

Haemophilia is a rare genetic disorder that prevents the blood from clotting properly. One in every 5,000 boys is born with it; girls are more rarely affected. A male cannot pass the gene for haemophilia to his sons, though all his daughters will be carriers of it. Each male child of a female carrier has a 50 percent chance of having haemophilia.

Human blood contains special proteins known as clotting factors. Identified by Roman numerals, these factors help stop bleeding and allow a blood vessel to heal after an injury. The last step in the clotting process is the creation of a 'net' that closes the torn blood vessel and stops bleeding. This part of the process involves clotting factors VIII and IX. People with haemophilia are deficient in one of those factors due to their abnormal genes, and as a result their blood cannot clot properly.

The symptoms of haemophilia vary, depending on severity of the factor deficiency and the location of the bleeding.

Very few babies are diagnosed with haemophilia because they are unlikely to sustain a wound that would lead to bleeding.

Types

- *Haemophilia A*, also known as factor VIII deficiency, is the cause of about 80 percent of cases.

- *Haemophilia B*, which makes up the majority of the remaining 20 percent of cases, is a deficiency of factor IX.

Patients are classified as mild, moderate or severe, based on the amount of factor present in the blood. A patient whose blood tests suggest severe haemophilia will usually bleed frequently, whereas a patient with a milder form will usually bleed only rarely.

Intuitive Remedies

I have found that gene work has had good results. Witness the Creator making changes in the genes.

Belief Work

Look at issues of communication and self-perception.

HAEMORRHOIDS

Haemorrhoids are inflamed painful veins in the rectum. They are very common.

Haemorrhoids are associated with constipation and straining at bowel movements. They can also be associated with pregnancy. It is considered that these conditions lead to increased pressure in the haemorrhoid veins, causing them to swell. Liver disease can also cause increased pressure in the veins and can also cause haemorrhoids.

Types

- There are two sets of veins that drain the blood from the lower rectum and anus. The internal veins can become swollen to form *internal haemorrhoids*. Unless these are severe, they cannot be seen or felt.

- Similarly, the external veins can swell to form *external haemorrhoids*. These can be seen and felt around the outside of the anus. They are not tumours or growths.

- A *prolapsed haemorrhoid* is an internal haemorrhoid that collapses and protrudes outside the anus, often accompanied by mucous discharge and heavy bleeding. Prolapsed haemorrhoids can become thrombosed, which means that they form clots that prevent them from receding.

Symptoms

The most common symptoms include:

- burning pain
- inflammation
- irritation
- itching
- seepage
- swelling

Belief Work

Since haemorrhoids are part of the digestive tract and are usually made worse by constipation and diarrhoea, the belief systems associated with them will pertain to the digestive system: anger, fear, guilt, old abuse, resentment and the inability to accept love.

Supplements and Other Nutritional Remedies

- CoQ10
- vitamin A
- vitamin C
- vitamin E

***

- Cleanse the liver using ALA and 'Cleanse and Build' from Lidtke Technologies. This is the key to helping haemorrhoids. Some things that help the liver are the juices from beetroot, carrot and celery.
- Drink *Aloe vera* gel.
- Drink plenty of water, avoid fatty foods and use one tablespoon of flaxseed oil a day.

HAIR LOSS

I'm going to tell you a secret: most hair loss, in both men and women, is caused by parasites. Conventional medicine contends that male pattern baldness is genetic. But I've taken men who were almost completely bald and suggested liver and parasite cleanses and in many instances their hair has grown back.

The other diseases that cause baldness are Graves' disease and thyroid problems.

Sudden hair loss can be caused by stress or be a reaction to a traumatic event that happened three months in the past.

Supplements and Other Nutritional Recommendations

If the thyroid is only slightly imbalanced, I would suggest using Irish moss for a week. This has worked with many clients; however, a person's belief system might be as such that they have to go to the doctor to be put on thyroid medication before there is an improvement. Then, in many instances, the thyroid medication will stop them from losing their hair.

Useful supplements:

- alpha-lipoic acid
- amino acids
- liver cleanses (*see the Liver*)
- mineral complex
- noni

For hair that does not grow back thickly after chemotherapy, use omega 3s.

HANTAVIRUS

Hantavirus pulmonary syndrome (HPS) is a disease contracted from infected rodents or their urine and droppings. It was first recognized in 1993. Although rare, it is potentially deadly.

The virus goes into the cell and disrupts the plural membrane. The lungs fill with water, which seems like pneumonia to a doctor. Survivors are puffed up and look as though they have Cushing's disease.

Rodent control in and around the home remains the primary strategy for preventing hanta virus infection. Don't sweep up mouse droppings; use a wet towel with a disinfectant on it.

Intuitive Remedies

Ask the Creator to show you and command it done. Witness it.

HASHIMOTO'S DISEASE

See Hypothyroidism.

HAY FEVER

See Allergies.

HEADACHES

A headache is defined as pain in the head that is located above the eyes or the ears, behind the head or in the back of the upper neck. Like chest pain or dizziness, it has many causes.

There are two types of headache: primary and secondary.

Primary Headaches

Primary headaches are not associated with other diseases. Examples are migraine headaches, tension headaches and cluster headaches. Causes of primary headaches are anxiety, eyestrain, general tension, muscle tension and stress.

Tension Headaches

These are the most common type of primary headache. As many as 90 percent of adults have had or will have tension headaches. They are more common among women than men.

Tension headaches are a constant pain in one area or all over the head, with sore muscles and associated trigger points in the neck and upper back. They cause lightheadedness and dizziness.

The causes are anger, anxiety, depression, emotional stress, food allergies, poor posture, shallow breathing and worry.

Bromelain, ginger, magnesium and primrose usually relieve this condition.

Migraine Headaches

These are the second most common type of primary headache. They affect children as well as adults. Before puberty, boys and girls are affected equally, but after puberty, more women than men are affected.

There are two types of migraine:

- A *common migraine* has severe throbbing pain along one side of the head accompanied by cold hands, dizziness, nausea, vomiting and sensitivity to light and sound. It is caused by excessive dilation or contraction of blood vessels of the brain.

- A *classic migraine* is similar to a common migraine, but it is preceded by hallucinations, numbness in the arms and legs, the smelling of strange odours or visual disturbances.

You should understand that a migraine is not exactly a headache, but is caused by the way the blood is flowing to the brain. Three things cause migraine headaches:

1. The neck may be out of place.
2. There may be a hormonal imbalance.
3. It may be just absolute total stress.

To relieve a migraine:

- If it's hormonal, based around a woman's menstrual cycle, you can suggest several different remedies. Dandelion is one that I recommend. I find that three to four cycles of liver cleanses also helps (*see the Liver*).

- Always go in and intuitively move the neck back to where it should be.

- If the cause is stress, a hot bath laced with Epsom salts or a massage is an excellent way to relieve a migraine.

- You can also give relief with either a coffee enema or with caffeine.

Belief systems associated with migraines have to do with the blood and the digestive system. Many of the programmes will be associated with feeling unloved, and old abuse and stress.

Cluster Headaches

These headaches are characterized by severe throbbing pain on one side of the head, causing flushing, nasal congestion and tearing of the eyes, and can occur up to three times a day for weeks and months. Some of the causes are alcohol and smoking. This is one of the most painful of headaches. In many instances, it is only relieved by sleep.

The supplement L. tyrosine is suggested, though not if you are taking an MAO inhibitor drug. The Stanley Burrows light therapy using blue light can help.

Go back in the person's timeline to find out when the cluster headaches began and work on the associated beliefs. Clear all free-floating memories (*see Alcoholism*) and use the 'Sending Love to the Baby in the Womb' exercise (*see Cancer*).

Secondary Headaches

Secondary headaches are caused by associated diseases. These may range from life-threatening conditions such as brain tumours, haemorrhages, meningitis and strokes to less serious but common conditions such as discontinuation of analgesics and withdrawal from caffeine. Other possibilities are anaemia, brain disorders, constipation, hypertension, hypoglycaemia, sinusitis and spinal misalignment.

Reaction Headaches

Headaches can also be a sign of an underlying health problem or allergy. People who suffer from frequent headaches may be reacting to certain foods and food additives such as alcohol, citric acid, chocolate, dairy products, fermented food, hot dogs, luncheon meat, marinated food, monosodium glutamate, nuts, sugar, sulphates and/or wheat.

Reaction headaches may also be caused by alcohol use, nutritional deficiencies and exposure to perfume, or pollution or other toxins.

Other Types of Headache

Arthritis Headaches

The pain is caused by inflammation of the joints at the shoulder and/or the neck. A feverfew supplement is good for this, but should not be used during pregnancy.

Beliefs associated with an arthritis headache are those associated with arthritis itself:

> 'I always have to be right.'
>
> 'I fear having to depend on other people.'
>
> 'I fear change.'
>
> 'I resent everything.'

Download:

> 'I can listen to the words of another person without rejection.'

Feelings to work on:

- fear
- guilt
- resentment

Bilious Headaches

A bilious headache has dull pain in the forehead and throbbing in the temples. This kind of headache is caused by indigestion and lack of exercise.

A colon cleanse and coffee enema can alleviate the problem.

Caffeine Headaches

These are caused by caffeine withdrawal because of blood vessels that have been dilated. The best treatment is to taper off from caffeine slowly.

Exertion Headaches

Headaches caused by physical exertion, these are usually related to migraine or cluster headaches.

Go into the person's space and ask the Creator what is causing the headache. If it is a serious problem, give the person a healing and suggest they get a check-up with their doctor. If it is not a problem, give the person a healing and witness the headache being released.

Hangover Headaches

A hangover headache has a migraine-like throbbing pain accompanied by nausea. It is caused by alcohol dehydration and the dilation of blood vessels in the brain.

The person should drink plenty of water, take a vitamin B complex supplement and apply ice to the neck.

Give them a healing.

Hunger Headaches

These headaches arise because of low blood sugar, muscle tension and the rebound dilation of blood vessels. The cause is an inadequate diet.

To avoid hunger headaches, the person should eat regular meals with adequate amounts of complex carbohydrates. Have them checked for hypo-glycaemia and suggest that they alter their diet.

Hypertension Headaches

These headaches are characterized by generalized pain over a large area of the head and are aggravated by movement or exertion. The cause is severe high blood pressure. The person should get their blood pressure under control.

Sinus Headaches

A sinus headache has a gnawing, nagging pain over the nasal sinus area, often increasing in severity as the day goes by. There may be a fever and discoloured mucus. The cause is blocked sinuses due to allergies, infections or nasal polyps.

The person should increase their intake of vitamins A and C and use moist heat to help the sinuses to drain.

Belief systems for the sinuses are associated with being irritated with someone in your life.

Temporal Headaches

A temporal headache has a jabbing and burning pain in the temple or around the ear when chewing. There can be associated problems with the eyesight and weight loss. If left untreated, a temporal headache can lead to a tear in the aorta, blindness, heart attack or stroke. It is caused by the inflammation of temporal arteries.

Conventional medicine uses steroid therapies. Use digging and belief work to find the cause.

Tumour Headaches

A tumour headache has progressively worsening pain with problems with equilibrium, speech and vision and personality changes.

Go into the person's space and shrink the tumour.

Vascular Headaches

Vascular headaches cause a throbbing on one side of the head, sensitivity to light and often nausea. They are related to cluster headaches and migraines. The causes are disturbances in the blood vessels. Remain calm to lower the blood pressure.

Intuitive Remedies

Check to see if the spine is straight and the person's hormones are balanced, as their oestrogen levels may be off-balance, which could be caused by birth control pills. Ask if they have been in the military. Check for waywards. Vessel dilation in the brain can be due to improper blood flow. There could be parasites present. Ask the Creator to show you the problem.

Supplements

For Primary Headaches
Depending upon the cause of the headache, the following are suggested:

- calcium–magnesium
- CoQ10
- D-phenylalanine
- hydroxy
- L. glutamine
- L. tyrosine
- tryptophan

- Clean the intestinal tract with intestinal cleanses.
- Organic coffee enemas can be used to relieve pain.
- Use parasite cleanses and change to an alkaline diet.

Herbs for Primary Headaches
- Cayenne pepper clears the blood, reduces pain and allows blood to flow.
- Chamomile tea relaxes the muscles.
- Ginger, peppermint and wintergreen oil rubbed on the neck and temples can relieve headaches.
- Goji juice is helpful to get rid of headaches.
- Guarana is used for cluster headaches.
- Skullcap is an anti-spasmodic agent and has sedative effects.

Supplements for Cluster Headaches
- potassium
- vitamin B complex
- vitamin C
- vitamin E

Results will vary according to the underlying cause of the headache.

HEARING IMPAIRMENT

The human ear consists of three sections: the outer ear, the middle ear and the inner ear. The outer ear includes the auricle (pinna), the visible part of the ear that is attached to the side of the head and the waxy, dirt-trapping auditory canal. The tympanic membrane (eardrum) separates the external ear from the malleus (hammer), the incus (anvil) and the stapes (stirrup). The cochlea and semicircular canals make up the inner ear.

The ears are in charge of collecting sounds, processing them, sending sound signals to the brain and also helping to keep equilibrium and balance.

Hearing impairment is defined as 'a partial impairment in hearing, whether permanent or fluctuating, that affects hearing performance'.

Deafness is defined as 'a hearing impairment so severe that the person is impaired in their hearing ability with or without amplification'. It is the complete loss of the ability to hear from one or both ears. It may be inherited or caused by infectious diseases such as meningitis, complications at birth, exposure to excessive noise and the use of ototoxic.

Around half of all deafness and hearing impairment can be prevented.

Types

There are various types of hearing impairment:

- *Conductive hearing losses* are caused by diseases or obstructions in the outer or middle ear (the conduction pathways for sound to reach the inner ear). They usually affect all frequencies of hearing evenly and do not result in severe hearing loss. A person with conductive hearing loss is usually able to use a hearing aid or can be helped medically or surgically.

- *Sensorineural hearing losses* result from damage to the delicate sensory hair cells of the inner ear or the nerves that supply them. These hearing losses can range from mild to profound. They often affect the person's ability to hear certain frequencies more than others. Thus, even with amplification to increase the sound level, a person with sensorineural hearing loss may perceive distorted sounds, sometimes making the successful use of a hearing aid impossible.

- *Mixed hearing loss* refers to a combination of conductive and sensorineural loss and means that a problem occurs in both the outer or middle and the inner ear.

- *Central hearing loss* results from damage or impairment to the nerves or nuclei of the central nervous system, either in the pathways to the brain or in the brain itself.

Causes

With deafness and hearing impairment, the first thing to do is to find the cause. This could be any number of problems or a combination of different things.

Hearing Loss in Children

In children the causes can be:

- Acquired hearing loss caused by any number of infections and exposure to loud noise.
- Genetic factors passed down from the parents.
- *Otitis media*, an inflammation in the middle ear that damages the delicate parts of the middle ear.

Hearing Loss in Adults

Age seems to be a major factor in the loss of the ability to hear the full range of frequencies in everyday communication. One third of people over the age of 65 have problems with their hearing.

As well as the aging process, hearing loss in adults can be caused by disease or infection, ototoxic drugs, trauma, tumours and exposure to noise, and may or may not be accompanied by tinnitus (ringing in the ears).

It can also be caused by certain prescription drugs, including antibiotics, aspirin taken over a long period of time, non-steroid-anti-inflammatory drugs, quinine and viral infection of the inner ear, not to mention wax build-up.

If hearing loss develops gradually, the individual experiencing it may be unaware of it until it reaches an advanced stage. Generally, family and friends notice it first.

With the advent of the industrial age, an increasing problem with 'noise pollution' has caused many individuals to have hearing loss. If you have ever walked away from a concert or worksite with a loud buzzing in your ears, you have experienced what is called temporary threshold shift. When this condition happens, overnight rest usually restores normal hearing, but this is a sign that damage has occurred to the hair cells in your inner ear. If this type of damage is repeated, permanent threshold shift is the result.

Researchers have ascertained that constant loud noise can impair your vision, make you impotent and give you heart disease, as well as cause other health problems.

Intuitive Insights

Are you keeping what you hear sacred? Do you understand what sacredness is? Do you understand what it feels like to be sacred? When someone comes to you and tells you something confidential, it is your responsibility to keep what they say sacred and to yourself. This will give you credibility with all your clients.

Do you hear what you should? The ears are an important processor for intuitive information. Do you have any blocks to hearing other people? Do you accurately perceive what is best for another person? As a healer, you must develop the ability to hear the person's truth and the highest truth from the Creator of All That Is. Set aside your own truth. Be clear in your thoughts and make sure the person that you work with understands what you are saying.

Mature people have a tendency to conveniently 'tune out' the world around them because they don't want to hear things that will hurt them. Sometimes they don't give the other people in their life a chance to be heard. This occurs in very stubborn, headstrong people and they will actually create their own hearing loss.

Intuitive Remedies

The ear is an incredible biological transducer of sound waves. When you intuitively heal the ear, it is useful to understand the working parts of the middle ear – the eardrum, hammer, anvil and stirrup – and the parts of the inner ear – the cochlea, auditory nerve and Eustachian tube. Knowing the different parts will assist you when you witness the Creator heal any of the parts that are damaged.

When you heal the ear, tell the damaged portion to regenerate. Tell the ear that it is young again and then witness the regrowth of the follicles or damaged portion. Command the hearing to be as the hearing of a 25 year old.

Many people have ongoing infections in the ear without even knowing it. When a person has problems with complications from a past infection, go in and watch the Creator pull off the memory of the infection and witness it being sent to God's light to permit them to heal.

Hearing loss and deafness occur when the brain or the ears have lost the cells that are needed to permit the ear to function. Teach the brain how to hear again and break the person into the world of sound gently.

If children do not learn how to hear before they are ten years old, the cells that teach the brain how to hear will be gone. If this is the case, the child will have a difficult time learning to speak. If a child has never heard before and is over 12 years of age, it is very likely that they will not be able to speak. This is because the receptors that teach speech patterns die away by 12 years old. Conventional theories say that if a child is deaf from birth and does not learn to speak by the time they are ten years old they will never learn how. I say, 'Never say never to the Creator.'

In the instance of a deaf child it is very important to command that the receptors that were there at birth be gathered again and reconditioned. Command that the foetal memory repairs the damage.

When working with children with hearing disabilities, always go up and ask the Creator to correct the hearing and to awaken the cells that teach the brain how to hear.

When working with an adult, watch the Creator take the cells back to the fetal memory and create new cells that learn to hear. In the fetus, the stem cells will become any cells that the brain needs. They are so intelligent that they will create only what the body needs. Doctors can take a fetal cell out of the heart of a fetus and a fetal cell out of another organ and change them around. These cells will actually become the cells of the new organ. Fetal cells know how to make what the body needs. This is why some children are able to grow back limbs that were lost; they don't know that they can't. There are many documented cases where children have actually grown back hands and arms.

It is important to witness the full reconstruction of the damaged parts of the ear. For instance, if it is the eardrum that is damaged, you will see what looks like little hairs start to pop up to receive sound. Continue to witness this process until the eardrum is fully reconstructed.

Sometimes deafness is caused by scar tissue, and when that pulls away you can witness the ear reconstruct itself.

The ears are related to the kidneys. When you work on the ears, you will be likely to end up working on the kidneys as well.

Belief Work

Some people have the belief that they will become deaf because their family has deafness in it, but the most prevalent belief system I see associated with hearing impairment is 'I'm afraid to hear what's going on'. Follow the fear to the bottom belief and download the feelings and knowledge associated with hearing. This alone can improve the hearing.

Download:

'I know what it feels like to hear the joy around me.'

'My hearing gets stronger and better every day.'

'I can hear the wind through the trees.'

'I can hear the voice of God, the voice of creation.'

'I know what it feels like to get close to God without giving up my hearing.'

'I know what it feels like to live without feeling that I will lose my hearing with age.'

'I know what it feels like to know my hearing is getting stronger each day.'

'My body is strong.'

'I know how to hear and perceive the truth.'

'I can hear birds singing.'

'I know what it feels like to hear without feeling overwhelmed.'

'I know what it feels like to hear my wife without it driving me crazy.'

'I know what it feels like to hear my husband without it driving me crazy.'

'I know what it feels like to hear others without it driving me crazy.'

'I know how to live without "tuning out" the world.'

'I am free to hear.'

'I am free to make good decisions.'

'I know how to live without having hearing loss.'

'I know how to respect another person's space and what they feel as truth.'

'I know how to recognize another person's truth.'

'I know how to respect another person's truth and still hold my own truth.'

'I understand how to hear truth.'

'I know how to live my own truth.'

'I understand what sacredness is.'

'I know how to hear God's truth.'

'I know how to accept God's truth.'

'I understand what it feels like to be sacred.'

'I am listened to.'

'I know how to live in my own truth.'

'I have the Creator's definition of being able to listen.'

See also *Kidney Disease.*

THE HEART AND CIRCULATORY SYSTEM

An experiment was once done to ascertain the effect of stress on living organisms. A dog was the test subject. It was given love from its master and good nutrients. Then it was taken away from its master's love, ignored and left alone. It developed leukaemia. What was interesting was that when it once more received its master's love, it got better.

The heart, blood and circulatory system react to love in a positive fashion, but can also react to negative influences with disease or dysfunction. So, if you cannot receive love, you will have problems in the circulatory system.

When a person comes to you with a challenge in the circulatory system, work with the way they receive feelings and thought forms. The more unbalanced a person is, the more they misjudge what is going on in their lives. If someone in their life is angry about something, they might misjudge the feeling and take it personally.

The whole circulatory system is about the ability to absorb food, absorb thoughts and absorb feelings that are helpful to the body. Happiness, anger and sorrow all serve you if they are in balance. Too much anger doesn't serve you, because you cannot absorb love if you are too angry.

Belief Work

The veins constrict when there is untruth and poor blood flow causes:

- poor self-nurturing abilities
- the inability to receive, accept and give love
- difficulties in going with the flow of life and hence fear of life

Check for beliefs in these areas.

Issues carried in the blood and arteries include:

- anger, due to thinking the world owes you or the people in your life owe you
- communication with others
- self-perception

The way in which we perceive ourselves is reflected back to other people. So people are seeing you in the way that you perceive yourself. How *are* people seeing you? Do you feel listened to? Do the people you come in contact with feel important to you? When they are in front of you, they should be the most important person in the world. The love, attention and compassion you give to others are the most important aspects of being a healer.

Do you know how to love yourself and receive love back? Download:

'I understand the Creator's definition of what it feels like to be nurtured.'

'I know the Creator's definition of how to nurture myself.'

Healers often have issues with the blood because they give to others all the time and do not nurture themselves. Because of this, the spleen can sometimes become tired and the blood sluggish.

See also Cardiovascular Disease.

HEART DISEASE

See Cardiovascular Disease; The Heart and Circulatory System.

HEARTBURN/GASTROESOPHAGEAL REFLUX DISEASE

Heartburn is a burning sensation and pain in the stomach and/or chest behind the breastbone. It may be accompanied by a sour taste in the mouth, bloating, wind and shortness of breath. It often occurs when hydrochloric acid (which is used by the stomach to digest food) backs up into the oesophagus, causing sensitive tissues to become irritated. Under normal conditions the oesophageal sphincter muscle pinches itself off and prevents the stomach acid from surging upward. However, if the sphincter is not functioning properly, the acid can slip past it into the oesophagus. Acid reflux disease can burn a hole directly through the oesophagus if left unchecked.

Antacids will give you relief, but they will mask an underlying problem. Some antacids contain aluminium, which is not beneficial, because aluminium is associated with Alzheimer's. Some of the harmful agents in antacids are:

- aluminium–magnesium mixtures
- aluminium salts and gels
- calcium carbonate
- calcium–magnesium mixtures
- magnesium salts or gels
- sodium bicarbonate

Belief Systems

Energy test for the following:

'I am overwhelmed.'

'I am always stressed.'

'I can never slow down.'

'I can never do enough.'

'I understand what it feels like to live in the now.' (Not living in the now goes against permitting your digestive system to do its job.)

'I am too busy.'

'I have too much to do.'

Supplements and Other Nutritional Recommendations

- bromelain
- calcium–magnesium
- MSM
- probiotics
- vitamin B

***

- *Aloe vera* juice helps in soothing the intestinal tract.
- At the first sign of heartburn, drink a large glass of water.
- Avoid caffeine, carbonated drinks, fried foods, peppermint, spearmint, spicy food and tobacco.
- Catnip, fennel, ginger and marshmallow in a mixture help to heal the problem.
- Chamomile tea is helpful with acid reflux.
- Drink a glass of carrot and celery juice a day.
- One tablespoon of apple cider vinegar mixed with water a day is beneficial.
- People with this disorder should not eat their food too quickly.
- Raw potato juice helps.
- Smaller meals four or five times a day will be beneficial, as will changing the diet to have less fried food and more fresh vegetables.

HEAVY-METAL POISONING

See Prologue; also Lead Poisoning.

HEEL SPURS

See Bone Spurs.

HEPATITIS

The liver is one of the body's powerhouses. It helps process nutrients and metabolizes medication. It also helps clear the body of toxic waste products. 'Hepatitis' means an inflammation of the liver and it can be caused by one of many things, including a bacterial infection, liver injury caused by a toxin (poison) and even an attack on the liver by the body's own immune system.

Types

Although there are several forms of hepatitis, the condition is usually caused by one of three viruses: hepatitis A, hepatitis B or hepatitis C. Some hepatitis viruses can mutate, which means they can change over time and can be difficult for the body to fight. In some cases, hepatitis B or C can destroy the liver. The patient may need a liver transplant to survive, which is not always available or successful.

- *Hepatitis A* is known as infectious hepatitis and is easily spread through contaminated food, person-to-person contact, water and even raw shellfish.

- *Hepatitis B* is referred to as serum hepatitis and is spread through contact with infected blood. It is contracted through sexual activity and blood transfusions.

- *Hepatitis C* is the most serious form of hepatitis. It is four times more prevalent than AIDS and 20 times easier to catch. About 85 percent of infections lead to chronic liver disease. People with hepatitis C have elevated levels of iron in the liver, which cause severe damage. The most common means of hepatitis C transmission is a blood transfusion, but it can also be transmitted by intravenous drug use and sexual contact and from mother to child during childbirth.

- *Hepatitis D or Delta hepatitis* occurs in some people already infected with hepatitis B. It is the least common of all the hepatitis viruses, but the most serious because there are two types of hepatitis working together. It can be transmitted through sexual contact or from mother to child at birth.

- *Hepatitis E* is rare in the West but more common in other parts of the world. It is usually spread through fecal contamination and appears to be dangerous for pregnant women but generally does not lead to chronic hepatitis.

- *Toxic hepatitis* develops because of exposure to certain toxins or alcohol and drug use, including the overuse of over-the-counter medications such as acetaminophen or ibuprofen.

Symptoms

The symptoms of hepatitis include:

- abdominal discomfort
- appetite loss
- dark urine
- drowsiness
- fever
- headache
- jaundice
- joint pains
- light-coloured stools
- muscle aches
- nausea
- vomiting
- weakness

The more liver damage, the more erratic the personality. This disorder causes the person to be moody and aggressive.

Intuitive Insights

Hepatitis C may appear to look like a spider or a robot, and the liver will be seen to have a smoky film over it with moving speckles.

Intuitive Remedies

We have experienced very good results with hepatitis. In most instances, simply telling the virus to leave the body has been enough.

A possible reason for this is that hepatitis C is one of the friendliest viruses that you will ever meet. When you first go in and make contact with it, it is polite and sends thought forms like 'please' and 'thank you'. It is happy to communicate with you, and when you tell it it is bad for the body, it says things like 'Whoops, I'm sorry!' It is sweet, kind, appreciative, adorable, it talks to you, it is polite and it has good manners. While this might seem bizarre, it is true.

Most of the healings that are done on hepatitis C are instant. They are achieved by contacting the virus and telling it it is bad for the body. In most instances, it simply changes to a form that is harmless to the body.

Belief Work

I have only worked on a few people whose hepatitis didn't clear immediately. They all had anger issues that needed to be released with belief work.

In such cases it is likely that the person has contracted the disease through sharing needles in drug abuse. This generally means that they need belief work pertaining to worthiness and domination issues.

They also need to work on the belief systems that they had during the time they were using the drugs. These may not be apparent in their life in the present. This is why it is important to do digging work to find the root beliefs at the time the disease was contracted.

Hepatitis C is about nurturing issues. It projects to the host thoughts of 'It's OK' and 'I'm incurable.' The person then thinks that consciousness is their own.

So, make the command to change the core beliefs that are associated with the host and download:

'I know how to take care of myself.'

'I know how to take in the breath of life.'

'I understand how to deal with confrontation.'

'I know how to interact with others.'

'I know when to fight for my right to be.'

'I know how to say no.'

'I know how to live without allowing people to take advantage of me.'

'I know how to have people honour my boundaries.'

'I know how to honour the boundaries of others.'

'I know how to feel the joy of life.'

'I know how to enjoy life.'

'I know how to learn easily and effortlessly.'

'I know what it feels like to assert myself.'

'I know how to live without allowing confrontation to frighten me.'

'I know how to confront someone in the highest and best way when it is necessary.'

'I know how to be aware of other people's feelings.'

'I know how to respectful.'

'I know how to be assertive and still be respectful.'

Supplements and Other Nutritional Recommendations

*   alpha-lipoic acid, 600–1,200 mg
*   amino-acid combinations
*   artichoke
*   beetroot juice, carrot juice and spirulina
*   calcium–magnesium
*   cat's claw
*   green tea
*   liquorice root
*   milk thistle (continue with it for an extended time)
*   noni
*   omega 3s, 6s, 9s
*   selenium
*   stinging nettle
*   vitamin B combinations
*   vitamin C, 2,000–5,000 mg
*   vitamin E 400 IUs

If the person is healthy enough, suggest a liver cleanse (*see the Liver*).

HERNIA

A hernia is the protrusion of an organ or tissue from its normal cavity. Brain tissue, for example, may protrude through a defect in the skull. The protrusion may extend outside the body or between cavities within the body, as when loops of intestine escape from the abdominal cavity into the chest through a defect in the diaphragm (the muscular partition between the two cavities).

The term is usually applied, however, to an external herniation of tissue through the abdominal wall. This may occur at any weak point in the abdominal wall. The common sites are the groin (inguinal hernia), the upper part of the thigh (femoral) and the navel (umbilical).

Hernias may be congenital or may be acquired later in life.

Intuitive Remedies

Witness the rupture healed.

Supplements

- vitamin B complex

HERNIATED DISK

When a disc herniation occurs, the cushion that sits between the spinal vertebra is pushed outside its normal position. This would not be a problem if it didn't intrude upon the spinal nerves that are very close to the edge of these spinal discs, causing pain and discomfort. When people have a herniated disk, they experience back pain, leg pain or weakness of the lower extremity muscles.

Intuitive Remedies

Ask the Creator to show you what to do and witness the work done. Watch as the muscles relax around the disk and it moves into the correct place.

Once the healing is done, you should tell the person that you have worked on the disk, but that they still have to relax and change their lifestyle to avoid further injury.

If rods have been surgically placed in the back, you can still do a healing, but do not pull or disturb the rods. Remember, the Creator is the healer.

Belief Work

You will have to do belief and feeling work on the person before they can truly be healed.

Fifty percent of back problems are because of vitamin and mineral deficiencies. Teach the person how to accept and receive love and this will help them with the absorption of their vitamins.

HERPES

Types

- The two main types of herpes virus are *herpes simplex type 1 (HSV-1)* and *herpes simplex type 2 (HSV-2)*. These look exactly the same under the microscope, sharing 50 percent of their DNA. Both can stay dormant in the nervous system for life or produce erratic symptoms. Both are spread the same way (direct contact orally and genitally). The main difference between the two types is their preferred part of the body while establishing dormancy. Either type can infect mucosal surfaces in the oral and genital areas, although generally HSV-1 occurs in the mouth area and HSV-2 below the waist.

HSV-1 usually affects the lips and inside of the mouth and may be the cause of Bell's palsy. It typically establishes latency in the trigeminal ganglion near the ears; thus symptoms occur in the facial region, with cold sores or fever blisters developing, and can spread to other parts of the body. HSV-1 is generally mild when it affects the lips, face and genitals, but can be serious when affecting the eyes and the brain.

HSV-2 generally causes genital herpes. The virus rests in the sacral ganglion at the base of the spine and, when activated, symptoms occur in the genital area. The lesions may be found in and around the vaginal area (e.g., vulva, cervix), on the penis, on the buttocks, around the opening of the anus and on the thighs. HSV-2 can be so mild it does not produce any obvious symptoms. It rarely causes complications and spreading to other parts of the body is very uncommon.

- There are other types of herpes. *The Epstein-Barr virus* is the virus that causes infectious mononucleosis. *Human herpes viruses six and seven* are suspected of triggering auto-immune disorders, including multiple sclerosis and rosella. *Human herpes type eight* is very closely related to the Epstein-Barr virus and may lead to cancer of the bone, chronic fatigue syndrome and infection of the lymphatic system.

Symptoms

More than half of the people who have some type of the herpes virus never develop serious symptoms. It is, however, especially dangerous to babies, who can be infected in the birth canal and face the risk of blindness, brain damage and death.

For those people whose symptoms do not remain dormant, genital herpes causes outbreaks of red sensitive skin, itching, burning and painful fluid-filled blisters that are highly infectious until they are completely healed, which takes up to three weeks.

Symptoms in a woman can be a mild tingling and burning in the genital area, followed in a matter of a few hours by blisters around the cervix, clitoris and rectum and in the vagina. In men there can be blisters on the groin, penis and scrotum, often with a discharge and painful urination.

The first attack of genital herpes usually comes within 20 days after exposure to the virus, but the symptoms may be so mild that they are not noticed.

Although a serious illness, herpes is not normally life-threatening. Those who have the virus should adjust their lifestyle to protect themselves and others.

Intuitive Insights

HSV-2 seems to be drawn to people who have high levels of heavy-metal poisoning. The lack of structure in their life and the feeling they are not supported makes them very vulnerable to this disease.

Intuitive Remedies

Look for the virus in the body. Sexual herpes hides in the lower spine. You have to work on the attitude of the virus, which will require a lot of belief work. In many instances, however, the removal of beliefs will be enough to be rid of the virus. Ask the Creator to show you and witness the changes.

Belief Work

Of all the viruses that I have worked with, herpes seems to have the highest number of belief systems attached to it.

It is essential to go back to where the person first contracted the disease and address their belief systems at that time in their life. These usually have to do with guilt and worthiness issues. They are a good indicator of why the person has herpes in the first place. Sometimes it was a boyfriend, sometimes it was a one-night stand, but whatever, it will generally be associated with the lack of feeling worthy within themselves. This is where you start in the digging process.

The unworthiness issue may well extend into present-day relationships. If the person does not tell their partner that they have herpes, the unworthiness issues will perpetuate because of the guilt involved in not telling their partner that they are in danger of contracting herpes. It is the fear of rejection that keeps the disease a secret.

Any downloads that you instill into the person should also be instilled into the herpes virus itself. People forget that viruses have belief systems, too.

One person I was working with said that if she got rid of her herpes she would have no excuse not to have sex with her husband, which she didn't want to do. As you can see, it was serving her. Her herpes had to do with various worthiness issues, because as soon as she got into doing God's work, she put her family aside. She had programmes such as 'I can only do God's work', 'It's wrong for me to have a partner and be close to God' and 'I am married to God', which are essentially worthiness issues.

So, teach the person *and* the virus what it feels like to be worthy of the Creator's love. The virus will then change into something completely different and leave the body. This is the most effective way that I've found to work on sexual herpes.

One healing can clear the disease completely, but if you have not found all the associated beliefs, there will be an immediate breakout of the virus. This is why it is essential to release all the associated beliefs from the time when the person first contracted the disease.

At one time, I used vibrations and tones to deal with viruses. I would ask the Creator for the tone to destroy the herpes and witness it being sent through the virus. The virus would go dormant, but the first time I saw herpes actually disappear was when I told the virus that it was worthy of being loved and showed it what it felt like to be loved. After that, it left the body.

So, pull:

'I'm not good enough.'

'I'm worthy, no.'

'God is punishing me.'

Replace with:

'I know what it feels like to have self-worth.'

'I know what it feels like to be worthy of being cherished.'

'I know what it feels like to be worthy of love.'

'I know what it feels like to be appreciated, accepted and adored.'

'I know what it feels like to be safe in a relationship.'

'I know how to let someone truly love me.'

'I know what it feels like to totally appreciate my body.'

'I know what it feels like to appreciate the love I receive.'

'I know what it feels like to live without degrading others in order to feel self-important.'

'I know what it feels like to live without elevating myself at the expense of others.'

'I know what it feels like to be worthy of the greatness of all I can be.'

'I know what it feels like to make other people feel appreciated and accepted.'

'I am worthy of a strong and healthy body.'

'My body becomes stronger and healthier day by day.'

'I know how to appreciate my mate.'

'I know what it feels like to be appreciated by my mate.'

'I know what it feels like to understand that sexual energy is the energy of creation.'

'I understand what it feels like to respect sexual energy.'

'I understand what it feels like to feel sacred, beautiful and sexy.'

'It is possible to have a wonderful love life and still be close to God.'

'I know what it feels like to live life without feeling I am condemned.'

'I know what it feels like to live without this virus and tell it no.'

'I understand how to tell this virus to leave my body.'

'I know what it feels like to live without fear of an outbreak.'

'I know how to eat good food, vitamins and mineral supplements without shocking my body.'

Supplements

- acidophilus
- cat's claw
- garlic
- goldenseal
- L. lysine with amino-acid complex
- Lecithin
- noni on both upper and lower sores
- olive-leaf extract
- raw thymus glandular
- shiitake mushrooms
- spirulina

- tea tree oil (applied directly onto the open mouth sore)
- vitamins A, B, C and E
- zinc

HIGH BLOOD PRESSURE

See Cardiovascular Disease.

HIGH CHOLESTEROL

See Cardiovascular Disease.

HIVES

When there is an allergic reaction to a substance, histamine and other chemicals are released into the bloodstream, causing itching, swelling and other symptoms. Hives are a common reaction, especially in people with other allergies like hay fever.

The severity of a hives outbreak can be different from person to person. Some people can break out in hives even if they come into just the slightest contact with an allergen.

When swelling or welts occur around the face (especially the lips and eyes), it is called angioedema. Swelling from angioedema can also occur in the hands, feet and throat. This is not necessarily considered to be hives.

Causes

Many substances can trigger hives:

- animal dander (especially that of cats)
- insect bites
- medication
- pollen
- shellfish, fish, nuts, eggs, milk and other foods

Hives also develop from:

- emotional stress

- excessive perspiration
- extreme cold or sun exposure
- infections from mononucleosis, auto-immune diseases and leukaemia
- itching
- swelling of the surface of the skin into red or skin-coloured welts (called weals) with clearly defined edges

Viruses also can cause hives. Hepatitis B and Epstein-Barr virus are the two most common causes.

Some bacterial infections can also cause outbreaks of hives, as can yeast infections.

Antibiotics such as penicillin and related compounds are the most common cause of drug-induced hives.

Following are some of the substances that are the most common causes of outbreaks:

- animals
- aspirin
- Allopurinol
- antimony
- Antipyrine
- barbiturates
- BHA or BHT (preservatives)
- bismuth
- cancer (leukaemia)
- chloral hydrate
- colognes and perfumes
- Cortiotropin
- eucalyptus
- exercise
- fluoride
- food allergies
- food colourings
- gold
- hyperthyroidism
- infections, especially strep infections

- insect bites
- insulin
- make-up
- menthol
- mercury
- morphine
- opium
- penicillin
- saccharin
- salicylates
- shampoo
- soap
- sulphates
- thorazine

Intuitive Remedies

Go into the person's space and witness the Creator bringing the body back into balance so that it does not react severely to the allergens. This generally brings the person's cortisone levels up and can have an immediate effect on the hives.

Belief Work

You need to find out what the person is allergic to. This can be associated with yeast. Yeast is generally elevated in people who break out in hives. Yeast is fungus and fungus is generally associated with resentment issues. So work with those. Download:

'I know how to live my day-to-day life without resenting myself and others.'

'I know how to live my life without being pushed.'

'I know how to say no.'

'I know how to use my words well.'

'I know how to live my life without blaming others for things that are my responsibility.'

'I know how to live my day-to-day life taking good care of my body.

'I know how to live my life without exposing myself to irritating people.'

'I know how to live my life without exposing myself to toxic substances.'

'I know what it feels like to live without being resentful of people who irritate me.'

'I know what it feels like to live without being irritated with myself.'

'I know what it feels like to live without being vulnerable and easily taken advantage of.'

'I know what it feels like to live my life without having to fight all the time.'

'I know how to allow my body to adjust to the influences of the outside world.'

Supplements

- ALA
- Quercetin
- vitamin B complex
- vitamin B12
- vitamin C, 5000 mg
- vitamin D
- vitamin E

Herbs

With any use of herbs, it is best to be careful that the person is not allergic to them.

Stinging nettle is the first herb that I suggest, because it is beneficial against allergic reactions.

Also try:

- *Aloe vera*
- cat's claw
- noni, applied directly to the skin
- red clover

- Avoid all alcohol and processed foods, especially foods high in saturated fats.
- Use skin products that are hypoallergenic.

HUNTINGTON'S DISEASE

Huntington's disease (HD) results from genetically programmed degeneration of brain cells, called neurons, in certain areas of the brain. This degeneration causes uncontrolled movement, loss of intellectual faculties and emotional disturbance.

HD is a familial disease, passed from parent to child through a mutation in the normal gene. Each child of an HD parent has a 50–50 chance of inheriting the HD gene. If they do not inherit the gene, they will not develop the disease and cannot pass it to subsequent generations.

Huntington's is a sad disease. People with this malady are usually angry. They will yell and scream and then forget they were angry. There is a genetic memory of anger that is unexpressed.

Huntington's can cause blindness and death. It responds well to healing.

Downloads

'I know what it feels like to enjoy my day-to-day life in every way.'

'I know how to be totally connected to God.'

'I know what it feels like to control my temper.'

'I know what it feels like to control my moods.'

'I know what it feels like to be free of this disease.'

'I know what it feels like to know I am safe.'

'I know how to love myself.'

'I know how to have balance in my life.'

'I know what it feels like to know I am balanced.'

The following downloads are useful for children with parents who have Huntington's:

'I know what it feels like to live without the fear of getting Huntington's because my parent has it.'

'I know what it feels like to control my temper.'

'I know what it feels like to control my moods.'

'I know what it feels like to be free of this disease.'

'I know what it feels like to know I am safe.'

'I know how to love myself.'

'I know how to have balance in my life.'

'I know what it feels like to know I am balanced.'

'I know what it feels like to live without being affected and made resentful by those around me.'

'I know how to control my temper without blaming it on something else.'

HYPERTENSION/HIGH BLOOD PRESSURE

See Cardiovascular Disease.

HYPERTHYROIDISM

The thyroid is a butterfly-shaped gland located at the base of the neck just below the Adam's apple. It has a vast impact on health. Every aspect of your metabolism, from your heart rate to how quickly you burn calories, is regulated by thyroid hormones. You cannot live without your thyroid gland or the thyroid hormone, thyroxine. If the thyroid secretes too much hormone, hyperthyroidism results; too little hormone will result in hypothyroidism.

Many instances of both hypothyroidism and hyperthyroidism are believed to be the result of abnormal immune responses.

One in eight women experiences some kind of thyroid problem at some point in their lives. Thyroid problems can cause many recurring illnesses and fatigue. Alcohol, drugs, endurance exercise, excessive consumption of saturated fats, fluoride in the water, pesticide residues on fruits and vegetables, poor diet and radiation from X-rays are all causes.

There is interconnectedness between the pituitary gland, the parathyroid glands and sex glands. All these glands work together and are influenced by thyroid function. If there is a problem in one place they may all be affected.

Hyperthyroidism affects women more than men.

There seems to be an association between Parkinson's disease and hyperthyroidism. Once the thyroid condition is treated, the Parkinson's disease improves dramatically.

Medical practitioners use anti-thyroid medications and radioactive iodine to slow the production of thyroid hormones. Sometimes doctors surgically remove part of the thyroid gland. Although hyperthyroidism can be fatal if ignored, most people respond well to conventional methods.

Symptoms

Hyperthyroidism can considerably accelerate your body's metabolism, causing:

- an enlarged thyroid gland (goitre), which may appear as a swelling at the base of the neck
- anxiety or anxiety attacks
- changes in bowel patterns, especially more frequent bowel movements
- changes in menstrual patterns
- difficulty sleeping
- fatigue
- increased sensitivity to heat
- irritability
- muscle weakness
- nervousness
- rapid heartbeat (tachycardia)
- sudden weight loss, even when your appetite and food intake remain normal or increase
- sweating
- tremor – usually a fine trembling in the hands and fingers

Older adults are more likely to have minor symptoms, such as an increased heart rate, heat intolerance and the tendency to become tired during ordinary activities.

Medications called beta blockers (used to treat high blood pressure and other conditions) can mask many of the symptoms of hyperthyroidism.

An undiagnosed thyroid condition can be mistaken for menopausal symptoms. Symptoms such as depression, fatigue and mood swings are often present in both circumstances. If you are experiencing menopausal symptoms, it is a good idea to have your thyroid function tested.

Causes

Hyperthyroidism can be caused by using too much conventional hypothyroid medicine.

One of the other causes can be a tumour on the thyroid gland, so it is a good idea for the Theta practitioner to go into the body and ask the Creator to show them the thyroid gland.

Intuitive Insights

Hyperthyroidism is associated with over-expression, and hypothyroidism is associated with not saying enough. Both conditions cause the person to become compulsive.

Intuitive Remedies

Hyperthyroidism is one of the easier thyroid problems to work on intuitively.

Go into the person's space and command the body to go back to a normal state. Witness as the Creator makes the changes to the thyroid.

This works almost instantly in most cases.

Supplements

Avoid dairy products for at least three months, discontinue use of caffeine and avoid white sugar as much as possible.

The following are beneficial:

- green vegetables
- Lecithin
- vitamin D
- vitamin E

Hyperparathyroidism

The parathyroid glands are positioned behind the thyroid and secrete a hormone called PHT, which controls calcium levels. Hyperparathyroidism is a rare disorder in which the parathyroid glands become enlarged and over-active, releasing excess PHT into the system. The result of this is excess calcium leaking out of the bones into the blood. If left untreated, this can lead to other problems such as bone pain and kidney stones.

HYPOGLYCAEMIA

Hypoglycaemia, also called low blood sugar, occurs when blood glucose (blood sugar) levels drop too low to provide enough energy for the body's activities.

To explain how this happens, we look at glucose, a form of sugar that is an important fuel for the body. Carbohydrates are the main dietary source of glucose. Rice, potatoes, bread, tortillas, cereal, milk, fruit and sweets are all carbohydrate-rich foods. After a meal, glucose molecules are absorbed into the bloodstream and carried to the cells, where they are converted to energy. Insulin, a hormone produced by the pancreas, helps glucose enter the cells. If you take in more glucose than your body needs at the time, your body stores the extra glucose in your liver and muscles in a form called glycogen. Your body can use the stored glucose whenever it is needed for energy between meals. Extra glucose is also converted to fat and stored in fat cells. When blood glucose begins to fall, glucagon, another hormone produced by the pancreas, signals the liver to break down glycogen and release glucose, causing blood glucose levels to rise toward a normal level. If you have diabetes, this glucagon response may be impaired, making it harder for your glucose levels to return to the normal range.

In adults or children older than ten years, hypoglycaemia is not common except as a side-effect of diabetes treatment. However, it can be the result of other medications or diseases, hormone and enzyme deficiencies or tumours. It is often an underlying cause of what is misdiagnosed as attention deficit disorder.

Over half the people with hypoglycaemia who are over 50 have thyroid problems.

Symptoms

Symptoms include:

- confusion
- difficulty speaking
- dizziness or lightheadedness
- feeling anxious or weak
- hunger
- nervousness and shakiness
- perspiration
- sleepiness

People with hypoglycaemia can become very aggressive and lose their tempers easily. Any or all of these symptoms may occur a few hours after eating sweets or fats. The onset and severity of symptoms are directly related to the length of time since the last meal was eaten and the type of food that the meal contained. This is why a proper diet is important for people with hypoglycaemia.

Types

- *Fasting hypoglycaemia* occurs as a result of abstaining from food for eight or more hours. This is generally caused by liver disease or a tumour of the pancreas.

- *Functional hypoglycaemia* is the over-secretion of insulin by the pancreas in response to a rapid rise in blood sugar or glucose.

- *Reactive hypoglycaemia* is when blood sugar drops to abnormally low levels two to five hours after eating a meal.

Causes

Hypoglycaemia is mostly caused by the body's inability to properly handle the large amounts of sugar that the average person in the western world consumes today. It's the overload of alcohol, caffeine, stress, sugar and tobacco that is the problem.

In medical terms, hypoglycaemia is defined in relation to what causes it. It can be inherited, but it is mostly caused by inadequate diet. It is usually caused by an allergic reaction to gluten and other dietary concerns. Many other bodily disorders can cause hypoglycaemic problems, such as adrenal insufficiency, pancreatitis and thyroid disorders. Immune deficiency and *Candida* are also strongly linked to hypoglycaemia. Other causes are chronic liver failure, smoking and the consumption of too much caffeine. Low blood sugar can also be an early sign of diabetes. Proper diagnosis is crucial, since the symptoms of hypoglycaemia mimic other diseases. The conventional way to diagnose hypoglycaemia is through a glucose tolerance test.

Belief Work

Individuals suffering from hypoglycaemia need to have joy in their life. They must believe that joy can be a lasting thing. Download:

'I believe that joy can last.'

'I know when my body needs energy.'

'I know how to take care of my body.'

'I know how to utilize the life force in the highest and best way.'

'I feel safe in a relationship.'

'I feel safe with others.'

'I know how to acknowledge my own physical needs.'

'I know how to cherish and care for my body with dignity.'

'I know what it feels like to be energized and accepted.'

'I know how to control my moods when I feel tired.'

'I know when I am getting tired.'

'I know when I need to eat.'

'My body saves energy.'

'My body is strong.'

'My body gets stronger every day.'

'With each passing day, the systems of my body become stronger.'

'I breathe the breath of life.'

'When I am tired, I find energy from the breath of life.'

'My body understands how to regulate my sugars.'

'I am amazing.'

'I am brilliant.'

'I am full of energy and strength.'

'I use my words wisely.'

'I understand what it feels like to live without the fear of becoming diabetic.'

Supplements and Other Nutritional Recommendations

- A diet high in proteins consisting of chicken breast, fish, grains, kefir, low-fat cottage cheese, low-fat yogurt and turkey is beneficial.
- ALA should be considered as a supplement, along with calcium–magnesium, manganese, vitamin D, vitamin E and zinc.
- Avoid high-carbohydrate foods such as pasta, breads and sugars. Foods that are best are high in fibre and high in minerals and vitamins, such as raw vegetables.

- Brewer's yeast is helpful.
- Chromium picolinate used for three or four months at a time is good for hypoglycaemia, but it should not be used continually, as this could cause other problems.
- Exercise is very important.
- Fruit is also recommended, especially apples, apricots, avocados, bananas, grapefruit and lemons.
- Glutathione treatments are one of the best things for hypoglycaemia, since they stimulate the whole body to produce more glutathione.
- Injections of vitamin B complex as well as vitamin B6 accompanied by liver extract have produced good results.
- It is suggested to eliminate white bread from the diet.
- People who are most prone to hypoglycaemia are those taking medication for high blood sugar or diabetes.
- People with hypoglycaemia should eat small meals four to five times per day, consisting of good wholesome foods low in carbohydrates.
- Use a protein powder supplement.

Herbs

- Dandelion root for small periods of time.
- Liquorice root can also be used, but not on a daily basis and not if you have high blood pressure or if you have female cancers.
- Milk thistle can be used to stimulate the liver.

HYPOTENSION/LOW BLOOD PRESSURE

See Cardiovascular Disease.

HYPOTHYROIDISM

Hypothyroidism is the opposite of hyperthyroidism. Whereas with hyperthyroidism the thyroid is producing too much thyroid hormone, with hypothyroidism it is not producing enough.

If congenital hypothyroidism in children is left untreated, it can lead to mental retardation. Generally, however, hypothyroidism is detected within a baby's first few months, when routine blood tests are performed.

A condition that stems from long-term undiagnosed hypothyroidism is myxedema coma. The result of this condition is a coma that occurs after an accident, during illness, from exposure to cold or as a result of the ingestion of narcotics and/or sedatives.

The trace mineral lithium, used to treat manic depressive disorders, can sometimes cause thyroid malfunction.

Symptoms

The most common symptoms of hypothyroidism are fatigue and intolerance to cold. Other symptoms include:

- constipation
- depression
- difficulty concentrating
- drooping, swollen eyes
- dry and scaly skin
- fatigue
- fertility problems
- goitre (a swelling of the thyroid gland)
- hair loss
- hoarseness
- loss of appetite
- migraines
- milky discharge from the breasts
- muscle cramps
- muscle weakness
- premenstrual period pain
- recurrent infections
- respiratory infections
- slow heart rate
- weight gain

Because menopause is similar to the symptoms of thyroid dysfunction, it is important to know the difference between the two. Taking thyroid medication while you are in the throes of menopause is not a good thing.

Hashimoto's Disease

A condition called Hashimoto's disease, or Hashimoto thyroiditis, is the most common cause of an underactive thyroid. In this disorder the body becomes allergic to thyroid hormone. It then produces antibodies against its own thyroid tissue. Hashimoto's disease is a common cause of goitre. Among adults, it can occur in association with other disorders, such as infections, lupus, pernicious anaemia and rheumatoid arthritis.

The conventional treatment for Hashimoto's disease is usually a prescription of a thyroid hormone that must be taken for the duration of one's life.

Hashimoto thyroiditis responds well to healings.

Wilson's Syndrome

Wilson's syndrome is a condition that results from a problem in the conversion of one thyroid hormone, T4, to one called T3. This causes symptoms of decreased thyroid function, such as allergies, anxiety and panic attacks, depression, dry skin, fatigue, frequent infections, headaches, insomnia, intolerance to cold, lack of energy and motivation, loss of concentration, low body temperature, memory loss, menstrual dysfunction, and unhealthy nails. The symptoms can be triggered by significant physical or emotional stress but persist even after the stress has passed.

Conventional Treatment

Since thyroid medication can interact with other pharmaceutical drugs, take them several hours apart from one another. Always let your doctor know of any medication you are taking before you start on another.

Applying a natural progesterone cream may increase thyroid activity.

Thyroid Tests

A blood test measuring the levels of the thyroid-stimulating hormone secreted by the pituitary gland can determine if the thyroid gland is working properly. An iodine absorption test may also be performed. This test involves ingesting a small amount of radioactive iodine. An X-ray then shows how much of the iodine has been absorbed by the thyroid. A low uptake indicates hypothyroidism.

For a self-test, keep a thermometer by your bed at night. When you wake in the morning, place it under your arm and hold it there for 15 minutes. Keep still and quiet. Any motion can upset your temperature reading. A temperature of 97.6° Fahrenheit or lower might indicate an underactive thyroid. Keep a temperature log for five days. If your readings are consistently low, consult your doctor.

Intuitive Remedies

People who have hypothyroidism seem to have an imbalance in their pituitary gland. The reason I say this is because every time I have witnessed healings on these individuals, I have been brought back to the pituitary gland.

In a healing for hypothyroidism, connect to the Creator and command a healing be done on the person. You will witness the energy being released from the pituitary gland and sent to the thyroid.

Gently rubbing the thyroid glands in a circular motion to stimulate them can help.

Hypothyroidism does not seem to heal as readily as hyperthyroidism. More often, there will be belief work to do.

Belief Work

Most of the belief systems of hypothyroidism pertain to how well the person expresses themself and communicates with others. They will be fatigued and irritable, so you must be very careful and gentle when you work on their beliefs. They have the belief that what they say is not going to be heard. They have a tendency to overcorrect, which means that by the time they decide to express themselves, they say too much.

In hypothyroidism, the perceptions are expanded more than normal. Little things that are everyday occurrences for most of us are terrible ordeals for people with hypothyroidism. They often become compulsive, consumed with feelings, and have a difficult time dealing with everyday affairs.

In both hypothyroidism and hyperthyroidism, the person is overwhelmed by small things.

Download the following:

'I know how to speak my truth.'

'I know my spiritual direction.'

'I know how to connect with the Creator.'

'I know I have my own opinion.'

'I know how to voice my own opinion.'

'It is easy for me to voice my own opinion.'

'I know how to live without being overwhelmed, too tired or overstressed.'

'I know what it feels like to have energy.'

'My body is energized.'

'I have good communication skills.'

'It is easy for me to be connected to balanced spiritual energy.'

'I know what it feels like to have tolerance and kindness and speak my truth.'

'I know how to create a life of joy.'

'I know how to create a life of respect.'

'I know what it feels like to be respected by my family.'

'I know what it feels like to be respected by my children.'

'I know how to live without being over or under-aggressive.'

'I am in perfect balance.'

'I am connected to the Creator.'

'The Creator is real.'

'It's easy for me to breathe.'

'It's easy to have energy.'

'I know what it feels like to have energy every day.'

'With each passing day, I become happier and joy surrounds me.'

Supplements and Other Nutritional Recommendations

- selenium 250 mcg
- vitamin A
- vitamin B complex
- vitamin C, 5,000 mg
- zinc, 50 mg

***

- A diet including apricots, egg yolks with raw milk and cheeses is recommended.
- L. tyrosine is used for people with hypothyroidism but does not work well with those with high blood pressure.
- Raw thyroid glandular works well for hypothyroidism.

Herbs

Many alternative practitioners will suggest that you use kelp. They believe the iodine in the kelp will help the person. I cannot understand why this is, since the iodine in kelp is different from the iodine that your body needs. The right herb would be Irish moss, which has the type of iodine that your body can break down. It will also break down the herb bladderwack, which also has iodine in it.

Parsley is also a good herb to consider.

I

IMPLANTS

In ThetaHealing today, we do not have an opinion as to the validity of implants or alien energies; we simply help the person heal.

When working on people with implants, make sure you find out if they have breast implants, heart implants or a pacemaker before you start commanding that any implants be removed. There are many medical implants that are used today.

Downloads

Psychic Implants

'I am safe.'

'My body is my own.'

'I know what it feels like to know that my body is my own.'

'Nothing can take advantage of my body.'

'The Creator of All That Is is the highest power.'

Surgical Implants

'I know what it feels like to accept the changes in my body easily and effortlessly.'

'I know how to accept the better and improved form that I have become.'

'Surgical implants that are in my body benefit me and are accepted easily by every cell in my body.'

'I can live and be happy.'

'I cherish every moment I have in this life.'

IMPOTENCE

Impotence (erectile dysfunction, ED) is a common problem among men that is characterized by the consistent inability to sustain an erection sufficient for sexual intercourse, the inability to achieve ejaculation, or both. It can involve a total inability to achieve an erection or ejaculation, an inconsistent ability to do so, or a tendency to sustain only very brief erections.

The risk of impotence increases with age. It is four times higher in men in their sixties than in those in their forties. It tends to be more prevalent in men with less healthy lifestyles due to a less healthy diet, alcohol abuse and little or no exercise. Physical exercise tends to lessen the risk of impotence.

Causes

Erections result from a complex combination of brain stimuli, blood vessel nerve function and hormonal reactions. Anything that interferes with any of these functions can lead to impotence.

The causes can be alcohol, arteriosclerosis, certain medications, tobacco use or a chronic illness such as diabetes or high blood pressure.

In the past, it was assumed that impotence was primarily a psychological problem. But doctors today believe that 85 percent of all cases have a physical basis. If there is another health condition that is causing ED, this must be addressed to clear the ED.

It has been recognized that over 200 drugs may cause impotence. Some of the most common are:

- alcohol
- antidepressants
- antihistamines
- antihypertensives/blood-pressure medication
- chemotherapy
- diuretics
- narcotics
- nicotine
- sedatives
- stomach acid inhibitors
- ulcer medications

Downloads

'It's OK to have sex.'

'I am attracted to my partner.'

'It's possible to be sexually attracted to my partner.'

'My partner is sexually attracted to me.'

'I release past resentments about my partner.'

'I release past resentments about the opposite sex.'

'I can be sexually stimulated.'

'I can relax from stress.'

'I am strong.'

'I am healthy.'

'I am beautiful.'

'I know what it feels like to deal with my anger towards my partner.'

'I am an intelligent, wonderful being of light.'

'I reflect joy in everything I do.'

'My body absorbs vitamins and minerals with ease.'

'I feel total love for my partner.'

'It is easy for me to feel love and be accepted by my partner.'

'It is easy for me to move with the flow of life.'

'Nothing blocks the energy that I feel from the Creator.'

'I feel the flow of life throughout all the veins of my body.'

'It is easy for me to accept and appreciate love.'

'I know what it feels like to express love in a sexual, sensual way.'

'I know what it feels like to satisfy my partner.'

'I know what it feels like to have my partner satisfy me.'

'I know what it feels like to be exhilarated by the energy of having sex.'

'My body is healthy and strong.'

'I feel happy to be alive.'

'I enjoy the energy that I share with my partner.'

'I can relax from stress and enjoy the moment.'

'I know how to live in the moment.'

'My partner loves to be with me.'

'I know what it feels like to live without the fear of disappointing my partner.'

Vianna's Magic Potion for Impotence

There are several pharmaceutical drugs that can be prescribed for impotence, but in my experience, if the person has no sexual appetite and the cause isn't emotional or psychological, then there is likely to be a shortage of vitamins. In this instance, the following recipe has worked well in the individuals that have used it.

To increase sex drive in both men and women, take:

- Damiana, 6 pills a day
- ginseng, dose on the bottle (take two weeks on and two weeks off)
- Lecithin, 1 pill
- selenium, 250 mcg
- vitamin E, 400IU
- zinc 100–150 mg

Also:

- Always use omega 3s, 6s and 9s for ED.
- The body needs certain vital nutrients to produce testosterone and one of these is zinc. Lecithin and zinc help to open capillaries.

Extra Herbs
- DHEA, 100 mg for men
- horny goat weed

***

- Saw palmetto is helpful in normalizing prostate function.
- The sexual vitality of men has been increased by using a combination of two herbs: green oats and stinging nettle.
- Wild yam can help ED because of the natural steroids in it.

INCONTINENCE

Urinary incontinence means that you can't always control when you urinate. As a result, you wet your clothes. This can be embarrassing, but it can be treated. It usually happens when the bladder has slipped and the kidneys are weak.

Types

There are four basic types of incontinence:

Functional incontinence: Incontinence that occurs when physical disabilities, external obstacles or problems in thinking or communicating prevent a person from getting to a bathroom before they urinate.

Overflow incontinence: Incontinence that occurs when the bladder is constantly full and reaches a point where it overflows and leaks urine. This condition can occur when the urethra is blocked due to kidney or urinary stones, tumours or an enlarged prostate. It may also be the result of weak bladder muscles, due to nerve damage from diabetes or other diseases.

Stress incontinence: Incontinence that occurs during coughing, sneezing, laughing, lifting heavy objects or making other movements that put pressure or stress on the bladder. This results from weak pelvic muscles or a weakening of the wall between the bladder and vagina. The weakness is due to pregnancy and childbirth or lower levels of oestrogen during menstrual periods or after menopause.

Urge incontinence: Incontinence after feeling a sudden urge to urinate while drinking water, sleeping or listening to water running.

Intuitive Remedies

Ask the Creator to show you what is causing the problem.

- If the bladder is out of place, witness the Creator pulling it up. Watch the muscles being strengthened and tightened to hold it.
- If the cause is the kidneys being weak, witness a healing being done on them.
- If the cause is a kidney stone, witness the stone disintegrating and being flushed from the system.
- If the cause is a tumour, witness it shrinking.
- If the cause is another disease in the body, it will be necessary to work on that.

I believe incontinence is another malady that can be improved with a liver cleanse (*see the Liver*). When the kidneys are in a weakened condition, they do not absorb calcium as readily as they should.

This challenge may take two or three healings to be completely overcome.

Supplements

- Build the kidneys up with the herb juniper berry.
- Calcium and magnesium can help.
- Vitamin A, zinc and sometimes potassium (if the potassium does not interfere with another medication) can be beneficial.

INDIGESTION

Indigestion can be anything from a bloating feeling after eating to chronic diarrhoea, constipation or even vomiting. Heartburn can also accompany it.

Specific indigestion is a challenge I do not work on very much. The only time that I get to work on it is when it is caused by something like *Giardia*, *Salmonella* or *E. coli*. Other maladies that are associated with indigestion that I work with are Crohn's or other digestive problems.

Causes

Hydrochloric acid (HCI) is produced by the glands in the stomach for the breakdown and digestion of food, and insufficient amounts of HCI can lead to indigestion.

You can determine if you need more hydrochloric acid with this simple test. Take a tablespoon of apple cider vinegar or lemon juice. If this makes your indigestion go away, you need more stomach acid. If it makes it worse, you have too much acid.

Other factors that can cause or contribute to indigestion are a lack of friendly bacteria, malabsorption, peptic ulcers and disorders of the gallbladder, liver or pancreas. There can also be an underlying parasite problem.

Belief Work

Work on:

- how to receive and accept love – the ability to process other people's affection

- old worthiness issues
- victimization issues from childhood

Supplements

Many commercial antacids have aluminium in them, which has links to Alzheimer's disease. Antacids contain calcium carbonate and magnesium as well, so it is best to build your system using supplements instead. The following will help the intestinal tract:

- acidophilus
- ALA
- *Aloe vera*
- amino-acid complex
- ginger (once a day)
- noni juice (once a day)
- omega 3s, 6s and 9s
- slippery elm
- vitamin B complex

Sometimes copper can be beneficial, but you can't use it if you have Wilson's disease.

INFERTILITY

Infertility can be defined as the failure to conceive after a year or more of regular sexual activity at the time of ovulation. It can also refer to the inability to carry a pregnancy to term.

Causes

In 40 percent of infertile couples, problems affecting the male partner are the cause. This is most often because of low sperm count. Many factors can cause a low sperm count, including acute illness, alcohol consumption, endocrine disorders, excessive heat, exposure to toxins, prolonged fever, radiation and testicle injury.

For women, the most common causes of infertility include blocked Fallopian tubes, endometriosis, ovulatory failure or defect and uterine fibroids. Some women develop antibodies to their partner's sperm, actually becoming allergic to them. Chlamydia, a sexually transmitted disease, also causes infertility.

The most prevalent reasons couples are unable to conceive are:

- The woman has endometriosis.
- The man has abnormal sperm, a low sperm count or erectile dysfunction.
- The woman's Fallopian tubes are blocked.
- Ovulation takes place rarely or irregularly.
- The cervical mucus attacks and kills the sperm.
- The woman does not manufacture enough progesterone to carry the baby to term.
- The woman is over 34.

Some artificial lubricants can prevent the sperm from reaching the cervix. Saliva may also have a detrimental effect on the sperm.

Ulcer medications such as Tagamet and Zantac may decrease sperm count.

Marijuana and cocaine lower sperm count.

Intuitive Insights

In my opinion, pregnancy is dependent upon when the baby wants to come. Sometimes we think that we can pick and choose the time, but the truth of the matter is babies will come when they want to, not when we will it. It is important to understand that your divine timing and the divine timing of the child can be in conflict.

Women come to me all the time telling me that they can't get pregnant. When I go up out of my space, I can see that the spirit of the baby is not ready to enter the mother's body. I go into the mother's space and ask the Creator when she will have her baby.

I remember one particular woman who came in and told me that she was going to go and be implanted in September. I went into her space and told her, 'No, you're going to get pregnant in August.' Sure enough, she came back in August and told me she was pregnant.

In my opinion, what happens is that even though the spark of life is in the embryo from the beginning, the larger spark of life of the spirit waits to be sure of the embryo. It watches the formation of the tiny body to make sure it is perfect. In most instances, if it is not perfect, the spirit does not stay.

Oddly enough, when a child is ready to come into the womb, the mother will suddenly want a child more than anything!

I have also noticed that there is much more fertility if the couple is in love.

Intuitive Remedies

If the woman has blocked Fallopian tubes, go into her space and witness the Fallopian tubes open and change. This simple healing works in all kinds of women who have been going to doctors for years trying to get pregnant.

Infertility can also be associated with stress. In many instances all you have to do is remove the stress from your life and like magic, you are pregnant!

Downloads

'I know what it feels like to be allowed to have children.'

'It's safe for me to have children.'

'My body is strong and functions perfectly.'

'My body is balanced and strong.'

'The eggs in my body are strong.'

'I am ready for the child that is to be mine.'

'I am fertile.'

'I trust my mate will be a good father.'

'I trust my mate will be a good mother.'

'I have enough love for everyone in my life.'

'I can love my partner and my baby.'

'I am special.'

'I am part of God.'

'I am completely functional and normal.'

'With each passing day, my body gets stronger.'

'With each passing day, my body prepares for my baby.'

'The time is now.'

'Every cell in my body is awake and alive.'

'I have enough nutrients for myself and my baby.'

'My ovaries are perfect.'

'My uterus is perfect.'

'My Fallopian tubes are perfect.'

'My body is a perfect place for my baby to grow.'

'I am ready to show the world how much I love my child.'

'I am prepared to bring up a child.'

'My body accepts my mate.'

'My hormones are perfectly balanced.'

Supplements and Other Nutritional Recommendations

- ginseng
- sarsparilla
- spirulina
- stinging nettle

***

- A woman can raise her progesterone levels just by using more omega 3s, 6s and 9s.
- A woman should also consider the use of Damiana, which will help with fertility. However, Damiana has oestrogen and testosterone all in one plant and some of these compounds can excite female cancers. If there is a history of cancer, Damiana should be avoided.
- Both sexes should avoid all alcohol, cigarettes, fried food, junk food and sugar.
- Fresh foods, herbal teas, fresh pineapple (or bromelain), freshwater fish and salmon are suggested.
- Royal jelly and bee pollen help the body to normalize.
- The transdermal use of natural progesterone cream may benefit infertile women.

INFLUENZA

Influenza (the flu) is a contagious respiratory illness caused by the influenza virus. It can cause mild to severe illness and at times can lead to death, but this is mostly in young children or older people. Older people, young children and people with certain health conditions are at higher risk of serious 'flu complications.

The symptoms of influenza begin much like those of the common cold. In many cases, a fever develops and the person feels unbearably hot one moment and chilled the next. Often, they are so weak and uncomfortable that they do not feel like eating or doing anything else. A common cold can last for about a week to 10 days, but the flu may last longer, up to 12 days or more.

Flu viruses spread mainly from person to person through coughing or sneezing. Sometimes people may become infected by touching something with a flu virus on it and then touching their mouth or nose. Most healthy adults are able to infect others from one day before symptoms develop to up to five days after becoming sick.

Symptoms

- dry cough
- extreme tiredness
- fever (usually high)
- headache
- muscle aches
- runny or stuffy nose
- sore throat

Stomach symptoms, such as nausea, vomiting and diarrhoea can also occur, but are more common in children than adults.

Complications include bacterial pneumonia, dehydration, ear infections, sinus infections and the worsening of chronic medical conditions such as asthma, congestive heart failure or diabetes.

Intuitive Remedies

When people come to me with influenza, I always suggest that they go to the doctor as well. In most instances, I will simply let their immune system take care of the influenza virus, because this is the natural order of things. The immune system was designed to build antibodies to combat most bacteria and viruses. It is only when it is compromised that I will do a healing to stop the influenza virus.

Healers often do not understand the ramifications of what happens when they go into someone's space and do a healing on influenza. Once the healing kills the virus, all the dead cells from the virus still need to be processed from the body. It may take up to three to four days for the body to balance completely. This is why many people feel worse after this kind of healing instead of better.

Supplements and Other Nutritional Remedies

- Avoid using any iron supplements, because iron actually feeds different bacteria.
- Avoid using zinc at the same time that you are drinking juices, as these stop the potency of zinc.
- Cayenne pepper helps to keep mucus flowing and aids digestion and the associated headaches.
- Echinacea is very effective at enhancing the body's own natural defences. Alcohol-free Echinacea extract can be given to children. Give four to six drops of extract with water or juice every four hours for three days.
- Elderberry has antiviral properties.
- For some strange reason, chicken and turkey soup seem to help with influenza.
- Get as much rest as possible.
- Increasing your vitamin C helps considerably.
- Many people use goldenseal. However, you should not use it for more than a week at a time and it is not recommended during pregnancy or for those who have diabetes.
- One of the best concoctions I have found is Old Indian Wild Cherry Bark cough syrup from Planetary Formulas.
- Purchase a new toothbrush so that you are not getting the same germs and reinfecting yourself.
- Tahhebo tea has antibacterial properties to it that can help with influenza.
- Thyme helps to rid the sinuses of mucus.

INSECT ALLERGY (FROM STINGS)

The stings of ants, bumblebees, honeybees, hornets, spiders, wasps and yellow jackets can all cause allergic reactions.

Symptoms

Symptoms include:

- diarrhoea
- hives
- itching
- nausea
- pain and swelling in the joints
- respiratory distress
- tightness in the throat
- vascular swelling
- wheezing

These symptoms vary from person to person and are dependent upon how severely the person is allergic. In the most severe cases, the person can go into anaphylactic shock.

If you have ever had a reaction to a sting, a good precaution is to have an epinephrine emergency kit on hand, prescribed by a doctor.

To avoid insect stings, wear light-coloured clothing and avoid wearing anything that is flowered or dark. Do not wear shiny jewellery or use hairspray, perfume, scented soaps or suntan lotion.

Intuitive Remedies

If you see that a person is having a reaction to an insect's sting, witness a healing done on them that brings the body back to balance and then immediately take them to hospital as a precaution.

As you witness the healing, you will see more adrenaline and cortisone being sent into the body to be not only utilized against the insect venom, but to normalize the allergic reaction. This will help to balance the flood of histamine coursing through the body.

Supplements and Other Nutritional Recommendations

- For those people who are allergic to bees, consider using a little bee pollen (only a tiny amount at first) to build up a resistance to bee venom. This should only be done by a certified health practitioner.
- Regular use of vitamin C (5,000 mg daily) will help those with allergic reactions.

INSECT BITES

When my granddaughter Jenaleighia was three years old, she liked to squish bugs, so I explained to her that they were alive. All of a sudden she decided she loved ants. She sat down right in the middle of a red ants' nest. She came in screaming and crying, with bites all over her body.

Her mother, Bobbi, rushed into the house to bring her to me. I immediately reverted to my old naturopathic training. I said, 'Quick, put her in the bathtub with some herbs!'

But when Bobbi began to prepare the tub of water, Jenaleighia rebelled against this and said, 'No, I want my grandma to fix it. She can fix anything.'

No pressure there!

So I put my hands on this little girl who had so much faith in me and I commanded that the bites be gone and she be out of pain now. This stopped the pain and swelling of the bites and immediately she was better.

Isn't it amazing how her faith was rewarded? My first reaction was fear; her reaction was: 'I want my grandma to fix it.'

Most insect bites are a nuisance, causing only a little itching and redness. However, others can be serious, such as tick bites, which can spread Lyme disease. Mosquito bites can transmit malaria and yellow fever. Spider bites (though spiders are not technically insects) can be detrimental as well. Black widow and brown recluse spider bites are extremely dangerous.

Intuitive Remedies

When you see an insect bite a person, do an immediate healing on them. Say to the body of the person, 'No, this did not happen. No, not today.' In many instances this stops the reaction immediately.

It is best to follow up with their doctor.

Supplements

Foods that are rich in vitamins B1, such as black strap molasses, brewer's yeast, brown rice, cayenne pepper or fish, can help prevent insect bites because of the odour and compounds exuded from the skin.

INSOMNIA

By definition, insomnia is 'difficulty initiating or maintaining sleep, or both'. It affects all age groups, and among older adults, it affects women more often than men. The incidence increases with age.

Stress most commonly triggers short-term, or acute, insomnia. If you do not address acute insomnia, however, it may develop into chronic insomnia. Many people remain unaware that there are behavioural and medical options available to treat insomnia.

Intuitive Remedies

Insomnia is usually caused by lack of magnesium. Sometimes the person may lack other vitamins, too, but ask the Creator. Go in and pull feelings of anxiety and fear and bring in those that are calming and soothing. Witness the stimulation of more serotonin and the release of melatonin.

IRRITABLE BOWEL SYNDROME

Irritable bowel syndrome (IBS) is a disorder characterized most frequently by abdominal pain, bloating, constipation, cramping and diarrhoea. It causes a great deal of discomfort and distress, but it does not permanently harm the intestines and does not lead to a serious disease such as cancer; although colitis, where the colon actually starts to deteriorate, and diverticulosis, where the intestine develops infected pouches or pockets in it, can develop.

Most people can control their symptoms with diet, stress management and prescribed medications. However, for some people IBS can be disabling. They may be unable to work, attend social events or even travel short distances.

IBS is one of the most common disorders diagnosed by doctors. It occurs more often in women than in men, and it begins before the age of 35 in about 50 percent of people.

Symptoms

Abdominal pain, bloating and discomfort are the main symptoms of IBS. However, symptoms can vary. Some people have constipation. Often these people report straining and cramping when trying to have a bowel movement but cannot eliminate any stool. If they are able to have a bowel movement, there may be mucus in it, which is a fluid that moistens and protect passages in the digestive system.

Some people with IBS experience diarrhoea with frequent, loose, watery stools. Others alternate between constipation and diarrhoea. Sometimes people find that their symptoms subside for a few months and then return, while others report a constant worsening of symptoms over time.

Causes

Researchers have yet to discover specific causes for IBS. One theory is that people who suffer from it have a colon that is particularly sensitive and reactive to certain foods and stress. The immune system may also be involved.

In watching people over the years, I have found that their colon problems are due to a shortage of magnesium and acidophilus.

I had irritable bowel syndrome for the first part of my life. My mother and my sisters have had it as well. I think that it is possible that it is a genetic disorder that in some instances gives people a predisposition to it.

Normal mobility may not be present in the colon of a person who has IBS. It can be spasmodic or even stop working temporarily.

In IBS, the lining of the stomach called the epithelium can be affected by disorders in the immune and nervous systems. The epithelium regulates the flow of fluids in and out of the colon. In IBS, the contents inside the colon move too quickly and the colon loses its ability to absorb fluids. The result is too much fluid in the stool. In other people, the movement inside the colon is too slow, which causes extra fluid to be absorbed. As a result, the person develops constipation and does not get enough nutrition. They are being mildly poisoned because of the constipation.

In yet other instances a person's colon may respond strongly to stimuli from certain foods or stress that would not bother most people. This means that the person may have food allergies.

Recent research has reported that serotonin is linked with normal gastrointestinal (GI) functioning. Serotonin is a neurotransmitter that delivers messages from one part of your body to another. Ninety-five percent of the serotonin in your body is located in the GI tract and the other 5 percent is found in the brain. Cells that line the inside of the bowel work as transporters and carry the serotonin out of the GI tract. People with IBS have diminished receptor activity, causing abnormal levels of serotonin to exist in the GI tract. As a result, they experience problems with bowel movement, motility and sensation, having more sensitive pain receptors in their GI tract.

Researchers have reported that IBS may be caused by a bacterial infection in the gastrointestinal tract. Studies show that people who have had gastroenteritis sometimes develop IBS, otherwise called post-infectious IBS.

Researchers have also found very mild coeliac disease in some people with symptoms similar to IBS. People with coeliac disease cannot digest gluten, a substance found in wheat, rye and barley.

The overuse of antibiotics, antacids or laxatives may also be a factor.

Intuitive Remedies

Because of the associated pain, diarrhoea, nausea and sometimes severe headaches, a person with IBS may dread eating. Because of this, malnutrition may result because nutrients often are not absorbed properly. People with IBS require as much as 30 percent more protein than normal as well as an increased intake of minerals and trace elements, which are quickly depleted by diarrhoea.

Diagnosis of genuine IBS requires ruling out disorders that can cause similar symptoms, such as coeliac disease, colon cancer, Crohn's disease, depression, diverticulitis, endometriosis, faecal impaction, food poisoning, infectious diarrhoea, lactose intolerance and ulcerative colitis. The practitioner must be sure that they have scanned the body for the possibility of these other disorders. It is very important that the person follows up with their healthcare practitioner to be sure they do not have any of these disorders.

Belief Work

Belief systems associated with IBS relate to mother and father issues. This means that most of them go back to childhood, with the possibility of sexual abuse.

Download:

'I know how to live without feeling the Earth is too much for me.'

'I know how to live without feeling like the world is caving in on me.'

'I know how to live without taking on other people's "stuff".'

'I know how to live without feeling the stress of others.'

'I am safe.'

'It is safe to be alive.'

'I can deal with any situation at any time.'

'I know what it feels like to feel safe in any situation.'

'It is easy for me to adapt.'

'It is easy for me to adjust.'

'I am assertive.'

'I can live without feeling overwhelmed.'

'I can live without feeling attacked.'

'I can live without being afraid.'

'I can live without being afraid of doing something wrong.'

'I know how to live without taking life so seriously that it makes me ill.'

'I know how to live making quick and decisive decisions.'

'Every day the Earth and its energy becomes easier for me.'

'Every day, in every way, I feel happier and lighter.'

'I know that my decisions matter.'

'I know how to make a decision.'

'I know how to make a decision that is right for my family and me.'

'I know how to live my life without bending to the thoughts and feelings of others.'

'I know what it feels like to live my life without being afraid of hurting the feelings of everyone around me.'

'I know how to use my words wisely.'

'I know how to let my body deal with stress easily and effortlessly.'

'I know what it feels like to be without pain.'

'I know what it feels like to live without having diarrhoea ruin everything.'

'I know what foods make me feel good.'

'I know how to find the foods that make me feel healthy.'

Supplements and Other Nutritional Remedies

- acidophilus
- ALA
- *Aloe vera* juice
- goji juice
- noni juice
- protein drinks

***

- One of the first things I suggest for a person who has irritable bowel syndrome is to discontinue the use of wheat and gluten products as well as dairy products.

- Avoid carbonated beverages, fried foods, grapefruit juices, spicy foods and alcohol and tobacco.
- Cut back on the use of red meat. Use protein drinks instead of red meat.
- Increasing fibre in the diet can help.
- Liver cleanses – 'Cleanse and Build' by Lidtke Technologies is good.

KIDNEY DISEASE (RENAL FAILURE)

The kidneys play key roles in the body, not only by filtering the blood of uric acid and getting rid of waste products, but also by balancing levels of electrolytes in the body, controlling blood pressure and stimulating the production of red blood cells. Chronic kidney disease includes conditions that damage the kidneys and decrease their ability to keep a person healthy by carrying out these functions. If kidney disease is severe, wastes can build to high levels in the blood and make a person feel terrible.

Complications that are caused by kidney disease are anaemia (low blood count), high blood pressure, nerve damage, poor nutritional health and weak bones. Kidney disease also increases the risk of having heart and blood vessel disease. These problems may arise slowly over a long time.

Early detection and treatment can often keep kidney disease from getting worse. If left untreated, it may eventually lead to kidney failure, which requires dialysis or a kidney transplant to maintain life. Kidney failure can be accompanied by many disorders, such as congestive heart failure, diabetes, hypertension, liver disease, lupus and sickle-cell anaemia.

With diabetes, high blood sugar, high blood pressure or a family history of kidney disease, you may be at higher risk for kidney disease.

Conventional tests for kidney dysfunction involve the levels of calcium, creatinine, haemoglobin, phosphorus, potassium, protein and urea.

Types

- *Bright's disease* is a kidney disease marked by the presence of blood protein in the urine and retention of water in the tissues.

- *Glomrulonephritis* is an inflammation of the tiny blood vessels within the kidney that filter out wastes from the blood. This can be the result of an infection such as a streptococcus throat infection.

- *Hydronephrosis* is a condition in which the kidney and renal pelvis become filled with urine and can cause obstruction of urinary flow.

- *Kidney stones* are mineral accumulations in the kidneys (*see Kidney Stones*).

- *Polycystic kidney disease* is an inherited disease in which cysts grow on the kidneys, rendering them incapable of functioning.
- *Pyelonephritis* is a kidney infection that may be caused by a birth defect.
- *Renal tubular acidosis* is a disease that occurs when the kidneys fail to excrete acids into the urine, which causes the blood to remain too acidic. Without proper treatment, chronic acidity of the blood leads to bone disease, growth retardation, kidney stones and progressive renal failure.

Symptoms

Symptoms of kidney problems include:

- abdominal pain
- appetite loss
- back pain
- chills
- fever
- fluid retention
- urinary urgency
- vomiting
- One key symptom is oedema. This results when the kidneys produce less urine because they are unable to excrete salt and other wastes properly. As a result, fluid builds up in the body. The hands and ankles swell, and the person becomes short of breath. Toxic wastes may accumulate in the bloodstream, also causing oedema.
- The urine may be cloudy or bloody.

Causes

Chronic kidney disease can be caused by diabetes, high blood pressure and other disorders; also heavy exposure to chemotherapy, drugs, heavy metals, poisons and other toxins.

High doses of the painkiller ibuprofen can lead to kidney dysfunction.

Lead and other metallic poisons are very harmful to the kidneys. Anyone who works with lead or who is exposed to lead regularly should take precautions to protect their kidneys from damage.

Belief Work

If the kidney dysfunction was caused by toxins, then a simple healing will clear the problem.

However, if it was not caused by toxins, it may require belief work. Resentment and old anger are stored in the kidneys. Kidney problems associated with emotions also arise when a person is very upset or over-judgemental.

Always look to clear old resentments and grudges to get the kidneys working again. This may take a little time because you must find the way that the resentment is serving the person in order to completely clear the disorder.

Download:

'I know how to live without resenting myself.'

'I know how to live without resenting others.'

'I know it is possible for me to communicate easily and effortlessly.'

'I know how to get rid of the destructive energies that are in my life.'

'I know how to live without taking on everyone else's emotions.'

'I know how to live without being judgemental of others.'

'I know what it feels like to have my body flow with happiness.'

'I know what it feels like to communicate with others without having old resentments.'

'I know what it feels like to follow through with ideas and plans.'

'I know what it feels like to know I am important to God and that I matter.'

'I know what it feels like to listen to others.'

'I know what it feels like to live without the fear that my body is failing me.'

'I live with the knowledge that my body is getting stronger every day.'

'I know how to live without accepting stress.'

'I know the difference between the emotions that are caused by the kidneys and those that are normal.'

'I know how to say no before a difficult situation begins.'

'I know what it feels like to live without others taking advantage of me.'

'I know how to be happy.'

'I can breathe the breath of life.'

'I know what it feels like to eat food that is good for me.'

'I know how to forgive my body.'

'I know how to be grateful that I am alive.'

'I know what it feels like to fill every cell in my body with gratitude and love.'

'I am in perfect harmony with my environment.'

Supplements and Other Nutritional Recommendations

- Celery and parsley are good natural diuretics. They help the body to get rid of uric acid. Be cautious of parsley, because it speeds up the metabolism.
- Corn silk tea can be helpful.
- Cranberry juice is amazing for the kidneys.
- Dandelion root tea helps the kidneys, but you should only use it for a few days at a time.
- Juniper berries can be used as a restorative.
- Marshmallow tea helps to clean the kidneys.
- Studies have proven that the use of spirulina can reduce the effects of kidney poisoning caused by mercury and drugs.

Kidney Infections

Act upon a kidney infection the same way as you would a bladder infection: witness the Creator scraping the infection out of the kidneys, pulling it down and out of the body.

Kidney Stones

Kidney stones are small solid masses that form when salts or minerals normally found in urine crystallize inside the kidney. In most cases, the crystals are too tiny to be noticed and pass harmlessly out of the body. However, they can build up inside the kidney and form much larger stones. A kidney stone can be one of the most painful experiences that you will ever have.

Kidney stones are much more common in the present day than they were at the beginning of the 20th century. This may be due to an increase in the levels of animal fats and proteins in an average western diet. I also believe that it is because our soil is high in calcium but does not have enough magnesium. Magnesium helps to balance out calcium build-up in the body. The chances are 50 percent that if you have had one kidney stone, you will have another in the next 10 years.

People who have Crohn's disease or irritable bowel syndrome may have an increased risk of kidney stones. This is also due to oxalate adsorption and excretion.

If a stone becomes large enough, it may begin to move out of the kidney and progress through the ureters, the tubes that carry urine from the kidney to the bladder. If it gets stuck in the ureter, it can cause an infection, which can lead to permanent kidney damage.

Types

There are four types of kidney stones:

- About 80 percent of all kidney stones are *calcium oxalate stones*. Calcium stones can run in families because of genetic factors. There seems to be a problem with the absorption of oxalate in these people. High blood calcium levels can also result from malfunctioning parathyroid glands, multiple myeloma and vitamin D intoxication.

- *Cystine stones* are caused by a rare condition where the stones are composed of the amino acid cystine.

- *Struvite stones* are unrelated to metabolism and are caused by infection. Women generally get these kinds of stones.

- *Uric acid stones* occur when the volume of urine excreted is too low or the blood levels of uric acid are too high.

All the kidney stones are composed of different minerals.

Depending on where they are located, kidney stones are also known as nephrolithiasis, renal calculi, urinary calculi, urinary tract stone disease, ureterolithiasis and urolithiasis.

Intuitive Remedies

I once had a woman call me up in intense pain because of her kidney stones. She was going to have an operation the next day and she was not sure she was going to make it through the night because of the pain. I went up, connected to the Creator and witnessed the stones being dissolved. She was out of pain immediately and did not require surgery the next day. Even though she did not like me that much (and still doesn't), her kidney stones still disappeared. This goes to show you that if you believe it will work, it will work.

Going in and imagining the kidney stones breaking up and dissolving into tiny pieces is a very effective way of removing them.

Belief Work

Kidney stones are caused by a lack of minerals in the body or an imbalance of minerals in the body. Anytime you have difficulties with minerals, it is likely to be associated with belief systems pertaining to communication and anger with the Creator.

Supplements and Other Nutritional Recommendations

- *Aloe vera* juice
- breakstone tea
- gravel root
- horsetail
- l-arginine
- magnesium
- marshmallow extract
- uva-ursi
- vitamin A
- vitamin B complex
- vitamin C
- vitamin E
- zinc – 100 mg daily can inhibit the formation of kidney stones

***

- Balance your calcium and magnesium intake.
- Increase your consumption of foods rich in vitamin A. Vitamin A is beneficial in the urinary tract and helps to discourage the formation of stones. Good sources of vitamin A include alfalfa, apricots, carrots, pumpkin and squash.
- Reduce your consumption of animal protein.
- Reduce your intake of potassium phosphate.

- Strangely enough, drinking coffee can lower your risk of kidney stones, while drinking grapefruit juice can raise the risk.

- To relieve kidney pain, squeeze half a lemon into a glass of water and drink it.

KNEE PROBLEMS

Knee problems create a substantial amount of work for healers. Ask the Creator where you need to go in the knee to put it back where it should be and witness it being put back in place. Scrape out any excess deposits if need be.

Always clarify which knee needs to be worked on, as you may be mistaken in which side of the body you are observing. Problems in the left knee may have something to do with the feminine side of the person. Problems in the right knee reflect their lack of desire to go forward.

You will find that there is a direct correlation between the knees and the kidneys. Healing disorders of the kidneys will heal disorders of the knees.

See also Kidney Disease.

LEAD POISONING

Lead, mercury and aluminium are three of the heavy metals that I see most often in clients. Lead is one of the most toxic metals known. It is a 'cumulative' poison that is retained in the body. When it finally leaves the bloodstream, it is stored along with other minerals in the bones, where it continues to build up over a lifetime. It can then re-enter the bloodstream at any time as a result of severe biological stress, such as menopause, pregnancy, prolonged immobilization or illness, or renal failure.

Lead reacts with selenium and sulphur-containing antioxidant enzymes in the cells, seriously diminishing the ability of these substances to protect against free-radical damage.

The body cannot distinguish between calcium and lead. Once it enters the body, it is assimilated in the same manner as calcium.

Lead is much more harmful to children than adults because it can affect their developing nerves and brains. The younger the child, the more harmful lead can be. Unborn children are the most vulnerable. Children get lead in their bodies when they put lead objects in their mouths, especially if they swallow them. They can even get lead poisoning from touching a dusty or peeling lead object and then putting their fingers in their mouths or eating food afterward. Testing has shown that many children have elevated levels of lead in their blood. Children living in cities or older houses are more likely to have high levels.

Sources

Lead is found in:

- Hobbies involving art supplies, jewellery making, pottery glazing, miniature lead figures, stained glass and soldering (always look at labels).
- House paint before 1978. Small children in particular often swallow paint chips or dust from lead-based paint. Even if the paint is not peeling, it can be a hazard. Lead paint is very dangerous when it is being stripped or sanded. These actions release fine lead dust into the air.

- Lead bullets, curtain weights, fishing weights.
- Pewter pitchers and dinnerware.
- Pipes and plumbing. Lead can be found in drinking water in homes whose pipes were connected with lead solder.
- Soil contaminated by decades of car exhaust or years of house-paint scrapings. Thus, lead is more common in soil near highways and houses.
- Some painted toys and decorations.
- Storage batteries.
- Toys and furniture painted before the early 1970s.

Symptoms

When a person swallows a lead object or inhales lead dust, some of the poison can stay in the body and cause serious health problems. A single high dose of lead can cause severe emergency symptoms. It is more common, however, for lead poisoning to build up slowly from repeated exposure to small amounts of lead. In this case, there may not be any obvious symptoms, but the lead can still cause serious health problems over time.

There are many symptoms of lead poisoning, as lead can affect many different parts of the body. Over time, even low levels of lead exposure can harm a child's mental development. The health problems get worse as the level of lead in the blood gets higher. Possible complications include:

- abdominal pain and cramping (usually the first sign of a toxic dose of lead)
- aggressive behaviour
- anaemia
- behavioural or attention problems
- constipation
- difficulty sleeping
- failure at school
- headaches
- hearing problems
- irritability
- kidney damage
- loss of previous developmental skills (in young children)

- low appetite and energy
- reduced IQ
- reduced sensations
- slowed body growth

Very high levels of lead poisoning may cause coma, muscle weakness, seizures, staggering gait or vomiting.

Preventative Measures

- Always check the labels when purchasing foreign-made products such as eye make-up. Some of these products may contain as much as 99 percent lead oxide.
- Be careful of drinking hot beverages from lead-glazed ceramic cups.
- Be careful when buying imported ceramics, toys and other painted goods.
- Do not turn bread bags inside out and use them, because the ink may be lead-based.
- Do not use lead glass crystal to store food.
- Have your water tested.
- If you drink wine, always wipe the mouth of the bottle with a damp cloth before pouring, due to the foil wrappers around the cork being made of lead.
- Look for food cans that are sealed without lead.
- Never boil water longer than necessary, because this will concentrate contaminants, including lead.
- Never use the first water drawn from your tap. Let it run for at least three minutes.
- Wash your children's hands and be careful where they play.

Considerations

- Any building 50 years or older should be inspected by a professional, and if there is lead-based paint on the walls, it should be removed by someone with the proper expertise and equipment.
- Anyone who grows crops or garden produce near busy roads or highways should check the lead level in the soil.
- Hair analysis is a method that can be used to detect heavy-metal toxicity.
- Many hair colours used by men are lead-based.

Intuitive Remedies

In a healing, never command all the lead to be pulled out of the body. Any heavy metal should be pulled out gently and gradually. If you pull out all the lead that is in the bones, it will be sent into the bloodstream to be flushed out with the urine and the shock to the system might be too great. It is best to use supplements to pull lead gently and easily from the system. Ask the Creator what to do and to show you.

Belief Work

Lead is drawn to people in need of nurturing. These people are only receiving artificial nurturing from the people around them and so they will have a tendency to be a little depressed. They desperately need real love and nurturing. This situation creates a kind of weakness and makes the person open to lead poisoning.

The key to avoiding lead poisoning in children is more love and more connection to the family. The child has to feel involved and nurtured.

Download:

'I know what it feels like to be supported and loved.'

'I know what it feels like to have structure in my life.'

'I know what it feels like to be totally connected to God.'

'I know I am important.'

'I know how to live without others taking advantage of me.'

'I know what it feels like to draw people who are for my highest good.'

'I know how to pick my friends wisely.'

'I know what it feels like to be always connected to the Creator.'

'I am always supported by the universe.'

'I know how to take vitamins, minerals and food that will make me strong.'

'My body absorbs calcium and magnesium in the highest and best way.'

'I know what it feels like to permit any lead to leave my body easily and effortlessly without any problems or stress.'

'I know what it feels like to build my body back to youth and vitality.'

'I can function without depression.'

'I know my body is strong and I can have joy.'

'With each day, I have patience in the knowledge that I am becoming stronger.'

'With each day I feel the Creator's love more.'

Supplements

- amino acids
- apple pectin
- calcium
- Lecithin
- magnesium
- selenium, 200 mcg daily
- vitamin C
- zinc, 80 mg daily
- Chelation with EDTA can prevent the accumulation of lead. However, EDTA will strip the body of minerals that are beneficial, so it is best to use supplements along with it.
- ALA is less invasive than EDTA and is very effective. It should be used with omega 3s.

LEGIONNAIRES' DISEASE

Legionnaires' disease is a serious lung and bronchial tube infection caused by bacteria. The bacteria live primarily in water and are transmitted through airborne vapour droplets. It is wise to have the heating and cooling systems checked in your home and in your workplace so that legionnaires' disease is not spread through the venting systems. The bacteria can also be found in newly ploughed soil.

The incubation period is from two to ten days after exposure. The disease does not spread from one person to another. The risk of contracting it is higher for those in poor health, the very young and the very old.

Symptoms

The first signs and symptoms may resemble those of the flu: aches and pains, fatigue, headache and moderate fever. The disease then progresses to include a high fever, chills, coughing, diarrhoea, disorientation, nausea and vomiting, severe chest pain, shortness of breath and, because of inadequate oxygen, a bluish tinge to the nails and skin.

Healing

I have worked on Legionnaires' disease a few times, both during and after the disease, and have witnessed a healing on the lungs and depleted systems of the body. Always ask the Creator what should be done. Witness the lungs heal.

Supplements

- Echinacea
- olive-leaf extract
- slippery elm tea

To help rebuild the structure of the lung:

- amino acids
- beta carotene
- proflavanols
- raw thymus glandular
- vitamin C

Change the diet to eliminate wheat and dairy products.

THE LIVER

The liver is responsible for over 500 functions in the body. It produces cholesterol and bile from the breakdown of dietary fat and old red blood cells. Using amino acids, it makes proteins and stores glycogen, iron and vitamins. It also removes substances such as poisons and waste products from the blood, excreting them or converting them to safer substances.

When the liver becomes inundated with toxins, it can no longer function correctly. This in turn will cause imbalances in the hormones that regulate growth, sexual behaviour and the flow of serotonin. The Taoists teach that if the liver and kidneys are clean, we will not age. Due to all of the toxins and pollutions in our environment, our livers are overworked.

To keep the gallbladder and liver functioning correctly, I offer you the excellent liver cleanse listed below. Read the instructions carefully and, of course, go up and ask the Creator if is this is right for you.

Gallbladder/Liver Cleanse!

This cleanse should not be used by those who have hepatitis or cirrhosis of the liver.

As with any cleanse, this is a suggestion only, and those who use it should be cautious, as it can be powerful.

1. Take an herbal laxative in the evening.

2. Each morning for the next three days, place 100 drops of Ortho-Phos (a brand name for orthophosphoric acid) in a quart of high-quality apple juice and drink it during the morning. During these three days you do not need to alter your diet. If for some reason you cannot drink apple juice, place 135 drops of Ortho-Phos in a quart of water and drink it during the morning. These drops are the basis of the cleanse.

3. On the evening of the fourth day, eat supper early. Then about an hour before your normal bedtime stir together and drink a cup of olive oil, a cup of Coke and 1 whole lemon squeezed. Use a high-quality olive oil, one that is cold pressed. The Coke is used to help swallow the olive oil. Without it, the olive oil is very hard to swallow. You will find that the Coke and lemon make the olive oil almost tasteless.

4. Immediately after drinking the olive oil mixture, go to bed. Put your knees up to your chest. Lie on your right side for half an hour. This will cause the oil to go directly to the gallbladder and liver. These organs will not know what to do with all that oil, so they will spasm and throw off stones. Then you are free to get up and do as you wish. By taking this oil mixture, you empty the system of its old bile, forcing it to make new bile without the old toxins.

5. Take an herbal laxative that evening so that you will eliminate the next morning. This will help flush the stones out of the colon.

6. Consider taking a colonic two days after the flush.

If you are very ill with a challenge (such as cancer), consider doing this once a month for a few months. Everyone's system is different, therefore there are no absolutes. For prevention, repeat this cleanse at least once a year.

Epsom Salts Variation

The Epsom salts keep the bowels moving, so any remaining toxins are removed from the body.

1. On the third day of the liver flush, two hours after lunch, dissolve two table-spoons of Epsom salts in three ounces of water and drink it. If you find the taste intolerable, add a little citrus juice.

2. Evening dose: five hours after lunch, dissolve one tablespoon of Epsom salts in three ounces of water and drink it.

3. The next morning, dissolve one tablespoon of Epsom salts in three ounces of water and drink it.

This cleanse is intended as an informational guide. The remedy, approaches and technique described herein are meant to supplement, not to be a substitute for, professional medical treatment. This cleanse should not be used to treat a serious aliment without prior consultation with a qualified healthcare professional.

The drops for this cleanse are available from a variety of healthfood stores.

Downloads

Many of the following downloads will be very beneficial to strengthen and cleanse the liver:

> 'I know what it feels like to live without other people's anger affecting me.'

> 'I know how to live without carrying old anger.'

> 'I know what it feels like to live without carrying old resentment.'

> 'I know what it feels like to recognize the things in my life that serve me.'

> 'I know what love feels like.'

> 'I know what joy feels like.'

> 'With each day, my body becomes stronger.'

> 'I love my body.'

> 'I know when to say no.'

'I know I am living in a world where I am responsible and accountable for my own connection to God.'

'I am accountable for my commitments to others.'

'I know how to live without my family members taking advantage of me.'

'I appreciate and love myself.'

'With each passing day, I appreciate and love life more.'

'I am totally connected to God.'

'My liver regulates all my hormones easily and effortlessly.'

'I respect and love my body.'

'I clean toxins from my body easily and effortlessly.'

'I love my liver.'

'I know how to live without illness.'

'I know how to live without illness as a challenge.'

'My immune system works in harmony.'

'I know how to live without being obsessed.'

LOU GEHRIG'S DISEASE

Lou Gehrig's disease is also called amyotrophic lateral sclerosis. It damages motor neurons in the brain and spinal cord. Motor neurons are nerve cells that control muscle movement. Upper motor neurons send messages from the brain to the spinal cord and lower motor neurons send messages from the spinal cord to the muscles. Motor neurons are an important part of the body's neuromuscular system. The neuromuscular system enables the body to move and is made up of the brain, many nerves and muscles. Things that we do every day such as breathing, walking, running, lifting and even reaching for a glass of water are all controlled by the neuromuscular system.

Intuitive Insights

I believe that a micro-plasma is going into the myelin sheath and the T-cells are attacking the mitochondria of the myelin sheath. The T-cells are doing their job, but causing an enormous amount of damage. Doctors can only try to suppress them before too much damage is done.

Aluminium poisoning is one of the key factors causing this challenge. Lack of vitamin E can also cause this disorder.

Intuitive Remedies

Witness a healing and ask the Creator to show you.

Belief Work

Every time I have worked with Lou Gehrig's disease, the most prevalent problem has been the spouse of the client. In order to successfully work with this disease you need to find the beliefs that are keeping the client blocked, but the spouse will always bring the client in and will be in utter denial, usually saying that life is good and everything is under control.

The client will not talk about any deep feelings around the spouse. The only thing that they will say is that they are perfectly happy and everything is fine. This is why you must somehow get them alone. Then they will reveal their deepest feelings.

Don't be surprised if you find anger, an enormous amount of resentment and out-of-control feelings. People with Lou Gehrig's are also very stubborn. Their beliefs are very close to those of people with MS.

Download:

'I know what it feels like to express my own feelings.'

'I know what it feels like to live without taking on the entire world.'

'I know what it feels like to live without believing that I have to take care of everyone close to me.'

'I know what it feels like to live without being responsible for everything that goes wrong.'

'I know how to live without pretending.'

'I know what it feels like to be accountable.'

'I know what it feels like to be responsible.'

'I know what it feels like to permit others to have their own responsibility and happiness.'

'I know what it feels like to express myself without pretending.'

'I know what it feels like to live without pretending that I am happy.'

'It is safe for me to be alive.'

'I have control of myself and my body.'

Supplements and Other Nutritional Recommendations

- Add vitamin E to the diet.
- Suggest a detoxification programme for heavy metals.

See also Multiple Sclerosis.

LOW BLOOD SUGAR

See Hypoglycaemia.

LUPUS

Lupus is a chronic inflammatory disease that can affect many of the body's organs. It is an auto-immune disease that occurs when the immune mechanism forms antibodies that attack the body's own tissues. This can damage the blood vessels, joints, organs and skin.

Types

There are many kinds of lupus:

- *Discoid lupus* causes a rash that doesn't go away.
- *Neonatal lupus*, which is rare, affects newborns.
- *Subacute cutaneous lupus* causes sores after being out in the sun. Another type can be caused by medication.
- The most common type of lupus, *systemic lupus erythematosus*, affects many parts of the body.

Anyone can get lupus, but women are most at risk.

Symptoms

Lupus has many symptoms:

- fever with no known cause
- joint pain or swelling
- muscle pain
- red rashes, often on the face (also called the 'butterfly rash')

This is a very painful disease.

Causes

The cause of lupus is not known to conventional medicine. Many experts believe that it is due to an unidentified virus. I believe that it is due to a micro-plasma of some sort that gets inside the cells and connective tissues. This causes the immune system to develop antibodies to resist the virus that in turn attack the body's connective tissue.

Conventional Treatment

Conventional medicine treats lupus with steroids. Unfortunately, this can sometimes be as detrimental as the disease itself. Cortisone treatment can cause the person to have problems with their heart, mental stability and auto-immune system.

Intuitive Insights

In lupus, the immune system is *not* attacking itself; it is attacking the micro-plasma that doctors can't see. This is caused by molecules from petroleum products. These products can be found in hair or nail chemicals, lead and nickel. Ask the person if they have inhaled fumes from petroleum products.

It is believed that the plastic in breast implants causes a new form of lupus. This is when the body is rejecting the plastic implants. In most instances I will tell the woman to have the breast implants removed, but for some this is not an option, so in that case I do a healing in Theta and tell their body to accept them.

I have noticed that people who do manicures tend to get lupus because of the cryo-acrylic glues used for the nails.

People with lupus should change their environment to one that is toxin-free. If they are nurses, they are going to have to wear masks more often when they are around plastic gloves. If they are fingernail technicians, tell them to get a hepa-filter for their working room (and a couple of other filters), so they don't have to breathe any fumes.

Intuitive Remedies

When I go into the body of a person who has lupus, I command an instant healing and watch the petroleum-based energies move out of the joints. You can actually go in and scoop them out of the joints.

Also, work on any DNA that may be damaged. The Creator will show you. Witness the work.

Belief Work

I believe that certain substances and diseases are drawn to us because of our beliefs. These beliefs do not need to be negative; they can be positive as well. This can be true in the case of those who have lupus. Lupus is one disease that is definitely drawn to the person because of their personality type.

Lupus comes with its own emotions, too, and actually takes over some of the emotions of the person who has it. If you work with somebody with lupus, good luck. They are the most stubborn and argumentative people I have ever seen. The reason for this is because the connective tissue is being attacked, which is keeping them from flowing with life. Teach them what it feels like to flow with life and that people are there to help them and do some work on love issues so their joints can stay clean.

People with lupus do not believe anything is their fault. They believe that they should have no physical problems and they have nothing to work on pertaining to emotional beliefs.

Test for:

- anger at the world and anger at people
- issues of communication, how to set boundaries and feelings about the Creator
- programmes of 'I am not good enough'
- worthiness issues

Teach them that they are worthy of change, worthy of healing, that healing is possible and that they can heal without guilt. Download:

'The past is cleared and I can go forward.'

'I know what it feels like to have strength in my body.'

'All my connective tissue is perfect.'

'All my joints are perfect.'

'I know what it feels like to live without being angry at the world.'

'I know what it feels like to live without having to fight for everything that I am.'

'I know what it feels like to live without being overly critical of others.'

'I know what it feels like to live without letting others irritate me.'

'I know what it feels like to take accountability for my life.'

'I know what it feels like to go with the flow of life and to allow others to love me.'

'I know what it feels like to live without having to argue all the time.'

'I know what it feels like to live without having to argue with myself.'

'I know what it feels like to allow life to move with me.'

'I know what it feels like to be flexible and enjoy life.'

'I am important.'

'I am strong.'

'I am healthy.'

'I know how to live without feeling guilty for other people's decisions.'

'I know what it feels like to live without carrying the responsibilities of others.'

'I can move forward.'

'I can receive love without falling apart.'

'I know what it feels like to receive health.'

'I know how to teach the people around me how to be accountable without falling apart.'

'I know how to accept help from others without being pushed into it.'

'I know what it feels like for my body to move easily and effortlessly.'

'I know how to live without feeling guilty for what others do.'

'I am worthy of change.'

'I am worthy of love.'

'With each passing day, my body gets stronger.'

'I know how to live without giving up hope.'

'I know how to live without accepting everything the doctor says.'

'I know how to live without expecting my body to fall apart.'

'I know how to use my creative will power.'

'I see possibilities in the highest and best way.'

'I move with ease and grace without pain.'

'I know what it feels like to live without pain.'

'I know what it feels like to live without being overly aggressive.'

'I know what it feels like to live without feeling threatened.'

Supplements and Other Nutritional Recommendations

People with lupus are low on lipids and need omega 3s. They should consider taking ALA. Their doctor may argue with them about this because it is an antioxidant, but most doctors will let them take it because they've found that it works well. They have also found that DHEA helps some people with lupus and MS. If a client is going to a doctor at the same time that I am seeing them, I will tell them to go to their doctor and ask if they can use ALA and DHEA with their cortisone treatment.

Things that stimulate the immune system will cause the body to go into detox. You have to get the person out of their lupus symptoms first, so you do not want to give them too many herbal supplements, but recommend:

- acidophilus
- amino acids
- cider apple vinegar
- calcium–magnesium
- copper and zinc
- CoQ10
- DHEA
- essential fatty acids
- grapeseed extract
- noni
- stinging nettle
- vitamin C
- vitamin E

No bread or dairy.

LYME DISEASE

One of the sickest people I have ever seen was a woman who had medically untreatable Lyme disease that caused her to have intense arthritis pain, adrenal dysfunction, blood clots, cancer, diabetes and more.

Lyme disease is caused by a bite from a deer tick that infects the host with the Borrelia bacteria of the spirochete class. People can become infected through ticks being carried by pets into the home. Once a tick bites a host, it becomes attached to the flesh, burrowing into tissue. The longer it is attached, the greater the risk of Lyme being contracted.

Lyme makes the infected person very ill and produces symptoms such as asthma, arthritis and overall body aches. In many instances, it is mistaken for fibromyalgia. The medical test for Lyme disease can be inconclusive in that it may not come up positive for Lyme the first time, or even the second.

If not diagnosed right away, Lyme disease causes swelling and can cause diabetes. It is treated by antibiotics – tetracycline. If caught in its early stages, before damage is done to the body's systems, it is medically curable, though the patient must take the full course of the treatment. Spirochete bacteria die off very slowly in the body even with antibiotics. There is a vaccine for Lyme, but it is not 100 percent effective.

The disease became obvious in 1975 when mothers of a group of children in Lyme, Connecticut, made researchers aware that their children had been diagnosed with rheumatoid arthritis. The unusual grouping of illness that appeared 'rheumatoid' led researchers to the identification of the bacterial cause of the children's condition, what came to be called 'Lyme disease', in 1982. Lyme disease has since been reported in every U.S. state, as well as China, Europe, Japan, Australia and the former Soviet Union.

Symptoms

A red circular lesion with a hole in the centre on the skin is the first indication of a tick bite. There may be an outer ring of brighter redness and a central area of clearing, leading to a 'bull's eye' appearance. This classic initial rash is called *erythema migrans*. More than one in four patients, however, never get a rash. Symptoms vary from person to person, but in general Lyme disease has several phases of symptoms:

- Early localized disease with skin inflammation.
- Early localized disease with fatigue, headache, joint and muscle stiffness and swollen glands.
- Early disseminated disease with heart and nervous system involvement, including palsies and meningitis.

- The later phases of Lyme disease can cause inflammation of the heart muscle, leading to abnormal heart rhythm and heart failure. The nervous system can develop Bell's palsy, meningitis and confusion. Inflammation in the joints can be accompanied by swelling, stiffness and pain, most commonly in the knees. The arthritis of Lyme disease can act like many other types of inflammatory arthritis and can become chronic.
- Lyme lowers the immune system, making the person susceptible to other diseases.

Intuitive Insights

I've found that to work on Lyme disease you've got to know it actually is Lyme disease. The disease is often mistaken for other disorders and a clear diagnosis is made only about 35 percent of the time.

I can tell someone has Lyme disease when they sit down in front of me and tell me nothing has worked for them. They also tell me that they are completely falling apart. The spirochete bacteria are giving them the feeling that there is no help and no cure for their condition. Because of this, they will not complete a course of antibiotics or herbs and the bacteria settle into a parasitic relationship with them. They will tell their healthcare professional that the medicine is not working, but if they were persistent and took the medicine, they would be better.

One of the tests that I use if I suspect Lyme is to go into the body and ask the Creator to show me the spirochete bacteria. Seen intuitively in the body, it will appear as a parasite-like bacterium that has funny little hooks as it floats through the bloodstream. Lyme also appears as a yellow colour on top of the blood plasma.

Belief Work

Once I believe it is Lyme, I will work on the 'Nothing ever works for me', 'I have no hope', 'I am falling apart' and 'No one can help me' belief systems.

In many instances, the person with Lyme either has no relationship or is in a relationship with a partner that they are incapable of loving due to the disease. They stay in the relationship because of the feeling that they cannot change anything in their life. I train them to use ThetaHealing on themselves and others and to do continual healings and belief work on themselves. Healing themselves and other people raises them out of the defeatist spiral they are in.

So, command Lyme to be gone – God will show you – and work on the beliefs of hopelessness. Download:

'I know what it feels like to have hope.'

'I know God's definition of hope.'

'I know how to live without falling apart.'

'I know how to live without giving up.'

'I have perseverance.'

'I know what it feels like to live my day-to-day life with joy, hope and love for myself.'

'I know how to set boundaries.'

'I know how to live without others taking advantage of me.'

'I am never trapped.'

'I can make my own decisions.'

'I have possibilities.'

'I know how to do things without being abused, hurt or taken advantage of.'

'I know what it feels like to be able to follow through with decisions.'

'I know how to live without the feeling of hopelessness.'

'I know what it feels like to live my life without the fear of doctors.'

'I know what it feels like to know what is going on with my body.'

'I know what it feels like to live without having to have a diagnosis to get better.'

'I know what it feels like to live without thinking that nothing ever works.'

'I know what it feels like to have a good relationship and to be loved.'

'I know what it feels like to have time for myself without my body falling apart.'

'I appreciate and love my body for its endurance.'

'I appreciate and love all that my body does for me.'

'With each passing day, I have more energy in every way.'

'I know what it feels like to be listened to.'

'I know what it feels like to live without expecting the most negative outcome.'

'With each passing day, I feel more positive about my life.'

'I respect and identify with the strength that is within myself.'

'I feel good when I help others.'

'I am allowed to help others.'

'I have good judgement.'

'I know how to live without listening to the Lyme disease.'

'I know how to follow through and take any vitamins and supplements that are good for me.'

'Nothing can deter me from becoming a success.'

Supplements and Other Nutritional Recommendations

- amino acids
- apple cider vinegar and water
- chlorophyll
- multiminerals
- multivitamins
- oregano capsules for an extended period of time
- the alkaline diet
- water of life copper

THE LYMPH SYSTEM

The lymph system is used to carry waste away from the cells, release fat and fight infections and parasites. It is the body's clearing and defence system, working hand in hand with the liver and the circulatory system.

Cancer, haemorrhoids, leukaemia and varicose veins are diseases of the circulatory and lymphatic systems. Any and all diseases of the immune system are held in the lymphatic system.

The tonsils, spleen and thymus form part of the lymph system. The spleen carries an extra reserve of red blood cells and destroys red blood cells that still have nuclei in them (rogue cells).

Vigorous movements pump the lymph system. If you do not move around enough, your lymph nodes become engorged and you can get more infections. Regular exercise prevents this. Weightlifters stay much healthier than others, because their muscles move the toxins out.

If you overwhelm your body with stress, the lymph system will get bogged down, which also means you are more prone to infection.

The lymph system has a very quick delivery to everything in the body, so lymph cancer can spread everywhere. The lymph system treats a cancer like a virus and swells to encapsulate it, but it gets through the encapsulation and spreads.

Intuitive Remedies

Do not use underwired bras that are too tight, as they cut off circulation to the lymph system. Avoid deodorants, as they are toxic to the system. If you drink a bit of chlorophyll every day you will not need deodorants. Body odour is a good indicator of how toxic your body is. When you do cleanses, you emit a bad odour (except for the olive oil cleanse). Cancers cause different types of odours to be emitted from the body. Overweight people have more odours because they are fighting a build-up of toxins.

If you get cancer in the lymph system, it spreads everywhere. If that is the case, do not give massages or lymphatic drainage, as that would spread it even further. A healing would be a better thing to do.

Belief Work

Many of the belief systems held in the lymph system have much in common with the beliefs of parasites, viruses and bacteria.

The lymph system can hold positive programmes such as the ability to set boundaries and know when to fight, but it can also hold the emotions of regret and confrontation, as well as the feeling of helplessness. People can become lost in regrets. Teach yourself the Creator's definition of forgiveness.

Help your immune system by downloading the Creator's definitions of:

'I know how to take care of myself.'

'I know how to take in the breath of life.'

'I understand how to deal with confrontation.'

'I know how to interact with others.'

'I know how to fight for my right to be.'

'I know how to say no.'

'I know how to live without allowing people to take advantage of me.'

'I know how to have people honour my boundaries.'

Confrontation

Some people think that they are under attack all the time. This can create immune diseases in the lymph system. When your brain is balanced and you have enough serotonin, however, confrontation is easily handled.

If you have too much mercury, it makes you combative and possibly suicidal.

Download the Creator's definition of:

'I know how to feel the joy of life.'

'I know how to enjoy life.'

'I know how to learn easily and effortlessly.'

'I know what it feels like to assert myself.'

'I know how to live without allowing confrontation to scare me.'

'I know how to confront someone in the highest and best way.'

'I know how to be aware of other people's feelings.'

'I know how to be respectful and assertive at the same time.'

Supplements and Other Nutritional Recommendations

Lymph Cleansers
- apple cider vinegar (1 tablespoon in water or a vinaigrette)
- half a lemon in water
- Stanley Burrow's lemon cleanse
- yellow light

You can pull out heavy metals in the lymphatic system with minerals:

- Calcium–magnesium pulls lead and cadmium.
- Selenium pulls mercury.
- Zinc pulls lead (but lowers copper levels if used in large amounts).

MACULAR DEGENERATION

Macular degeneration that is related to age is a chronic eye disease that occurs when tissue in the macula deteriorates. The macula is the part of the retina that is responsible for central vision. The retina is the layer of tissue on the inside back wall of the eyeball. Degeneration of the macula causes blurred central vision or a blind spot at the centre of the visual field. The condition usually develops gradually, but sometimes progresses rapidly, leading to severe vision loss in one or both eyes.

Because macular degeneration affects the central vision but not peripheral vision, it does not cause total blindness. Nevertheless, it is the leading cause of severe vision loss in people aged 60 and older.

Dry Macular Degeneration

Most people with macular degeneration have the dry form. This occurs when the cells of the pigmented layer of retina, or retinal pigment epithelium (RPE), begin to atrophy and lose their pigment. The normally uniform reddish colour of the macula takes on a mottled appearance because of the patchy loss of pigment. Drusen, fatty-like deposits that look like yellow dots, appear under the light-sensing cells in the retina.

Symptoms
- The need for increasingly bright illumination when reading or doing close work.
- Increasing difficulty adapting to low levels of illumination, such as when entering a dimly lit restaurant.
- Increasing blurriness of printed words.
- A decrease in the intensity or brightness of colours.
- Difficulty recognizing faces.
- Gradual increase in the haziness of the overall vision.
- A blurred or blind spot in the centre of the visual field, combined with a profound drop in the central vision acuity.

Wet Macular Degeneration

Wet macular degeneration develops when new blood vessels grow from the choroid underneath the macular portion of the retina. These new vessels are called choroidal neovascularizations (CNVs). They leak fluid or blood, which is why it's called wet macular degeneration. This causes the central vision to blur.

Eyes with the wet form of macular degeneration almost always show signs of the dry form, too, the drusen and mottled pigmentation of the retina. In addition, what should be straight lines become wavy or crooked and blank spots appear in the field of vision.

Symptoms
The following symptoms may progress rapidly:

- A central blurry spot.
- A decrease in or loss of central vision.
- Visual distortions, such as straight lines appearing wavy or crooked, a doorway or street sign that seems out of whack, or objects appearing smaller or farther away than they should.

Intuitive Remedies

Go up to the Seventh Plane and witness an instant healing.

If there is not an instant healing, use the belief work.

Belief Work

To work with this disorder, find out what the person is afraid of seeing in their life. Ask them, 'What is the worst thing that could happen to you if you could see perfectly?'

Work on their self-esteem issues about how they feel about themselves. Download:

'I know what it feels like to see.'

'I know what it feels like to see clearly.'

'I know that I'm safe.'

'I have good judgement about what I see.'

'Every organ in my body is working in perfect harmony.'

'I am always rejuvenating.'

'It is safe for my eyes to heal.'

'I'm ready for my eyes to be better and stronger.'

'It is possible for me to be back to perfection with my eyesight.'

'I appreciate perfection.'

'I appreciate everything the Creator does.'

'I know how to live without the fear of losing my sight forever.'

'I am connected to the Creator.'

'With every day in every way my body is stronger, happier and full of life.'

MANIC DEPRESSION

See Bipolar Disorder.

MEMORY LOSS

In our busy lives, we all forget things at one time or another. As we age, this can happen more frequently. Some older people have little or no change in memory, but in others, forgetfulness can begin to interfere with their lives in a noticeable way.

Short-term memory is what becomes impaired most often with aging. Long-term memories tend to remain vivid, even in the case of Alzheimer's disease. In most instances, changes in memory develop gradually over time.

Causes

Memory problems can be due to many conditions. These include Alzheimer's disease, depression, Parkinson's disease, strokes and thyroid disease. Medicines, either prescribed or herbal in nature, can also cause memory problems. Alcohol and drug addictions too can cause memory loss.

Intuitive Insights

I have found that many people who have memory problems have a high level of yeast in their system. The memory problems stem from a toxic by-product of yeast called acetaldehyde, which can get into the bloodstream, brain, joints and lungs. Aldehyde, a by-product of alcohol, can cause memory loss as well.

Lack of vitamins such as magnesium can also cause memory problems. Short-term memory loss can be caused by beta-carotene deficiency.

In addition, brain function depends upon neurotransmitters, the chemicals that act as electrical switches in the brain. If there are not enough nutrients to produce these chemicals, the brain will short-circuit, causing problems in the messages that are sent. Vitamin deficiencies can cause this condition.

Belief Work

Many people are told from the time that they are children that they are stupid and cannot remember things. These programmes can be carried into adulthood, cycling in the brain and making a person believe they cannot remember well.

Many people can benefit from the following downloads:

'I know what it feels like to remember everything that I see, hear and read.'

'I know how to gain access to the memory of everything I have ever experienced.'

'I know what it feels like to like myself.'

'I know what it feels like to remember easily.'

'My mind absorbs information like a sponge.'

'I have the infinite capacity to remember.'

'I know how to remember vividly.'

'I can recall information for tests easily.'

Supplements

- amino-acid complex
- DHEA (for those who cannot break down DHEA, use 7 Keto)
- magnesium
- molybdenum, 300 mcg, moving up to 500 mcg for a few months, to flush acetaldehyde and aldehyde from the system
- vitamin A
- vitamin B

See also Candida.

MENINGITIS

Meningitis is an inflammation of the membranes called the meninges and the cerebrospinal fluid surrounding the brain and spinal cord. It is usually due to the spread of an infection. The severity of the inflammation and the best treatment depend on the cause of the infection.

Due to vaccines that prevent this condition in young children, most meningitis cases now occur in young people between the ages of 15 and 24. Older adults also tend to have a high incidence of meningitis.

Types

Most cases of meningitis are caused by a viral infection, but bacterial and fungal infections can also lead to the disorder.

Bacterial Meningitis

Bacterial meningitis usually occurs when bacteria enter the bloodstream and migrate to the brain and spinal cord. However, it can also occur when bacteria invade the meninges directly, due to an ear or sinus infection or a skull fracture. Bacterial meningitis can be fatal and is generally much more serious than viral meningitis.

The strains of bacteria that can cause acute bacterial meningitis include:

- *Haemophilus influenzae-haemophilus:* Before the 1990s this bacterium was the leading cause of bacterial meningitis, but childhood immunizations have greatly reduced the number of cases of this type of meningitis.

- *Listeria monocytogenes-listeria:* These bacteria can be found almost anywhere. Most healthy people exposed to them don't become ill, although pregnant women, newborns and older adults tend to be more susceptible.

- *Neisseria meningitides-meningococcus:* Meningococcal meningitis commonly occurs when bacteria from an upper respiratory infection enter the bloodstream. This infection is highly contagious and may cause local epidemics in boarding schools and colleges and on military bases.

- *Streptococcus pneumoniae-pneumococcus:* This bacterium is the most common cause of bacterial meningitis in infants and young children in the United States. This strain can be deadly, causing brain damage, coma and hearing loss.

Chronic Meningitis

Acute meningitis strikes suddenly, but chronic meningitis develops over four weeks or more. The signs and symptoms are similar to those of acute meningitis: fever, headaches, mental cloudiness and vomiting. This type of meningitis is rare.

Fungal Meningitis

Fungal meningitis is uncommon. Cryptococcal meningitis is a fungal form of the disease that affects people with immune deficiencies, such as AIDS.

Viral Meningitis

Viruses cause a greater number of cases of meningitis each year than do bacteria. Viral meningitis is usually mild and often clears on its own in under 10 days. The most common symptoms are rash, sore throat, joint aches and headache.

Causes

As well as being the result of infections, meningitis can also be due to non-infectious causes, such as drug allergies, some types of cancer and inflammatory diseases such as lupus.

Symptoms

Symptoms can be confused with the flu and include:

- a high fever
- a stiff neck
- confusion
- lack of interest in drinking and eating
- seizures
- sensitivity to light
- severe headache
- sleepiness or difficulty waking up
- vomiting or nausea with headache

Newborns and young infants may not have the classic symptoms. They may cry constantly, seem unusually sleepy or irritable and eat poorly.

Intuitive Remedies

A person with meningitis will need extensive belief work pertaining to the programmes of bacteria and why they may be drawing diseases to them.

It is recommended that they use the internal exercises described by Stephen Chang in his book *The Great Tao*.

In a healing, command that any damage that has been done to the brain or hearing be repaired. Command that all past trauma be released from the body.

Supplements

When a person is recovering from meningitis, they need to take vitamins, but nothing too harsh. The following are suggested:

- amino acids, multivitamins, multiminerals and protein shakes
- vitamin A
- vitamin B complex
- vitamin C, 5,000 mg

If they have used antibiotics, it is good to use acidophilus.

MENOPAUSE

Menopause is a natural process in a woman's life when her monthly menstrual cycles stop, most often after the age of 45. It occurs because the ovaries stop producing the hormones oestrogen and progesterone.

Menopause is not a disorder, and most women do not need treatment for it, though afterwards they can be more vulnerable to bone loss and heart disease because of the under-production of oestrogen and progesterone.

A woman has reached menopause when she has not had a period for one year. Changes and symptoms can start several years earlier, however, because of lower progesterone and oestrogen.

Symptoms

The symptoms include:

- a change in periods
- changes in sexual appetite
- hot flushes

- irritability
- memory problems
- mood swings
- night sweats
- trouble focusing
- trouble sleeping
- vaginal dryness

Hormone replacement therapy is often prescribed, but it has a tendency to heighten the risk of certain cancers.

Intuitive Insights

The Taoist Chinese believed that when a woman went through menopause she ceased to age. They believed that the only reason that menopause was not a smooth transition was because the liver was congested.

In my experience, menopause is not a problem for most women if their liver is clean.

After menopause, the adrenals generally produce enough hormones for the needs of the body, unless there is a problem with the liver. This is why a liver cleanse is so important for individuals who are going through menopause (*see the Liver*). It may be beneficial to use oestrogen and progesterone creams until the liver is clean.

The process can be helped along by telling the body to go into full menopause instead of letting it fight itself.

Belief Work

Many women have the belief that they will fall apart when they go through menopause. Belief work should be centred on releasing beliefs that their life is ending.

It is important to convince women that they can become even sexier during this transition. They need to understand that they will not necessarily lose their sexual appetite, and no longer having their period to contend with will give them incredible freedom.

Download:

'I know what it feels like to live without thinking I am falling apart.'

'My body is young and regenerating.'

'I feel wonderful.'

'My body is still sexy.'

'I still have the desire to be with my partner.'

'I have new freedom.'

'I understand what it feels like to know that I am vital and important to God.'

'My moods are stable.'

'I am happy.'

'With each passing day, my life gets better.'

'I still enjoy being a woman.'

'My body is becoming stronger and more beautiful.'

'I understand the freedom and excitement that is coming into my life.'

'I always have the Creator's definition of hope.'

'I have endurance and energy.'

Supplements

Maca evens out the hormonal levels, and the good thing about it is that the body only uses what it needs, unlike black cohosh, which can provide too much oestrogen.

The following can be beneficial:

- boron
- calcium–magnesium
- Damiana
- DHEA
- essential fatty acids
- Lecithin
- selenium
- silica
- vitamin B
- vitamin C
- vitamin E
- zinc

The woman going through menopause should also drink plenty of water to stay hydrated, avoid stress and get plenty of exercise.

Male Menopause

Many people joke about male menopause. Nevertheless, men do actually go through a period in mid-life when they undergo hormonal changes.

When a man goes through menopause, he can experience anxiety and decreased sexual appetite.

DHEA and extra zinc are helpful to balance the hormones.

MENSTRUAL CRAMPS

For menstrual cramps and most other cramps, I suggest chelated calcium and magnesium, also potassium and vitamin E.

Damiana can be used for menstrual cramps and it has a lot of healthy calcium in it, plus it balances the hormones; however, it will deplete the iron in your system, so if you take it, you should do so with black strap molasses.

MERCURY POISONING

Mercury is one of the most toxic metals known to man. It is even more toxic than lead. It can be found in the soil, water and food supply. It is used in herbicides and pesticides and because it contaminates water, it can be found in high levels in fish. It is also used in batteries, cosmetics, dental fillings, fabric softeners, industrial instruments and even medication. In fact, it is so commonly used that it has been found in a series of flu and immunization shots.

The presence of mercury in the nervous system can prevent the normal entry of nutrients into the cells and the removal of waste from the cells. It can bind to immune cells and interfere with normal immune responses. This may be one factor behind some auto-immune disorders. Mercury can also cause permanent cardiac, kidney and respiratory problems. Because it is a cumulative poison, there is no barrier that prohibits it from reaching the brain cells. Significant amounts of it in the body can cause arthritis, depression, dermatitis, diarrhoea, dizziness, fatigue, gum disease, headache, insomnia, joint pain, memory loss, muscle weakness, nausea, slurred speech and vomiting. Mercury poisoning can also mimic the symptoms of multiple sclerosis and Lou Gehrig's disease. It is suspected to be one of the causes of autism.

Symptoms

Signs that indicate the presence of toxic mercury levels indicate behavioural changes, depression, confusion, hyperactivity and irritability. People with this toxicity may also experience allergic reactions or asthma. They may complain about a metallic taste in the mouth and their teeth may be loose.

Causes

According to the World Health Organization, amalgam dental fillings are a prime source of mercury exposure. These contain 50 percent mercury, 25 percent silver and 25 percent other materials. One amalgam filling can release 7 to 13 mcg of mercury each day. Many people have suffered for years from various health problems that have cleared up after they have had their amalgam fillings removed. Having amalgam fillings removed is almost as dangerous as leaving them in, however, unless they are removed properly. Very few dentists are trained to remove mercury correctly and safely. Make sure you find one who knows how to handle mercury before you let anyone touch your teeth.

After releasing the mercury from the system, you will find that you no longer have such unpredictable mood changes.

Intuitive Insights

Mercury poisoning is fairly difficult to clean up, because mercury attaches itself to the cells. People die every day from it. More than one doctor has noted the link between mercury, Alzheimer's and Parkinson's disease. It is also my belief that at least one third of the cases of depression and suicide are linked to heavy-metal poisoning of some kind, with mercury being the most prevalent. It is interesting to note that dentists have one of the highest rates of suicide of any profession.

Mercury poisoning is, I admit, a sore subject to me because I was told by the Creator that one of the causes of my cancer was mercury. This was before I had learned how to deal with mercury poisoning using energy healing. I spent many hours in an infra-red sauna as well as using herbal cleanses before I experienced instant healing.

Mercury has a tendency to attach to people who have a predisposition for depression and feel they are not good enough. It makes people easily angered and more depressed and raises the tendency for suicide. These thoughts and feelings are caused by the mercury filling these emotional receptors.

When you are working with someone who has questions or complaints about depression, check to see if they have amalgam fillings. Amalgam-mercury poisoning is quite common. At least 20 percent of the clients I speak to have it. The percentage is probably higher than that, but at least that many have this problem. When I do readings, I always check whether mercury poisoning is the cause of blood disorders, leukaemia and lymphoma.

Intuitive Remedies

Ask the Creator how to clear the body in the highest and best way. When you detoxify from heavy metals, you pull out old memories attached to them and these flood your system, so it is best to do this gradually.

You should not command all heavy metals from the body to be gone, since elements such as calcium and zinc are a vital part of our molecular structure. It is best to ask the Creator what to do, since everyone is different and toxins should be pulled out of the body at a rate tailored to the individual.

Downloads

Many people who have mercury poisoning tend to be too trusting in a way that might be considered naïve. They need discernment of who can be trusted and who cannot.

'I know what it feels like to live without depression.'

'I live my day-to-day life with joy.'

'With every day, my body becomes stronger.'

'I know what it feels like to live without my body falling apart.'

'I can see others the way they are.'

'It is easy for me to connect to the Creator of All That Is and know that I am worthy.'

'I know how to live without resentment, anger and regret pertaining to the past.'

'I am worthy of being connected to the Creator at all times.'

'I can distinguish between good and evil.'

'I know how to live my life without interference from the negative thoughts of others.'

'I know how to pursue the goals in my life with ease.'

'I know how to control my temper and my moods.'

'I am financially stable.'

'I am mentally stable.'

'My spiritual strength grows every day.'

'I know what it feels like to love without being critical.'

Supplements and Other Nutritional Recommendations

The Creator has said that if we change one atom in the molecule of mercury, we can make it into a harmless substance. Until you get to this point of Theta perfection, I would suggest that you use coriander to pull it out of the body.
   Also:

- ALA and liver cleanses will help to clear mercury out of the system.

- Chelation therapy is used to remove heavy metals from the system. It is recommended that you use ALA before deciding to use chelation, as this therapy can be rather difficult.

- Selenium, coriander or pectin will leech out mercury from the body. They will bind to the mercury in amalgam fillings and leech it out. For this reason, it is best to take out the amalgam fillings first, then do the cleanse.

- Spirulina and blue-green algae will pull out mercury.

MIGRAINE

See Headaches.

MULTIPLE SCLEROSIS

Multiple sclerosis (MS) is a nerve disorder caused by the T-cells attacking the insulating layer surrounding the neurons in the brain and spinal cord. This insulation, called the myelin sheath, helps electrical signals pass between the brain and the rest of the body. When it is damaged, nerve messages are sent more slowly and less efficiently. Patches of scar tissue can form, disrupting nerve communication to the body. Generally, the body rebuilds the damage that is caused by this attack just enough to keep ahead of the problem. The person may be losing the myelin sheath, but the body is continually replacing it or they would be dead in hours.

Women are almost twice as likely to get MS as men and rates are higher in the United States, Canada and northern Europe than in other parts of the world.

Symptoms

MS causes a wide variety of symptoms and can affect balance, bodily functions, co-ordination, sensation, strength and vision. They occur when the brain and spinal cord nerves no longer correspond properly with other parts of the body. Most people have their first symptoms between the ages of 20 and 40.

Symptoms vary wildly in severity from person to person and are likely to include:

- dizziness
- double vision or blurring of vision
- electric-shock sensations that occur with certain head movements
- fatigue
- numbness or weakness in one or more limbs
- partial or complete loss of vision
- tingling or pain in parts of the body
- tremor, lack of co-ordination or unsteady gait

They can also include:

- mental changes, such as forgetfulness or difficulties with concentration
- muscle stiffness or spasticity
- paralysis
- problems with the bladder or bowel
- sexual dysfunction – the person either wants sex all the time or has no desire
- slurred speech

MS can be a devastating disease or never cause any symptoms at all. At its worst, the person can become blind and paralyzed, a prisoner in their own body. Only a small percentage of those with MS become debilitated, however; 60 percent live normal lives. It is important for people to know this, since the fear of MS causes many problems.

Causes

Doctors are not certain why MS occurs, but they do know that white blood cells attack the myelin sheath as if it were a foreign substance.

Chlamydia is thought to be a possible cause.

Intuitive Insights

Seen intuitively, the nerves look like frayed cords. If I were to plug in a vacuum cleaner and roll over the electrical cord a couple of times, the cord would become frayed and I would have a short circuit. This is similar to what happens in the body. The brain of a person with multiple sclerosis sends a message through the nervous system for the arm to move. But because there is a short circuit in the nervous system, something else moves instead.

People with MS feel as if they are on fire. They will use the MS in an attempt to control the people around them.

When doctors do an examination for MS, they find things like lesions in the frontal lobe of the brain. These lesions are actually preventing communication to different parts of the brain and body. The person who does a lot of Theta work needs to be aware that if they are tested in the same way, electrical pulses in the frontal lobe of the brain that could be perceived as unusual could show up.

When you intuitively look at MS, you might at first confuse it with brain cancer, but if you focus you will see scar tissue or lesions. You might also see the erratic electrical currents shooting through the body.

It is my opinion that multiple sclerosis is triggered by a micro-plasma or heavy-metal poisoning. There are new kinds of MS appearing that I feel are coming from the same virus or micro-plasma that causes non-Hodgkin's lymphoma. The doctors aren't sure what to call it, but they know that it is some form of MS. When I go into the body, I can see that the immune system is attacking some kind of micro-organism that's in there. I think that some of this could also be caused by petroleum-based bacteria that are attacking the mitochondria in the cell.

Intuitive Remedies

It was quite an adventure when I first began to do healings on MS. I would witness strange things happening in the body and when I witnessed the healing, it would get some results, but the person wouldn't get completely better. When I asked the Creator about this, I heard the voice say, 'They believe that their lives are out of control.'

From this message I assumed that I had to do belief work and instil 'I have control over my life' and 'I know what it feels like to have control over my decisions', but even with these programmes, my clients only improved a little. So I asked the Creator again and I heard, 'They feel that they are not in control of their lives.'

In frustration I asked a major question: 'What do I do?!'

I heard the Creator say, 'Teach them how to do the healing on themselves.'

So I started teaching people with MS how to go up with me and command their own healing. I explained to them that some kind of virus or micro-plasma was causing part of their sickness and showed them how to command that their body completely heal. Then I told them to witness the healing take place and I showed them how to do the belief and feeling work on themselves.

The funniest thing happened: I started getting letters from people saying, 'I can get out of bed' and 'I can get out of my wheelchair.'

So, to work with someone with multiple sclerosis you must give them back their power. First, ask them if they want to change the reality that they are in. If so, ask the Creator what caused the MS. Give light and energy to all the muscles and give love to every part of the body. Ask the Creator if there is gene work that needs to be done and if so, witness it done.

Then give the person the responsibility of doing their own healing. Teach them how to go into Theta and show them how to change their virus and heal the myelin sheath. Give them the process going through their own spine, meridians and electrical systems with the energy of the Creator. If they accept healings in the first stages, they will get rid of the virus and be back in control of their life.

Bear in mind that they may enjoy receiving the extra love that they get from you and become co-dependent on you as the healer. This co-dependency could stop their own healing process, but you still have to let them know you are always there for them, while teaching them to take on their own power.

I not only tell the people with MS to work on themselves but also give them assignments to work on others. This helps them to see that other people have challenges instead of focusing completely on their own situation. You see, when the disease is at its worst, they are so absorbed in the fact that they can't control their own life that they try very hard to control the people around them. And the more out of control that they feel, the worse the MS becomes. So, in a weird sort of way, the solution to MS is not only giving them responsibility for their own life but also teaching them to be in the service of others.

After watching a couple of people die from MS I got really discouraged. But once I found out how to give back to people with MS responsibility for their own healing and allowed them to do healings on others, the changes were remarkable. These people became some of the best healers I have ever seen.

Belief Work

Belief work is very effective with MS. Some people with MS do not know how to change because they are so afraid of it. Download:

'I know how to change.'

'I can see all my possibilities.'

'I know how to live without feeling helpless.'

'I know what it feels like to have control over my life.'

'I believe that I can have control over my life.'

'I believe I know how to help other people.'

'I know how to live without the fear of MS.'

'My body can and will recover.'

'I know how to live without the stereotype of this disease.'

'I know what it feels like to ask for a second, third and fourth medical opinion.'

'I see my body heal every day.'

'I see my nerve endings working perfectly.'

'My myelin sheath is strong.'

'I feel happy about life.'

'I know I can succeed.'

'I know what it feels like to live my life without obsessing over things that doctors tell me.'

'With each day, I appreciate life more.'

'I feel life all around.'

'With every moment of every day, I appreciate what my body does for me.'

'I appreciate myself, God and others.'

'It is easy for me to help others.'

'It is easy for me to step out of my own fear paradigm.'

'I know how to bring incredible people into my life.'

'I know how to create the life I want.'

'I know how to be successful.'

'I know what it feels like to be with people who appreciate and love me.'

'I know how to live without discouragement.'

'I know how to live without pushing my will onto others.'

'I know how to live without controlling other people's lives.'

'I am totally connected to God.'

'I have good judgement about what is right and what is wrong.'

'I can control my emotions.'

'I know how to live with the Creator's definition of complete hope.'

'I know how to live without feeling overwhelmed.'

'My body is returning to strength.'

'My immune system is completely balanced.'

'I am deserving of change.'

'I know how to live without resenting others.'

'I know how to live without upsetting myself.'

'I am free to enjoy my life.'

Supplements and Other Nutritional Recommendations

With the person who has MS, there is always an excuse not to take their vitamins!

The following will be beneficial:

- Alpha-lipoic acid is good because the person doesn't detoxify too fast.
- I feel that you have to pull out some of the toxins from the body.
- I recommend DHEA if the person's doctor recommends it.
- Noni juice can be beneficial.
- One thing that you can suggest for MS is vitamin B. People with it are really low on it.
- People treated with honeybee venom have shown marked symptomatic improvements.
- Omega 3s mixed with cottage cheese also help in the production of natural interferon in the body.

- Sibu berry juice is beneficial.
- Switch to the alkaline diet.
- The person should exercise as much as possible.
- The person will need CoQ10, calcium–magnesium and lipids.
- Vitamin C helps in the production of natural interferon in the body.

THE MUSCLES

Muscles think they are the most important part of the body. It is the muscles that pump the lymph system. They are proud of their job. Their consciousness is of courage and bravery. They also have a lot to do with how you feel about yourself.

Muscles have a very strong energy. The jaw is the strongest muscle in the body. As well as being strong, the muscles can be stubborn and have tension locked into them. They are very controlling and hold on to stubbornness issues.

Along with much of the body, muscles think they are indestructible. If they are in an accident, there is a moment of shock when they realize they are not unbreakable. They may store the memory of an injury in the area of trauma. This is why it can be important to release the trauma of an accident that is held in the muscles with a healing.

Cardiovascular exercise is good for the muscles and weightlifting clears wastes from the system. If you exercise the muscles regularly, you will produce more antioxidants. Muscles also produce cortisone. Exercise triggers the body to produce more mitochondria too. Pilates and yoga move the muscles in a positive fashion. People with cancer should stimulate the muscle groups, as this can help send cancer into remission. Muscles relieve stress from the body when they are exercised. A deep full body massage is the equivalent to exercising all the muscles.

The muscles require protein. Weightlifters can develop diabetes or become hypoglycaemic if their diet doesn't have enough protein, as the muscles will steal the protein from the body's organs.

The muscles love to be babied and talked to.

Belief Work

Test for the following:

'I am stubborn.'

'I have to learn the hard way.'

'It's hard for me to learn.'

Also look at issues of confidence (not superiority), self-esteem and vulnerability. Download:

'I know the Creator's definition of what flexibility is.'

'I know how to live without allowing others to manipulate me.'

'I know how to live without manipulating others.'

'I know how to live without allowing people to intimidate me.'

'I know the Creator's definition of what it is to be charismatic.'

'It's OK to be strong.'

'It's OK for a woman to be strong.'

'I have the strength of the Creator within me.'

'It's OK to be who you want to be.'

'I have the Creator's definition of what it feels like to be physically strong.'

'I know the Creator's definition of what it is to rest.'

'I have the Creator's definition of how to relax.'

'I know what it feels like to be confident.'

Muscle Cramp

A muscle cramp is a sudden contraction of one or more of the muscles. The result can be intense pain and an inability to use the affected muscles.

Some muscle cramps occur during rest and a common variety occurs in the calf muscles or feet during sleep.

You can develop muscle cramps in your hand or arm after spending long hours gripping a tool. Writer's cramp affects the thumb and first two fingers of the writing hand and comes from using the same muscles for long periods of time.

Causes

The most common causes of leg cramps in athletes are overuse and dehydration during sports played in warm weather. Injury, muscle strain or staying in the same position may also cause muscle cramps. Other causes can be circulatory or nerve problems.

If cramping occurs after walking and ceases when you rest, the problem may be impaired circulation.

Supplements

When people complain to me that they have muscle cramps, I suspect that they have mineral deficiencies, usually magnesium and calcium, or potassium or vitamin E. Naturally, the cramps can also be due to the electrolyte imbalances that are the result of a lack of potassium.

Consider the use of more magnesium and vitamin C to help the body to get rid of toxins. Calcium tightens the muscles and magnesium relaxes them. Alpha-lipoic acid should be used when exercising to help clean up the toxins from the body and give more energy.

Also helpful are:

- Lecithin
- vitamin B complex
- zinc to help break down the vitamin Bs for good absorption

MUSCULAR DYSTROPHY

Muscular dystrophy (MD) is a genetic disorder that weakens the muscles that help the body move. People with MD have incorrect or missing information in their genes, which prevents them from making the proteins they need for healthy muscles. People are born with the problem. It's not contagious.

MD weakens muscles over time, so children, teenagers and adults who have the disease can gradually lose the ability to do the things most people take for granted, like walking or sitting up. Someone with MD might start having muscle problems as a baby or their symptoms might start later. Some people even develop MD as adults.

People with MD have an amazing way of trying to care for everyone else before themselves. The first healing that I saw of it was some years ago in Australia. A young lady came to class with the problem. Even though she was leaning on a staff in order to walk, when I asked her how I could help her, she said, 'Please help my sister.' I talked her into accepting a healing for herself. She had an amazing instant healing at that class.

Types

There are two types of MD:

- *First kind:* Strikes boys, not girls. Most don't make it to adulthood. It is passed on through a chromosome.
- *Second kind:* Caused by micro-plasma or viruses.

MD is seen as a genetic defect due to toxins. It can be caused by electrical currents and radiation.

Intuitive Insights

It never ceases to amaze me the incredible compassion that people with muscular dystrophy have. The little boys I have met with it have had a wonderful capacity for love.

When you work on muscular dystrophy you will find that when you ask the Creator to show you what it is and how to heal it, you will go into the mitochondrial DNA of the client. You may watch some different viruses die off there.

As you continue witnessing, you will be taken to the skeletal system. This is because the skeletal system feeds all the muscles. Even though people think that muscular dystrophy is a muscular disease, it starts in the skeletal system. So don't be upset and think you are in the wrong place. Witness the Creator making the changes that will guide the brain and DNA to heal.

Finally, witness the rebuilding of the muscles and the connective tissue. Say 'Creator, show me' and witness the work.

Remember that even though you may work on someone and they say they feel better, their muscles will still have deteriorated due to the MD. You have to go in and reconstruct some of the muscles. Make sure that their body has enough fuel to support this.

Belief Work

From the standpoint of the healer, muscular dystrophy can be one of the most frightening diseases to witness. It is a good idea for the healer to release their fear of the disease so that they are not blocking the healing. The very thought of these people being so helpless and yet so pure in spirit can have a profound effect on the healer. I advise you to pull your fear and get with the programme.

For the client, pull the belief that muscular dystrophy is incurable due to a DNA problem. Replace with:

'The Creator can heal me.'

'I know what good health feels like.'

'I deserve to be healed.'

Teach them how to live without the disease.

Other downloads:

'I enjoy life in every way.'

'I know how to love the people around me without being ill.'

'I am important.'

'My body is important.'

'It's safe for me to be strong, healthy and support myself.'

'I know what it feels like to support others.'

'I know what it feels like to be totally connected to the Creator.'

'I am worthy of healing.'

'I appreciate myself.'

'I am completely appreciated by others.'

'I don't have to die to prove myself to the Creator.'

'I am in good standing with the Creator of All That Is.'

'I have the strength to be here on this planet.'

'I have the will to be here on this planet.'

'I am not offended by this world.'

'I know how to live my life without taking on the sorrow of this planet.'

'I am unaffected by the grief, sorrow and maliciousness of those around me.'

'My psychic abilities are accepted.'

'I can teach others around me to have patience and conditional love without being ill.'

'Every day, in every way, I draw the support of the universe.'

'I believe in myself.'

'I believe that my body will become stronger and stronger.'

Downloads for the parents:

'I have hope that my child can heal.'

'With the Creator, everything is possible.'

Pull the fear that this disease is totally incapacitating.

Supplements

- A person with MD will need a little alpha-lipoic acid to clean up their system.
- They will also need to take amino acids to rebuild their muscles. Enzymes and zinc will rebuild the structures of their muscles. If they don't have enough zinc, they aren't going to break down the vitamins A, B, C and many of the other vitamins.

NARCOLEPSY

Narcolepsy is a chronic neurological disorder caused by the brain's inability to regulate sleep–wake cycles normally. At various times throughout the day, a person with narcolepsy experiences the fleeting urge to sleep. If the urge becomes overwhelming, they fall asleep for anything from a few seconds to several minutes. In rare cases, they remain asleep for an hour or longer. Narcolepsy is like a short-circuit in the brain.

Intuitive Remedies

Intuitively work on the hypothalamus and restructure the sleep–wake cycle.

THE NERVOUS SYSTEM

The nervous system is our electrical connection to the outside world. Along with the brain, it acts as the transponder, receiver and interpreter of outside energy.

The nervous system is connected to the whole body. When you work on it, you work with the neurons that are the electrical messengers of the body.

The best healer is the one who can step out of their own world and into another's paradigm to relate to them from their own point of view. This is done by having a balanced nervous system.

Travelling through the brain and body, neurons pick up thought forms instantly. This is the fastest computer known to man.

Types

The Autonomic Nervous System

The autonomic nerve fibres form a subsidiary system that regulates the iris of the eye and the smooth-muscle action of the bladder, blood vessels, colon, glands, heart, lungs, stomach and other visceral organs not subject to willful control.

Although the autonomic nervous system's impulses originate in the central nervous system, it performs the most basic human functions more or less automatically, without the conscious intervention of higher brain centres. Because it is linked to those centres, however, it is influenced by the emotions. Anger, for example, can increase the heartbeat.

The Sympathetic and Parasympathetic Nervous Systems

Autonomic nerve fibres exit from the central nervous system as part of other peripheral nerves but branch from them to form two more subsystems: the sympathetic and parasympathetic nervous systems, the actions of which usually oppose each other. For example, sympathetic nerves cause arteries to contract, while parasympathetic nerves cause them to dilate.

Sympathetic impulses are conducted to the organs by two or more neurons. The cell body of the first lies within the central nervous system and that of the second lies in an external ganglion. Eighteen pairs of such ganglia interconnect by nerve fibres to form a double chain just outside the spine and run parallel to it. Parasympathetic impulses are also relayed by at least two neurons. The cell body of the second generally lies near or within the target organ.

The Nervous System and Reflexes

In general, nerve function is dependent on both sensory and motor fibres, with sensory stimulation evoking motor response. Even the autonomic system is activated by sensory impulses from receptors in the organ or muscle. Where especially sensitive areas or powerful stimuli are concerned, however, it is not always necessary for a sensory impulse to reach the brain in order to trigger motor response. A sensory neuron may link directly to a motor neuron at a synapse in the spinal cord, forming a reflex arc that performs automatically. Thus, tapping the tendon below the kneecap causes the leg to jerk involuntarily because the impulse provoked by the tap, after travelling to the spinal cord, travels directly back to the leg muscle. Such a response is called an involuntary reflex action. Commonly, the reflex arc includes one or more connector neurons that exert a modulating effect, allowing varying degrees of response, depending on whether the stimulation is strong, weak or prolonged. Reflex arcs are often linked to other arcs by nerve fibres in the spinal cord. Consequently, a number of reflex muscle responses may be triggered simultaneously, as when a person shudders and jerks away from the touch of an insect. Links between the reflex arcs and higher centres enable the brain to identify a sensory stimulus, such as pain, or to note a reflex response, such as withdrawal, and to inhibit that response (as when the arm is held steady against the prick of a hypodermic needle).

Reflex patterns are inherited rather than learned, having evolved as involuntary survival mechanisms. But voluntary actions initiated in the brain may become reflex actions through continued association of a particular stimulus with a certain result. In such cases, an alteration of impulse routes occurs that permits responses without mediation by higher nerve centres. Such responses are called conditioned reflexes, the most famous example being one of the experiments Ivan Pavlov performed with dogs. After the dogs had learned to associate the provision of food with the sound of a bell, they salivated at the sound of the bell even when food was not offered.

Habit formation and much of learning are dependent on conditioned reflexes. To illustrate, the brain of a student typist must co-ordinate sensory impulses from both the eyes and the muscles in order to direct the fingers to particular keys. After enough repetition the fingers automatically find and strike the proper keys even if the eyes are closed. The student has learned to type; that is, typing has become a conditioned reflex.

Downloads

'I understand when I am receiving true communication from others.'

'I understand how to live without allowing negative thought forms to interfere with my progress.'

'I understand the difference between the Creator's perspective of truth and that of another person.'

'I understand how to see others from the Creator's perspective.'

'I have the Creator's definition of how to interact with others.'

'I am connected to the Creator of All That Is.

'The Creator of All That Is is connected to me.'

'I have the Creator's definition of how to recognize the highest truth.'

'I have the Creator's definition of how to discern the highest truth.'

'I have the Creator's definition from the Seventh Plane of what it feels like to be important.'

Supplements

* ALA and liver cleanses (to prevent healing crises in the skin)
* omega oils (3s, 6s and 9s)
* selenium
* vitamin E

OBESITY

Obesity means having too much body fat in ratio to muscle tissue. It is different from being overweight, which means weighing too much. Being overweight may be due to bone, fat and/or body water. Both of these terms, however, mean that a person's weight is more than what is considered healthy for their height.

In most people, obesity occurs over time when more calories are consumed than are used. The balance between calories in and calories out differs for each person. Factors that might cause obesity include the genetic make-up, overeating, eating high-fat foods and not being physically active. Obesity increases the risk of arthritis, diabetes, heart disease, stroke and some cancers.

Not everyone who is obese is eating too much food. Thyroid problems can cause obesity, as can psychological disorders. Certain types of medication, such as prednisone, and anti-depressants (MAO inhibiters) can also cause obesity.

In one study, it was found that American teenagers who ate breakfast every day weighed on average 15 pounds less than those who did not eat breakfast. One theory is that when people fast and then consume large amounts of food all at once, they have a tendency to store fat. More small meals spaced throughout the day are better than large meals all at once.

Intuitive Insights

Many people who are overweight have a tendency to be pushy, argumentative and critical of others (particularly with others who are overweight) and can be angry at the world. These feelings are caused by imbalances in their organs such as the liver and kidneys. Strict monitoring of the carbohydrate consumption (not calories) will help in an overall diet plan.

Intuitive Remedies

When you are overweight, you will always get the 'exercise lecture'. However, it is difficult for those who are obese to exercise when they can't breathe, let alone move without the danger of falling or injury. This is why it is best for them to do exercise that is simple such as walking, using a rowing machine, or riding a stationary bicycle at a slow pace.

The unfortunate thing that is likely to happen when someone begins to exercise after a long period of abstinence from it is that the exercise will release toxins that have been stored in the tissues. This can make the person feel terrible until these toxins are gone. This is why it is always best to start any exercise regime slowly.

People who have heavy-metal poisoning have a tendency to be overweight because the fat cells attempt to encapsulate the toxins. Release the heavy metals and the person will be likely to lose weight.

Also, intuitively stimulating the pituitary to make the correct hormones can help obesity.

The 'Sending Love to the Baby in the Womb' exercise and belief work seem to bring the best results.

Belief Work

For the most part those who are obese have their own special reason why it is serving them. Energy test for:

'If I am fat, I will not cheat on my spouse.'

'If I am heavy, I will not get involved in a relationship.'

'I fear being emotionally hurt.'

'I am afraid of love.'

'Food is bad.'

'Food is my enemy.'

'If I lose weight, I will not belong.'

Then, make sure that you programme the person to be thin. Don't programme them to 'lose' weight, because if you do, they will look for the weight and find it again. Always programme them to 'release' weight.

It is best to also release them from any judgement or criticism from others because they are overweight. The feelings that other people project to those who are overweight can cause them to become depressed, especially if they are intuitive.

Check the history and genetic levels for the belief that being overweight means being wealthy and for issues with power or safety. Many of the issues you will face with women will revolve around abuse, ancestral programmes that sex is shameful and feelings of guilt dealing with sexual energy. These need to be changed and put back into perspective.

Download:

'I love my body.'

'I enjoy the food that I eat.'

'I know when I am full.'

'I eat less.'

'I am young.'

'I am strong.'

'I enjoy exercise daily.'

'I feel good about myself.'

'I am important.'

'I avoid fatty foods.'

'I enjoy taking my vitamins.'

'My stomach is shrinking.'

'The mirror is my friend.'

'I take responsibility for what I eat.'

'I like water.'

'I enjoy good protein foods.'

'Smaller portions of food are satisfying.'

'Less bread is better.'

'I like fruit.'

'I like raw vegetables.'

'I exercise every day.'

'I am confident about releasing weight.'

'I am patient with myself.'

'I live without the fear of failing.'

'I eat slowly.'

'I am calm and collected.'

'I am thin and attractive.'

'If I am thin, people will still love me for who I am.'

'I understand what it feels like to absorb nutrients from food.'

'Every bite of food I eat is full of love and I become content easily.'

Supplements and Other Nutritional Supplements

You can make a major change in a person's weight just by taking them off all white bread and gluten.

I would also recommend for your further studies on this subject a book by Dr Peter J. D'Adamo called *Eat Right 4 Your Type*. This book deals not only with weight loss, but also with what you should and should not eat according to your blood type.

The American Cancer Society found that people who used artificial sweeteners actually gained weight instead of losing it. Artificial sweeteners are far worse than regular sugar on the body.

Chocolate, used judiciously, can actually be an aid in weight loss.

Many of the herbs that benefit those who are obese can be dangerous, due to the strain they place on the other organs of the body.

Those who are obese due to medication have a tendency to skip regular, nutritious meals. Fruit and vegetables are a must for these people, as they need something to clean the intestinal tract.

On the flip side of the coin, you have the obese person who cannot stop eating because their body cannot absorb the nutrients from the intake of food.

Parasite infections cause obesity in many people, so a parasite cleanse might be suggested.

Eating is not bad. In most people, eating the right foods will help in weight loss.

Just Like Sugar is an amazing supplement. Other useful supplements:

- ALA
- *Aloe vera* juice for the digestive tract
- amino-acid complex
- DHEA
- flaxseed oil
- grapeseed extract (though watch for contradictions with medication)
- omega 3s, 6s and 9s

- Lecithin
- vitamin E (in low doses)

A Diet for Obesity

This diet comes from the Sacred Heart Memorial Hospital and is used to help overweight heart patients lose weight rapidly, usually before surgery.

BASIC FAT-BURNING SOUP

12 green onions/scallions, chopped

2 green peppers

1 or 2 cans of chopped tomatoes

1 bunch of celery

1 large head of cabbage, chopped

1 packet of Lipton onion soup mix

Optional: I added cilantro or parsley, bundle-chopped.

Seasonings: Salt, pepper, curry, bouillon or hot sauce (Tabasco)

Cut vegetables in small to medium pieces, add the Lipton onion soup mix, canned tomatoes and seasonings, cover with pure filtered water, boil for 5–10 minutes and then let simmer until vegetables are tender.

This soup can be eaten anytime you are hungry and you can eat as much as you want.

This soup will not add calories. The more you eat, the more you will lose. Fill a thermos in the morning if you will be away during the day.

Warning! This diet, if eaten alone for indefinite periods, could cause malnutrition.

Day One

Eat only the soup and fruit (except bananas). Cantaloupe and watermelon are lower in calories.

Drink unsweetened tea, cranberry juice or purified water.

Day Two

Do not eat any fruit. Eat, along with the soup, all vegetables – fresh, raw or canned. Green leafy vegetables are better than beans, corn and peas. At dinner time, reward yourself with a baked potato.

Day Three

Eat all the soup, fruit and vegetables that you want. Have a baked potato.

Day Four

If you have eaten for three days as above and have not cheated, you will find on the morning of the fourth day you will have lost 5–7 pounds.

On the fourth day eat bananas and skimmed milk. Eat as many as three bananas and drink as many glasses of purified water as you can. Bananas are high in calories and carbohydrates, and so is the milk. Today your body will need the potassium and the carbs, proteins and calories to lessen your cravings for sweets. Eat the soup at least twice today.

Day Five

Beef and tomatoes. You may have 10–20 oz of beef and a can of tomatoes or as many as six fresh tomatoes today. Try to drink at least 6–8 glasses of purified water so to wash away the uric acid in your body. Eat the soup at least once today.

Day Six

Beef and veggies. Eat to your heart's content of beef and vegetables today. You can eat two or three steaks if you like. Eat green leafy vegetables. No baked potatoes. Be sure to eat the soup at least once today.

Day Seven

Brown rice, unsweetened fruit juice and vegetables. Stuff yourself! Be sure to have the soup at least once today.

Definite No Nos
   alcohol

   bread

   carbonated drinks (including diet) (Stick with purified water, unsweetened tea, black coffee, unsweetened fruit juice, cranberry juice and skimmed milk.)

   fried foods

   skin on chicken

You can eat broiled or baked chicken or broiled fish instead of meat only on one of the beef days. You need the high protein in the beef on the other days.

The basic fat-burning soup can be eaten anytime you feel hungry. The more you eat, the more you will lose. Eat as much as you wish.

Any prescribed medication will not hurt you on this diet.

By the end of the seventh day or the morning of the eighth day, if you have not cheated you will have lost 10–17 lbs and will have an abundance of energy. If you have lost more than 15 lbs, stay off the diet for two days before resuming the diet again at day one.

This seven-day eating plan can be used as often as you like. As a matter of fact, if correctly followed, it will clean your system of impurities and give a feeling of well-being as never before. Continue this plan as long as you wish and feel the difference. This diet is fast, fat-burning and the secret is that you will burn more calories than you take in.

This diet does not lend itself to drinking any alcoholic beverages at any time because of the removal of fat build-up in your system. Go off the diet at least 24 hours before any intake of alcohol.

Because everyone's digestive system is different, this diet will affect everyone differently. After day three you will have more energy than when you began. After being on the diet for several days, you will find your bowel movements have changed. Eat a cup of bran or fibre. Although you can have black coffee with this diet, you may find that you don't need the caffeine after the third day.

Continue this plan for as long as you wish, but in the short term only – it should not be used continually.

OESTROGEN IMBALANCES

We need oestrogen to absorb calcium. Too much, however, causes cancer, cysts, heart conditions and weight gain. Too little causes cysts, depression and weight gain.

Intuitive Remedies

Command the hormones to balance.

Check the person for relationship issues and thyroid problems.

Supplements

- Damiana
- liquorice root
- maca
- suma

Avoid these herbs if there has been an oestrogen-related cancer.

OSTEOMALACIA/RICKETS

Osteomalacia is softening of the bones. These softer bones have a normal amount of collagen, which gives them their structure, but are lacking in calcium. In children, the condition is called rickets.

Osteomalacia is most likely to occur in pregnant women and nursing mothers, whose nutritional requirements are higher than normal, or people with malabsorption problems. If left undiagnosed, it can cause renal failure.

Symptoms

Early signs include:

- cramps and numbness in the extremities
- nervousness
- painful muscle spasms

Bone malformations may develop due to softening of the bones. This may cause:

- a narrow rib cage
- a protruding breast bone
- bending at the ends of the ribs
- bowed legs
- delayed walking
- irritability
- knock knees
- profuse sweating
- restlessness
- scoliosis

Causes

There are numerous causes of osteomalacia, including:

- cancer
- hereditary or acquired disorders of vitamin D metabolism
- kidney failure and acidosis
- liver disease
- malabsorption of vitamin D by the intestines
- not enough exposure to sunlight, which produces vitamin D in the body
- not enough vitamin D in the diet
- phosphate depletion associated with not enough phosphates in the diet
- the side-effects of medication used to treat seizures

The use of very strong sunscreen, limited exposure of the body to sunlight, short days of sunlight and smog are factors that reduce formation of vitamin D in the body.

Risk factors for osteomalacia are related to the causes. In the elderly, there is an increased risk among people who tend to remain indoors and those who avoid milk because of lactose intolerance.

Intuitive Remedies

Go in to the person's space and command the body to return to health and accept vital nutrients.

Supplements

Essential nutrients are:

- boron, calcium, phosphorus, silica and vitamin D3 used together so that they can be metabolized together
- a good multivitamin and mineral combination, plus extra vitamin B12

A diet high in calcium is essential.

OSTEOPOROSIS

Osteoporosis is a condition characterized by the loss of the normal density of bone, resulting in fragile and abnormally porous bones and an increase in the risk of bone fracture. It is always associated with a lack of calcium; however, the body's inability to digest calcium causes the calcium itself to contribute to the osteoporosis.

Intuitive Insights

Osteoporosis looks like dark spots on the bones.

Go through the body and ask the Creator if the person has too much calcium in their blood. If they do, the parathyroid is not working correctly. This gland is responsible for telling the body to absorb calcium either in the muscles or the bones.

Always make sure the kidneys are functioning correctly.

Intuitive Remedies

Command a healing in the highest and best way. The Creator will show you.

Belief Work

If the bones do not actively respond to the healing process, there are beliefs blocking the healing. These will be concerned with accepting love, bearing the burdens of the world and either the inability to receive support or giving too much support to others.

If there are problems with the parathyroid, as with the thyroid there will be beliefs about having to defend yourself and not being able to speak up and say how you truly feel. Go in and programme the person to understand what they truly feel, what they should say and how to express it in the highest and best way.

Supplements and Other Nutritional Recommendations

- boron
- chelated calcium–magnesium
- MSM for flexibility
- vitamin C

OVARIAN CYSTS

A cyst is a fluid-filled sac. In most cases a cyst on the ovary does no harm and goes away by itself. Most women have these cysts at some point during their lives. They are rarely cancerous in women under 50. They sometimes hurt, but not always. Often, a woman finds out about a cyst when she has a pelvic examination.

Intuitive Insights

Ask the Creator if the cysts are caused by too much or too little oestrogen. Change any genetic tendency. Watch the Creator shrink the cysts.

Supplements and Other Nutritional Recommendations

- Calcium–magnesium will help with the cramps associated with cysts.

- Maca also helps get rid of cysts.

See also Oestrogen Imbalances.

PAGET'S DISEASE

Paget's disease as it pertains to the bone is a condition that affects the normal biological processes of the bones. The disease is named after a mid-19th-century English surgeon, Sir James Paget, who also identified Paget's disease of the breast. However, the two conditions are unrelated.

The bones are living tissues that are engaged in a continual process of renewal. This process is called remodelling. In Paget's disease, it is disrupted. Paget's causes the old bone to begin breaking down faster than new bone can be built. Over time, the body responds by generating new bone at a faster than normal rate. This rapid alteration produces bone that is softer and weaker than normal bone, which can lead to bone pain, deformities and fractures. It usually affects the skull, the spine and the bones in the arms, legs and pelvis.

Symptoms

Paget's disease of the bone affects each person differently. Most people have no symptoms. When symptoms do occur, they are typically present in specific areas affected by the disease, although they may be widespread and include:

- Bone deformities, such as bow legs and enlarged head size.
- Bone fractures.
- Bone pain that is most severe at night.
- Enlarged bones compressing the spinal cord or the nerves exiting the brain and spinal cord. Pain resulting from nerve compression can be severe and pressure on a nerve can cause double vision, hearing loss, numbness, tingling and weakness.
- Joint damage in the cartilage lining the joints near the affected bones. This wear and tear often leads to osteoarthritis.
- Neurological problems, such as hearing loss and headache.
- Warmth in the skin over the affected area.

Treatment is available in the form of medication or surgery.

Causes

No definite cause has been established for Paget's disease of the bone, although several genes have been discovered that appear to be linked to the disorder. It is believed that Paget's is related to a viral infection in the bone cells that may be present for many years before problems appear. Hereditary factors seem to influence a susceptibility to the disease.

Intuitive Remedies

Use the gene work and witness the changes.

I find that in some instances Paget's disease can be triggered by heavy-metal exposure. Pulling out the heavy metals can be beneficial.

Belief Work

With Paget's disease, belief systems cycle around how the person receives and accepts love and how they feel about the Creator. Download:

'I am totally connected to the Creator.'

'I feel completely supported by the Creator of All That Is.'

'The Creator and I are connected as one.'

'I understand I am creating my own reality.'

'I know that there are miracles every day.'

'I am ready for miracles in my life.'

'I am ready for my body to be strong and healthy.'

'Everything in my body becomes perfect when I am connected as one with the Creator.'

'Every day in every way I am getting stronger.'

PANCREATITIS

Pancreatitis is an acute inflammation of the pancreas. This is a large gland behind the stomach, close to the duodenum, the higher part of the small intestine. It releases the hormones insulin and glucagon into the bloodstream to help the body use the glucose it takes from food for energy. It also secretes digestive enzymes into the small intestine through a tube called the pancreatic duct. These enzymes digest fats, proteins and carbohydrates from food. Under normal conditions, they do not become active until they reach the small intestine. If they become active inside the pancreas itself, they cause damage to it.

Types

- *Acute pancreatitis* occurs suddenly, lasts for a short time and usually resolves itself.

- *Chronic pancreatitis* does not resolve itself and results in the slow destruction of the pancreas.

Either form can cause serious problems. In severe instances, bleeding, infection and tissue damage may occur. Pseudocysts, which are accumulations of fluid and tissue debris, may also develop. In addition, enzymes and toxins may enter the bloodstream, injuring the heart, lungs, kidneys or other organs. Acute pancreatitis occurs more often in men than women.

Conventional treatment depends on the severity of the attack. If no kidney or lung complications occur, acute pancreatitis usually improves on its own. Treatment is tailored to support vital bodily functions and prevent complications. A hospital stay will be necessary so that fluids can be replaced intravenously.

Symptoms

Acute pancreatitis usually begins with pain in the upper abdomen that may last for a few days. The pain may be severe and constant and can reach to the back and other areas. It may be sudden, intense or begin as a mild pain that gets worse when food is eaten.

Other symptoms may include:

- a swollen and tender abdomen
- fever
- nausea
- rapid pulse
- vomiting

Severe cases may cause dehydration and low blood pressure. The heart, lungs or kidneys may also fail. If the pancreas begins to bleed, shock and sometimes even death will follow.

Causes

Acute pancreatitis is usually caused by gallstones or too much alcohol. However, if these are ruled out, other possible causes should be carefully examined so that appropriate treatment can begin. Hepatitis A can cause pancreatitis, as can certain forms of medication, including some for seizures and arthritis. Certain cancers and chemotherapy can also trigger this disorder.

Intuitive Insights

Most of the people that I have worked on with this disorder have passed.

Make the command that the pancreas go back to health. Witness as light enters it from the Creator, filling it with energy and love.

Belief Work

Pancreatitis creates the fear of defeat. Issues will cycle around:

> 'I am defeated.'
>
> 'I will never be healthy.'
>
> 'I can never win.'

Supplements

- ALA
- burdock root
- chromium
- dandelion root
- grapeseed extract
- milk thistle
- multivitamin
- noni
- olive-leaf extract
- red clover
- vitamin C

PARALYSIS

Paralysis is the complete or partial loss of function, especially involving the loss of motion or sensation in a part of the body due to loss of nerve function. A paralyzed area no longer has an electrical current running through it.

Intuitive Remedies

Command new synapses to be made and connected. Ask the Creator to show you as this takes place.

If the paralysis is the result of the spinal cord being severed, you do not need to know exactly what to do. Simply ask the Creator to reconnect it. If it is partially severed, there is a good chance of reconnecting it.

If it is fully severed and someone has already told the person they won't walk again, ask the Creator to take you back to before that and change what they have heard.

Before any surgery, always ask the surgeon not to say anything. A person will even pick up thoughts from people during surgery. If there has already been surgery, ask the Creator to take you back to the surgery and change anything negative the person has heard or picked up during the surgery. Teach the body to be better than it was before the surgery, or before any accident that resulted in the surgery.

Belief Work

Energy test for the fear of being healthy. Check to see if the person knows what the Creator feels like and if they are afraid of beginning normal life again.

PARASITES

See Prologue.

PARKINSON'S DISEASE

Parkinson's disease is one of a larger group of neurological conditions called motor system disorders. Historians have found evidence of the disease as far back as 5000 BC. It affects more men than women. It was first described as 'the shaking palsy' in 1817 by British doctor James Parkinson. Because of his early work in identifying symptoms, the disease came to bear his name.

In the normal brain, some nerve cells produce the chemical dopamine, which transmits signals within the brain to produce the smooth movement of muscles. In Parkinson's patients, 80 percent or more of these dopamine-producing cells are damaged, dead or otherwise degenerated. This causes the nerve cells to fire wildly, leaving patients unable to control their movements.

Symptoms

Symptoms include:

- dementia
- depression
- poor balance and co-ordination
- slowness of movements
- stiffness of the arms, legs and trunk
- trembling of hands, arms, legs, jaw and face

Stress makes the symptoms more prevalent.

Intuitive Insights

Many young people come to me with Parkinson's. I find aluminium, mercury and lead in everyone with Parkinson's.

As for the genetic tendency towards Parkinson's, a person may have a father and grandfather with Parkinson's, but what you might see is that Grandma has been cooking with aluminium pans for 40 years and the whole family has been drinking out of lead pipes. That's where the genetic tendency lies. The effects of lead and aluminium can be passed down in the genes as the predisposition for Parkinson's. There is also the likelihood that as a child, the person ate food and drank water at Grandpa's house that was poisoned with heavy metals.

The brain will continue to learn as long as we use it. We can learn well past the age of 100 if we keep out heavy metals and yeast.

I believe that some of the people who are diagnosed with Parkinson's are actually suffering from mad cow disease. I think this is more prevalent than people know. I also think that exposure to certain viruses in the brain can trigger Parkinson's.

Intuitive Remedies

People with Parkinson's are very receptive to healings. They may have a fear of getting better, but they usually do whatever they can to get rid of the Parkinson's.

The thing I've seen work best with Parkinson's is asking the Creator to do a healing and watching the dopamine levels change. Intuitively witness the reconstruction of the master cell and the cells that create dopamine.

If the heavy metals are not cleared, the disorder will recreate itself, so ask the Creator to pull out the metals slowly, as is highest and best for the person.

Belief Work

People with Parkinson's have a tendency to be very critical of others. I am unsure as to why this is, but I suspect it is because their adrenals are overworked in the attempt to give the body the hormones it needs.

Look at issues of Parkinson's as incurable and test for:

'The world is falling apart.'

'I have no say-so in my life.'

'I need pity.'

'I may as well give up. But I don't want to give up.' (The client seems to be fighting with themselves.)

As well as pulling these programmes, also pull those that say we're supposed to forget things as we grow older.

Download:

'I know what it feels like to be strong and healthy.'

'My body is returning to total health.'

'I can remember.'

'I can remember easily and effortlessly.'

'I can move easily and effortlessly.'

'My body produces the right amount of dopamine.'

'My receptors are awake and alive.'

'I can receive impulses from the brain to the body.'

'My receptors are perfect.'

'I will gain control of my life.'

'I know what it feels like to move without pain.'

'I know what it feels like to live without stiffness.'

'I know what it feels like to move without shaking.'

'I know how to be still.'

'I know what it feels like to believe in myself.'

'I'm totally connected to the Creator of All That Is.'

'I am stronger and healthier every day.'

'With each passing day my body and mind become stronger.'

'I will no longer be taken advantage of.'

'Others believe in me.'

'I know what it feels like to live without resenting God.'

'I know what it feels like to live without resenting my life.'

'I can live without regret.'

'I know what it feels like to be in control of my emotions.'

Supplements and Other Nutritional Recommendations

- The best supplement I've ever found for Parkinson's is alpha-lipoic acid. Glutathione injections and alpha-lipoic acid will clean up heavy metals fast and pull toxins out of the brain.

- Liver cleanses are also beneficial and can make a client stop shaking (*see the Liver*), though some older people can't use the intensive liver cleanses, so in these cases ask the Creator to help clean up their liver and you'll see a huge difference. If you can, take three or four oil liver cleanses to pull out heavy metals.

- For memory loss, magnesium and beta carotene are needed.

- For those with a predisposition for Parkinson's disease, DHEA can be used as a preventative.

- amino acids such as tyrosine and creatine
- burdock
- calcium–magnesium
- cayenne pepper
- CoQ10
- dandelion root
- hawthorn
- milk thistle
- red clover
- vitamin B complex

- vitamin C, 3,000–5,000 mg a day
- vitamin E

PELVIC INFLAMMATORY DISEASE

See Chlamydia.

PEPTIC ULCERS

A peptic ulcer is a pustule in the lining of the stomach or small intestine tissues that has been eroded by stomach acid, leaving an internal open wound. It can be the result of an infection of *Helicobacter pylori* or of drugs that weaken the lining of the stomach or duodenum. Aspirin, non-steroidal anti-inflammatory drugs (NSAIDs) and corticosteroids can all irritate the stomach lining and cause ulcers. However, most people who take NSAIDs or corticosteroids do not develop peptic ulcers.

Discomfort caused by peptic ulcers tends to come and go. A conventional diagnosis is based on symptoms and on the results of an examination called an endoscopy. Antacids and other drugs are given to reduce acid in the stomach, and antibiotics are given to eliminate the *Helicobacter pylori* bacterium.

Complications of peptic ulcers are bleeding or rupture accompanied by dizziness, fainting and low blood pressure.

Types

Duodenal ulcers occur in the first few inches of the duodenum.

Gastric ulcers, which are less common, occur along the upper curve of the stomach.

Marginal ulcers can develop after stomach surgery, at the point where the remaining stomach has been reconnected to the intestine.

Stress ulcers can occur as a result of the stress of severe illness, skin burns or trauma.

Causes

Ulcers develop when the normal defence and repair mechanisms of the lining of the stomach or duodenum are weakened, making the lining more likely to be damaged by stomach acid.

People who smoke are more likely to develop a peptic ulcer and their ulcers to heal more slowly.

Although psychological stress can increase acid production, no link has been found between psychological stress and peptic ulcers.

Intuitive Insights

Seen intuitively, a peptic ulcer should not be mistaken for stomach cancer. Cancer grows and expands, whereas *H. pylori* creates a sore in the stomach lining.

Sometimes *H. pylori* 'sets up shop' when a person is physically weak and the immune system is compromised. This is why it is important for us all to make time to rest.

Belief Work

Since bacteria generally cause peptic ulcers, you need to work on guilt issues, including feeling guilty about not taking time for yourself.

Since the disorder is in the stomach, you also need to work on issues of digestion. These cycle around feeding yourself, taking in food and loving yourself.

Download:

'I love myself.'

'I understand what it feels like to say no and mean it.'

Supplements and Other Nutritional Recommendations

- acidophilus
- *Aloe vera* juice, four to five ounces a day
- amino acids
- bromelain
- catnip tea
- cat's claw for the liver
- essential fatty acids
- noni juice
- pectin
- vitamin complex
- zinc

- A diet of green leafy vegetables is beneficial to help with the *pylori* bacterium.
- Stay away from coffee and alcohol.
- Whenever possible, avoid salt and sugar.
- Cow's milk neutralizes stomach acid, so it is best not to use it.

See also Stomach Ulcers.

PLEURISY

Pleurisy occurs when the double membrane (pleura) that lines the chest cavity and surrounds each of the lungs becomes inflamed and is pulled away from the lungs by the person coughing. Also called pleuritis, pleurisy typically causes sharp pain, almost always during the act of breathing.

Intuitive Remedies

Always work on healing the coughing problem before you work on the pleurisy itself.

Pleurisy can be rectified by commanding that the inflammation goes away and witnessing the lining of the lungs reattaching.

Supplements

Suggest the herb pleurisy root.

PNEUMONIA

Pneumonia is a symptom, not a disease. It is an inflammation of the lungs caused by infection with bacteria, viruses, fungi or other organisms.

Pneumonia is of particular concern for older adults, people with chronic illnesses or impaired immune systems and the very young. Pneumonia that is contracted while in hospital can be particularly dangerous.

Symptoms

Pneumonia often mimics a cold or the flu and begins with a cough and a fever. Symptoms include:

- chest pain

- chills
- cough
- fever
- shortness of breath

They can, however, vary greatly, depending on the type of organism causing the infection.

Causes

Bacteria

Many types of bacteria can cause pneumonia. Signs and symptoms include a high fever, chest pain, chills, shaking, shortness of breath, sweating and a cough that produces thick greenish or yellow phlegm. Bacterial pneumonia is often confined to just one area (lobe) of the lung. This is called lobar pneumonia.

Antibiotics are used to treat bacterial pneumonia, but there are now antibiotic-resistant strains that are a growing problem. Be sure to take the full course of antibiotics. Failure to do so could result in the bacteria becoming resistant to the antibiotic.

Viruses

Viruses cause half of all pneumonias. Symptoms start with a dry cough, fatigue, fever, headache and muscle pain.

Mycoplasma

This tiny organism causes symptoms similar to those of other bacterial and viral infections. This type of pneumonia is often called walking pneumonia.

Fungi

Certain kinds of fungus cause pneumonia, although these types are less common.

Pneumocystis carinii

Pneumonia caused by *P. carinii* affects people with AIDS or those with compromised immune systems.

Intuitive Insights

One of the reasons why bacteria are able to enter the system is because of unbalanced emotions. If you are angry or afraid all the time, your immune system has to work harder. If these feelings continue, they have a tendency to exhaust the immune system. This is how emotions deplete the body. Fear and anger can be beneficial as survival reflexes – this is what they were designed for. They were not designed for continual, compulsive overuse. It can make you ill if you never express your anger and hold it inside. The ability to express your anger in a positive fashion is beneficial.

Intuitive Remedies

Bacteria are easy to get rid of intuitively. Make the command: *'Creator, heal this and show me.'* Witness the healing as done.

In a healing, go up and ask the Creator to get rid of the infection. Understand that after the healing, the body still has a natural process to go through and has to recuperate from the sickness. The benefits of the healing will not become fully apparent until later. Healings have a subtle effect in the body. Do not doubt the healing.

Belief Work

Guilt issues hold bacteria in the body, so check for these. Download:

> 'I know what it feels like to live without guilt.'
>
> 'I know how to live without holding on to guilt.'
>
> 'I know how to live without feeling guilty about who I am.'
>
> 'I know how to live without feeling guilty about the way my body looks.'
>
> 'I know how to live without feeling guilty about everything my parents have taught me.'
>
> 'I know what a friend is.'
>
> 'I know how to have friends.'
>
> 'I know how to be a friend.'

Supplements and Other Nutritional Recommendations

- cayenne pepper
- essential fatty acids
- ginger
- goldenseal, but not if you are diabetic
- proflavanols

- pycnogenols
- raw thymus gland
- vitamin A
- vitamin C, 4,000–8,000 mg a day (only use 1,000 mg at a time – space out the doses through the day)
- vitamin B
- vitamin E
- zinc 80 to 100 mg a day

**

- Air purifiers are helpful.
- Drink plenty of liquids to flush the system and use 'green drinks' that contain chlorophyll. Green Magic is a good choice.
- Humidifiers in the room help.
- To prevent and help pneumonia, you can use Echinacea.

POLIO

Types

Polio is a viral illness that in about 95 percent of cases actually produces no symptoms at all (called asymptomatic polio). In the cases in which there are symptoms (called symptomatic polio), the illness appears in three forms:

- a mild form called abortive polio
- a more serious form associated with aseptic meningitis called non-paralytic polio
- a severe, debilitating form called paralytic polio (this occurs in 0.1 percent to 2 percent of cases)

People who have abortive polio or non-paralytic polio usually make a full recovery. However, paralytic polio, as its name implies, causes muscle paralysis and can even result in death. In paralytic polio, the virus leaves the intestinal tract and enters the bloodstream, attacking the nerves (in abortive or asymptomatic polio, the virus usually doesn't get past the intestinal tract). The virus may affect the nerves governing the muscles in the limbs and the muscles necessary for breathing, causing respiratory difficulty and paralysis of the arms and legs.

Intuitive Remedies

Once your body knows how to fight polio, you can carry polio and survive.

As you get older, post-polio syndrome can manifest in the body. This is devastating and actually shrivels people up. One way to prevent it from happening is to ask the Creator to change the marker for polio in the body. Remember, this is *change* and not *pull* the marker, because you still need the antibodies.

I know people who have survived polio and have never developed post-polio syndrome. They don't have the marker. They have cleared their body completely.

I also know people who were given the 'sugar pill' (which was the first inoculation for polio) who have post-polio syndrome. When the antidote for polio first came out, they made a lot of sugar cubes. The first batch had more virus in it and so some people who took it are now going through post-polio syndrome. It's being misdiagnosed as a strange form of muscular dystrophy.

For polio, use the basic healing.

POLYPS

In conventional medicine, a polyp is a growth projecting from the wall of a cavity lined with a mucous membrane. The most common locations of polyps in the human body are the nose, the urinary bladder and the gastrointestinal tract, especially the rectum and colon. Women with diabetes have a higher than normal chance of developing polyps.

Usually, polyps are simple, benign growths, but a small percentage can be precursors to cancers or may actually contain cancers. For that reason, it is advisable, when possible, to have all polyps removed and examined microscopically.

Types

A polyp may have a broad base, in which case it is called sessile, or it may be a pedunculated polyp, i.e., one with a long narrow neck.

The surface of a polyp may be smooth, irregular or multilobular.

Symptoms

Symptoms of polyps depend upon their location and size. There may be no symptoms, or there may be symptoms resulting from pressure or from mechanical obstruction of all or part of a channel, such as that of the nose or the bowel.

Polyps may occasionally bleed.

Causes

The causes of polyps are allergies, cancer, parasites and smoking.

Intuitive Insights

Intestinal polyps respond very well to healings, whereas nasal polyps respond well to vitamin C therapy.

Supplements and Other Nutritional Recommendations

- *Aloe vera* juice
- calcium–magnesium
- cayenne pepper
- garlic
- green tea
- mustard seed
- vitamin A to protect the membranes
- vitamin E, but start slowly at 400 IUs and increase to 600 IUs

***

- A diet high in fibre can help.
- Alcohol and caffeine will irritate polyps.
- High doses of vitamin C (5,000–10,000 mg daily) can reduce or eliminate polyps.
- Increase water intake.
- Live foods, fresh fruit and vegetables are beneficial.

PREGNANCY-RELATED PROBLEMS

Most of the discomforts that occur during pregnancy are the result of nutritional deficiencies and profound anatomical changes. These include haemorrhoids, heartburn, insomnia, leg cramps, oedema (swelling of the hands and feet) and wind, also:

Anaemia

Anaemia occurs because there is a decrease in the proportion of red blood cells in the blood and also a decrease of the proportion of haemoglobin during pregnancy. The result can be anaemia. It is most likely to develop in the second trimester of pregnancy. It is unlikely to affect the developing baby. It is the fetus that depletes the mother's resources of iron.

Asthma

Many women who have asthma reduce their use of asthma medication when they become pregnant. As a result, their asthma symptoms become worse. It has been found, however, that there is more danger to the developing fetus from frequent asthma attacks than from the mother taking the asthma medication. Women with asthma who are pregnant should discuss their medication with their doctor and avoid anything that might trigger an asthma attack. Air purifiers in the home are a good way of relieving the air of viruses, bacteria and moulds.

Backache

Backache is common during pregnancy because of the anatomical changes and stresses on the body. Recommendations:

- Be sure your mattress is firm enough to support you and sleep with a pillow supporting your back.
- Do not wear high-heeled shoes.
- Include two to three minutes of gentle stretching exercises a day.
- Learn how to lift correctly.
- Swimming is a good way to relieve the strain on the back and on other parts of the body.

Bladder Discomfort

During pregnancy, the expanding uterus presses upon the bladder. This can result in the bladder not emptying completely. This is why infections of the bladder are very common at this time. To avoid this:

- Avoid sugary foods.
- Do not douche.
- Eat natural yogurt every day.
- Increase fluid intake.
- Wear cotton underwear.

Colds

Coughs and colds are more common during pregnancy. Once a pregnant woman has a cold, there is little she can do but let it run its course. She should never use cold and cough medication.

Depression

Because of shifting hormone levels, it is not uncommon to experience at least one bout of depression during the 40 weeks of pregnancy. Mood swings are common and it is not unusual to be more emotional and volatile during pregnancy.

The effect of antidepressants on the foetus are well known. A woman should talk to her doctor about taking antidepressants when pregnant.

Try the following:

- Acupuncture can be useful in treating depression.
- Do not isolate yourself if you begin to feel depressed; have someone to talk to about your feelings.
- Exercise can help lessen depression.

Ectopic Pregnancy

An ectopic pregnancy is also called a tubular pregnancy. It occurs when a fertilized egg becomes implanted in the Fallopian tube instead of the uterus. This can happen if the Fallopian tube is blocked because of endometriosis, inflammation and scar tissue. If you see an ectopic pregnancy in a reading, you should do a healing immediately and send the woman to the doctor.

Gestational Diabetes

Gestational diabetes occurs only during pregnancy. It affects 3 to 5 percent of women. It occurs because insulin does not work as effectively during pregnancy because of hormones secreted by the placenta. It can cause a woman to develop diabetes later on in life.

Symptoms of gestational diabetes may include excessive thirst, frequent urination and increased fatigue. There may be no symptoms at all.

This disorder responds very well to healing because it is caused by an imbalance in the body and not by emotions. There may be an instant healing.

Miscarriage

Spontaneous abortion is the technical term for a miscarriage. It is defined as the loss of a pregnancy before 20 weeks. The most likely reason is a chromosomal abnormality in the fetus that makes it unlikely that it will survive. Other reasons include cervical incompetence, diabetes, ectopic pregnancy, glandular disorders, infection and pregnancy-induced hypertension. Miscarriages are generally not caused by exercise, falls or sexual activity.

In many instances I have anticipated a miscarriage before it has happened. It is possible to do a healing that will stop it. However, this may be dependent on the choice of the baby. It may be that the baby does not want to stay.

Supplements

The kinds of supplements that a pregnant woman can use are limited:

- Alfalfa is a good source of vitamins and minerals, especially vitamin K.
- Blue cohosh, false unicorn and squaw vine are beneficial in the last four weeks of pregnancy, but should not be used in the beginning.
- Burdock root, dandelion, ginger and nettle help to enrich the mother's milk.
- Red raspberry leaf tea helps the uterus contract more effectively. It also helps to enrich mother's milk.
- Stinging nettle is also a good source of vitamins and minerals.

Herbs to Avoid
Avoid the following herbs in pregnancy:

- *Aloe vera*
- angelica
- Arnica
- barberry
- black cohosh
- blood root
- cat's claw
- celandine
- cottonwood bark
- dong quai

- Ephedra
- feverfew
- ginseng
- goldenseal
- lobelia
- myrrh
- Oregon grape
- pennyroyal
- rue
- sage
- saw palmetto
- tansy
- turmeric

Use any herbs with caution, especially in the first 12 weeks.

Other Substances to Avoid
- Avoid the sweetener NutraSweet, as it contains high levels of D. phenylalanine.
- Avoid taking any kind of shark cartilage.
- Do not use castor oil to start a delivery. Castor oil is a volatile substance!
- Do not use mineral oil. It blocks the absorption of vitamins.

The following substances can cause birth defects:

- Certain ACE inhibitors.
- Certain acne medications
- Certain antibiotics, e.g., ampicillin and tetracycline
- Certain blood-thinning medications.
- Certain cancer drugs.
- Certain hormone preparations.
- Certain thyroid treatment drugs.
- Chronic alcohol intake.
- Cocaine.

- Dilantin (used to control epileptic seizures) creates four times the risk of producing a baby with heart defects.

- The excessive intake of vitamin E has been linked with cleft palate, heart defects and other congenital defects.

Concerns

Folic acid, manganese and zinc deficiencies and amino-acid imbalances have been linked to fetal deformities and retardation. All women who are thinking of becoming pregnant should take a daily supplement of folic acid and vitamin B complex.

Both partners should give up alcohol, tobacco and illicit drugs at least three to six months before they decide to conceive. Marijuana, heroin, morphine and tobacco all reduce levels of male sex hormones and increase the risk of birth defects.

Men should take adequate amounts of selenium, zinc, vitamin C and vitamin E.

For a healthy pregnancy and birth, it is necessary to consult a qualified healthcare professional.

PROSTATITIS

Prostatitis is the inflammation or infection of the prostate gland. It can cause a variety of symptoms, including a frequent and urgent need to urinate and pain or burning when urinating, often accompanied by groin, lower back or pelvic pain. It can be difficult to diagnose, in part because its signs and symptoms often resemble those of other conditions, such as bladder infections, bladder cancer or prostate enlargement due to benign or cancerous growth.

Types

Prostatitis is classified by the National Institute of Health (NIH) into four types.

Type 1 is acute bacterial prostatitis.

Type 2 is chronic bacterial prostatitis.

Type 3 includes the conditions previously known as non-bacterial prostatitis, prostatodynia and chronic pelvic pain syndrome.

Type 4 is asymptomatic inflammatory prostatitis.

Pain-relievers and several weeks of treatment with antibiotics are typically needed for Type 1 and 2 prostatitis, which are bacterial infections.

Treatment for Type 3 prostatitis (non-bacterial) is less clear and mainly involves relieving symptoms.

Type 4 prostatitis is usually found during examination for another reason and often doesn't require treatment.

Symptoms

The symptoms vary, depending on the type of prostatitis.

Type 1: Acute Bacterial Prostatitis
Symptoms of this form of prostatitis usually come on suddenly and may include:

- fever and chills
- flu-like symptoms
- pain in the prostate gland, lower back or groin
- painful ejaculation
- urinary problems, including increased urinary urgency and frequency, difficulty or pain when urinating, inability to empty the bladder and blood-tinged urine

Type 2: Chronic Bacterial Prostatitis
The symptoms of this type of prostatitis develop more slowly and usually aren't as severe as those of acute prostatitis. In addition, they have a tendency to wax and wane in severity. They include:

- a frequent and urgent need to urinate
- a slight fever
- difficulty starting to urinate or diminished urine flow
- excessive urination during the night
- occasional blood in semen or in urine
- pain in the lower back and genital area
- pain in the pelvic area
- pain or a burning sensation when urinating
- painful ejaculation
- recurring bladder infections

Type 3: Chronic Non-Bacterial Prostatitis
The symptoms of non-bacterial prostatitis are similar to those of chronic bacterial prostatitis, although there may not be a fever. The only way to determine whether prostatitis symptoms are caused by bacterial infection or are non-bacterial is through lab tests to find out whether bacteria are present in the urine or prostate gland fluid.

Belief Work

Most issues are with relationships, so download:

'I know how to express myself in relationships.'

'I know how to feel good about myself.'

'I know when to fight for who I am.'

'I can change my life.'

'I love myself.'

'I know what it feels like to be completely loved.'

'I know what it feels like to change my life.'

'I know how to express myself in relationships.'

'I know how to feel good about myself.'

'I know when to fight for who I am.'

Supplements

* Echinacea
* glutathione
* olive-leaf extract
* omega 3s, 6s and 9s
* regular exercise

***

* Chelated zinc deficiency is linked to enlargement of the prostate, so zinc supplements should be an option.
* Horsetail is astringent and can be used for prostate enlargement in small amounts.
* Saw palmetto has been used to treat prostate enlargement and inflammation, painful ejaculation, difficult urination and enuresis.

It reduces prostatic enlargement by reducing the amount of hormonal stimulation of the prostate gland.

- Siberian ginseng is a tonic for the male reproductive organs.
- Stinging nettle is good for the prostate.

PSORIASIS

Psoriasis is an inflammatory skin condition. It usually causes some discomfort. The skin often itches and may crack and bleed. In severe cases, the itching and discomfort may keep a person from sleeping and the pain can make everyday life difficult.

Psoriasis is a chronic condition because there is currently no medical cure. People often experience flare-ups and remissions throughout their life. Controlling the signs and symptoms can require lifelong conventional therapy.

Psoriasis occurs equally in men and women. Recent studies show that there may be an ethnic link. Psoriasis is most common in Scandinavia and in northern Europe. It appears to be far less common among Asians and is rare in Native Americans.

There also is a genetic component with psoriasis. Approximately one third of people who develop it have at least one family member with the condition.

Research shows that psoriasis usually appears between 15 and 35 years of age, but it is possible to develop it at any age. After the age of 40, a peak onset period occurs between 50 and 60 years of age. About 1 in 10 people develop psoriasis during childhood and it can begin in infancy. The earlier it appears, the more likely it is to be widespread and recurrent.

Types

There are five types of psoriasis, each with their own symptoms:

- *Erythrodermic psoriasis* is typified by widespread redness, severe itching and pain.
- *Guttate psoriasis* is typified by small red spots on the skin.
- *Inverse psoriasis* is typified by smooth red lesions that form in skin folds.
- *Plaque psoriasis* is the most common type of psoriasis. About 80 percent of people who develop psoriasis have this kind, which appears

as patches of raised reddish skin covered by silvery-white scale. These patches, or plaques, frequently form on the elbows, knees, lower back and scalp. They can occur anywhere on the body.

- *Pustular psoriasis* is typified by white pustules surrounded by red skin.

Psoriatic Arthritis

Between 10 percent and 30 percent of people who develop psoriasis get a related form of arthritis called psoriatic arthritis, which causes inflammation of the joints.

This usually first appears between 30 and 50 years of age, often months to years after skin lesions first occur. However, not everyone who develops psoriatic arthritis has psoriasis. About 30 percent of people who get psoriatic arthritis never develop the skin condition.

Causes

Scientists still do not fully know what causes psoriasis, but research has appreciably advanced our understanding of it. One important breakthrough began with the discovery that kidney-transplant recipients who had psoriasis found it cleared up when they were taking cyclosporine. Cyclosporine is a potent immunosuppressive medication and this indicates that the immune system is involved. The condition may be caused by faulty signals in the body's immune system.

It is believed that psoriasis develops when the immune system tells the body to over-react and accelerate the growth of skin cells. Normally, skin cells mature and are shed from the skin's surface every 28 to 30 days. When psoriasis develops, the skin cells mature in three to six days and move to the skin surface. Instead of being shed, they pile up, causing the visible lesions.

Researchers have identified genes that can cause psoriasis or another immune-mediated condition, such as rheumatoid arthritis or Type 1 diabetes. The risk of developing psoriasis or another immune-mediated condition, especially diabetes or Crohn's disease, increases when a close blood relative has psoriasis.

The skin is the largest organ in the body and it eliminates an incredible number of toxins through perspiration. This is why it is imperative that the liver stays clean.

Research indicates that a trigger is needed for psoriasis to develop. Alcohol and drug abuse, skin injuries, strep infection, stress and sunburn are some of the known potential triggers. Certain forms of medication can trigger psoriasis, including anti-malarial drugs, beta-blockers and lithium.

Conventional Treatment

Treatment depends on the severity and type of psoriasis. Some psoriasis is so mild that the person is unaware of the condition, while a few people develop such severe psoriasis that lesions cover most of the body and hospitalization is required. These represent the extremes. Most cases fall somewhere in between.

- A systemic medication is a prescription medication that affects the entire body and is usually reserved for patients with moderate to severe psoriasis.
- Phototherapy (UVB, PUVA and lasers) involves exposing the skin to wavelengths of ultraviolet light under medical supervision.
- Topical treatments – agents applied to the skin – are usually the first line of defence in treating psoriasis.

Many people choose to treat their psoriasis in non-traditional ways, including dietary supplements, mind and body therapies, and sunlight.

Intuitive Remedies

When I work on psoriasis, I make the changes on a genetic level because I believe that psoriasis is caused by a miasm (*see Prologue*).

So, go back in time to eliminate it and bring that healing into the present.

Belief Work

Belief systems associated with the skin all have to do with beauty. Energy test for:

'People don't like me because I'm different.'

'I have to hide.'

Download:

'I know what it feels like to be beautiful.'

Supplements

If the liver is clean, the skin is also clean. I work with psoriasis as though it were a fungus and suggest a person uses ALA in suggested doses of 600 mg moving up to 900 to 1,500 mg a day for about three or four months, along with omega 3s, 6s and 9s, and it seems to clear the body up quickly.

Vitamin B complex, vitamin C and vitamin E can also clear up psoriasis. Other helpful herbs and supplements:

- amino-acid complexes
- blood purifiers such as Echinacea and red clover
- coal tar and black walnut salve applied topically
- coffee enemas and liver cleanses
- folic acid
- fungi cleanses for three months and vitamin D ointment
- Lecithin
- milk thistle for clearing the liver
- noni
- sarsaparilla
- selenium
- Sibu berry juice
- vitamin B6

RENAL FAILURE

See Kidney Disease.

THE REPRODUCTIVE SYSTEM/SEXUAL SYSTEM

The major function of the reproductive system is to ensure the survival of the species. An individual may live a happy life without producing offspring, but if the species is to continue at least some individuals must reproduce.

The reproductive system has four functions within the paradigm of reproduction:

1. The production of egg and sperm cells.

2. The transportation and continuance of these cells.

3. The nurturing and the development of offspring.

4. The production of hormones.

These functions are divided between the primary and secondary reproductive organs:

*   *The primary reproductive organs*, or gonads, consist of the ovaries and testes. These organs are responsible for producing the egg and sperm cells and hormones.
*   All other organs, ducts and glands in the reproductive system are considered *secondary reproductive organs*.

Belief Work

Abundance flows best when the first and the second chakras are open and negative programmes are cleared from these areas. Programmes held in this area of the body can stem from old stored anger or sexual abuse. Sexual abuse is registered any time anything is said to a child that diminishes them and their esteem.

When you clear those chakras, you will have more abundance and the pelvic floor muscles will become tighter in women. There might also be issues from childbirth and being on this Earth. Those beliefs will be different depending on the person's cultural background.

The issues may also be ones of intimacy. Some people think that if you do not have sex all the time you are not loved and you are not intimate.

Check to see if a divorced person feels free of any commitment to a prior mate.

Download:

'I know the Creator's definition of and perspective on what it feels like to be intimate.'

I know the Creator's definition of and perspective on what it feels like to be nurtured.'

'I know the Creator's definition of and perspective on what it feels like to be listened to completely.'

'I know the Creator's definition of and perspective on what it feels like to listen to my mate completely.'

'I have the Creator's definition of intimacy.'

'I know what it feels like to live my daily life without being victimized.'

'I have the Creator's definition of what it feels like to receive and accept love from a mate.'

'It's OK to feel sexual, sensual and sexy and still have good discernment.'

'I have the Creator's definition of what it feels like to enjoy sex with my mate.'

'I can receive and accept sexual love.'

'It's OK to be sexy.'

'It's OK to have sex and be spiritual.'

'I know what it feels like to live without being married to God.'

'I know what it feels like to live without my previous marriage.'

'I know and understand my partner completely.'

'I know what it feels like to live without it being my duty to have sex.'

'I know what it feels like to live without having to be a sacrifice.'

'It's OK to enjoy sex.'

'I know what it feels like to live without perceiving sex as dirty.'

'I know how to live without the fear of sex in the dark or in any other environment.'

'It's OK to show sexual emotion.'

'It's OK to be sensual.'

'I know what it feels like to live without being embarrassed about sex.'

'I respect my body.'

'It's OK to be in my body.'

'It's OK to be a girl or a boy.'

'I know how to be present in a relationship.'

'I know what it feels like to live without having sex all the time.'

'I know what it feels like to live without sex being my duty.'

'It's OK to show emotions during sex.'

'I know how to live without guilt.'

THE RESPIRATORY SYSTEM

When you are doing a body scan, listen to the songs the organs sing to each other, similar to the tones from a harp. Observe the lungs laugh and giggle with the joy of existence. The lungs are full of joy as they gather the pure life force of the air and convert oxygen into energy.

There are three molecules that we carry with us in all of our embodiments: one master cell in the brain, one in the heart and one at the base of spine. When we breathe, we activate and connect all three.

Any sickness associated with the lungs has to do with sorrow, pain and fear. Fear often breeds sorrow. When someone comes to you with problems in the respiratory system, talk to them to find out how you can help them to release some of the grief.

Intuitive Remedies

One thing that physically affects the lungs probably more than anything is a lack of water. This can cause major problems in the lung area and contribute to a person being asthmatic. Make sure you suggest that a person with lung problems uses enough water to hydrate themselves. Unfortunately, some of the water that we drink will not hydrate us, since its molecular structure is changed as it travels through our plumbing. This is caused by the water spinning in the wrong direction as it goes through the plumbing.

To counter this effect, hold a glass of water in your hands before you drink it and see the molecules move in a different direction. This will allow you to absorb the water with less difficulty.

Belief Work

You may not be able to completely change a person's sorrow, but you can pull out the programme that they have to have grief and that love hurts. Changing these things in their lungs will change their life immediately.

Download:

'I know what it feels like to live without being a victim.'

'I have the Creator's definition of what it is to cry.'

'I know what it feels like to live without regret.'

'I know what the Creator's definition of forgiveness feels like.'

'I know how to live in joy.'

Also acknowledge that you have compassion for the people you work with without taking on and storing their pain and sadness. Test yourself for 'It's OK to cry if I want to' and 'I know what compassion feels like.'

See also Asthma.

REYE'S SYNDROME

Reye's syndrome (RS) is chiefly a children's disease, although it can occur at any age. It affects all the organs of the body but is most harmful to the brain and the liver, the outcome of which is an acute increase of pressure within the brain. Often there are substantial accumulations of fat in the liver and other organs as well.

Symptoms

RS is defined as a two-phase illness because it generally occurs in conjunction with a viral infection, such as the flu or chicken pox. The disease commonly occurs during recovery from a viral infection, although it can also develop three to five days after the onset of the viral illness. It is often misdiagnosed as diabetes, drug overdose, encephalitis, meningitis, poisoning, psychiatric illness or sudden infant death syndrome.

Symptoms of RS include:

- convulsions
- delirium
- disorientation or confusion
- listlessness
- loss of consciousness
- persistent or recurrent vomiting
- personality changes such as irritability or combativeness

If these symptoms are present during or soon after a viral illness, medical attention should be sought immediately.

The symptoms of RS in infants do not follow a typical pattern. For example, vomiting does not always occur.

Causes

The cause of RS remains a mystery. However, studies have shown that using aspirin or salicylate-containing medication to treat viral illnesses increases the risk of developing it. A doctor should be consulted before giving a child any aspirin or anti-nausea medicines during a viral illness, which can mask the symptoms of RS.

Conventional Treatment

There is no known medical cure for RS. Successful management depends on early diagnosis and is primarily aimed at protecting the brain against irreversible damage by reducing brain swelling, reversing the metabolic injury, preventing complications in the lungs and anticipating cardiac arrest.

Recovery from RS is directly related to the severity of the swelling of the brain. Some people recover completely, while others may sustain varying degrees of brain damage. Those cases in which the disorder progresses rapidly and the patient lapses into a coma have a poorer prognosis than those with a less severe course.

Statistics indicate that when RS is diagnosed and treated in its early stages, the chances of recovery are excellent. When diagnosis and treatment are delayed, the chances are severely reduced. Death is common, often within a few days.

Intuitive Remedies

RS reacts well to a simple healing. Go up and say to the Creator, *'Change this and show me.'*

Generally there are no belief systems to work on, because children do not have that many.

Supplements

It is very important to be careful when giving a child supplements. Be certain that the child is on the way to recovery before you consider any supplementation. Discuss any supplements with a healthcare professional before using them.

RHEUMATIC FEVER

Rheumatic fever is a serious inflammatory condition that can affect many parts of the body, including the heart, joints, nervous system and skin. Although it can occur at any age, it most frequently occurs in children between the ages of 6 and 15 years. It is twice as common in boys as it is in girls.

Symptoms of rheumatic fever generally appear within five weeks after an untreated streptococcal (strep throat) infection. Only a small percentage of people with strep throat develop rheumatic fever.

In many cases, rheumatic fever affects the heart valves and interferes with normal blood flow through the heart.

There is no known medical cure for rheumatic fever, but it can be prevented by prompt and thorough treatment of a strep throat infection with antibiotics.

Rheumatic fever is not as common in the West today as it was before the widespread use of penicillin, though outbreaks do occur periodically. It is still common in developing countries.

Symptoms

Common symptoms of a strep infection include:

- fever
- headache

- muscle aches
- red and swollen tonsils
- sore throat

Symptoms of rheumatic fever include a combination of:

- chest pain
- fatigue
- painful swollen joints
- shortness of breath

In diagnosing rheumatic fever, doctors generally look for the presence of either two of the following major criteria or one major plus two minor criteria. In all cases, evidence of a preceding strep throat infection is key to making a diagnosis of rheumatic fever.

Major Criteria
- broad pink or faint-red non-itching patches on the skin (uncommon)
- inflammation of the heart, sometimes indicated by weakness and shortness of breath or chest pain
- involuntary jerky movements of the limbs and face or more slight movement difficulties, such as deterioration in handwriting, which usually disappear over several weeks
- lumps under the skin (uncommon)
- painful arthritis, most often affecting the ankles, elbows, knees and wrists, and often migrating from joint to joint

Minor Criteria
- a blood test indicating inflammation
- abnormal heartbeat on an electrocardiogram
- fever
- joint pain without inflammation
- new heart murmurs
- previous rheumatic fever or evidence of rheumatic heart disease

Causes

The exact causes of rheumatic fever are not clear. In a few people, it seems that when the body fights a strep throat infection, other parts of the body develop inflammation. For example, the heart valves are not necessarily infected with the streptococcal bacteria, but they can be injured or inflamed as the body fights strep throat.

Medical research has focused on an abnormal immune system response to the antigens produced by specific types of streptococcal bacteria. One possible cause for this is the similarities between streptococcal antigens and heart valve proteins and heart muscle cells. In addition, researchers are studying whether some people have a greater genetic disposition for an abnormal immune system response to streptococcal antigens.

Intuitive Remedies

Most of the time I do not work with people when they have rheumatic fever but after they have had it. It is the problems caused by the disease that I work with. These are generally arthritis, heart arrhythmias (and other problems with the heart), kidney problems and skin problems.

You have to go back into the past to find out what was happening when the person first contracted the disease. Talk to them about the emotions that were going on at that time (if they can remember). Use belief work to follow the trail to the bottom issues.

If the person can't remember the past, go back in time and witness as the Creator does a healing on the disease. Then bring the energy of healing back to the present. This has a tendency to relieve the overall symptoms.

Supplements

It is very important to be careful when giving a child supplements. Be certain that the child is on the way to recovery before you consider any supplementation. Discuss any supplements with a healthcare professional before using them.

If the person is over 18 years old, I suggest:

- ALA
- amino acids
- chondroitin sulphate for the joints
- omega 3s, 6s and 9s
- vitamin C

RICKETS

See Osteomalacia.

S

SALMONELLA

Salmonella isn't food poisoning, but a live bacterium. It is found wherever animals live. It can withstand hot and cold weather, even rain and drought. During slaughtering and processing, it may contaminate animal carcasses.

In recent years, fresh fruit and vegetables, for example, tomatoes and cantaloupes, have been implicated in outbreaks of salmonellosis. Investigations of these incidents did not identify the source of contamination. It could have occurred in the fields where the produce was grown, during processing after harvest or during handling in the distribution system.

Person-to-person transmission occurs when a carrier's feces, unwashed from their hands, contaminate food during preparation or through direct contact with another person. Usually the illness comes from animal feces found on or in raw meat, eggs, fish, shellfish and, most commonly, poultry.

Symptoms

Salmonella can make you so ill that you can bleed intestinally. Symptoms include:

- chills
- dehydration
- diarrhoea
- fever
- headache
- muscle aches
- nausea
- vomiting

Intuitive Insights

The first healings that I did to stop *Salmonella* were a bit harsh. I would go up and make the command: *'Creator, heal this and show me what has to be done. Get rid of this right now.'* This caused the person to throw up off and on for 30 or 40 minutes and then they felt better. Over time these healings became instantaneous.

If a person has *Salmonella* and they are not open to healings, use this little short cut: give them thyme. *Salmonella* dies at the first stroke of thyme. So, you may want to take Listerine with you when you travel, because it has thyme in it. You may not be able to take certain herbs with you when you go to other countries because of custom restrictions, but if you can, travel with thyme.

Intuitive Remedies

Use the healing, *'Creator, change this and show me.'*

If healing is not instant, give the person a tablespoon of Listerine, then another in one hour and another in about two hours.

SAUDI SYNDROME

I believe that people serving in the first Gulf War (in Kuwait) were injected with anthrax and exposed to radiation and all sorts of toxins, which resulted in Saudi syndrome, or Gulf War syndrome, as it is also known. Partners can also be exposed to this through semen.

Intuitive Insights

This syndrome shows up as greyish energy in the body.

Intuitive Remedies

Witness the toxins being pulled from the body and sent to the Creator's light. Use belief work to find the emotions and beliefs at the time of exposure.

Supplements and Other Nutritional Recommendations

- Aqua Chi foot bath soaks are recommended.
- Do liver cleanses (*see the Liver*).
- Sit in a sauna for an hour a day to relieve the body of toxins.
- Take alpha-lipoic acid (1,200–1,600 mg), selenium and zinc.

SCABIES

Scabies is an infestation by the mite *Sarcoptes scabiei*. Mites are small eight-legged parasites. They are tiny, and burrow into the skin to produce intense itching, which tends to be worse at night. The mites that cause scabies are not visible to the naked eye but can be seen with a magnifying glass or microscope.

Scabies mites are very sensitive to their surroundings. They can only live off a host body for 24 to 36 hours under most conditions. Transmission of the mites involves close person-to-person contact of the skin-to-skin variety. It is hard, if not impossible, to catch scabies by shaking hands, hanging your coat next to someone who has it, or even sharing bedclothes that had mites in them the night before. The physical contact required to contract scabies may be sexual. This is the most common form of transmission among sexually active young people. However, other forms of physical contact, such as mothers hugging their children, are enough to spread the mites. Over time, close friends and relatives can contract them this way too. School settings typically do not provide the level of close personal contact necessary for transmission of the mites.

Diagnosis of scabies is usually through a scraping of skin taken by a doctor that is then examined under a microscope.

When the rash first appears you may see fine wavy lines emanating from some of the lumps if they are observed closely. These can become dry and begin itching, especially at night. The rash seems to affect the armpits, buttocks, genitals and nipples in particular, as well as the skin between the toes and fingers.

Scabicides are commonly prescribed but are not recommended for children under the age of six or for pregnant women. In such cases a mild solution applied to the hair is usually recommended.

Calendula salve, cold compresses and cool oatmeal baths are natural alternatives to alleviate the swelling and itching.

Herbal Remedies

- *Aloe vera* has excellent healing properties. Apply the gel topically to the affected area as directed on the product label.
- Comfrey applied topically to the skin can help scabies.
- Foods high in zinc can be helpful.
- Melaleuca oil applied topically to the affected area can help as well. However, be careful with it in more sensitive places such as the groin and nipples and avoid putting it directly on open wounds, as it will burn.

SCARS

People will sometimes tell me that they don't like a certain scar on their body. I know that if they put vitamin E on it and use a little extra selenium, it is likely to fade.

It is interesting how people will become compulsive about a scar and do all they can to make it disappear. This is because it's the incident that created the scar that they are really trying to get rid of.

I go into the tissue and witness the scar being healed through the Creator of All That Is and use the belief work on the emotions and beliefs at the time that the scar was created.

When healings are done on a scar, the client must understand that it can take three months or so for all the skin layers to heal completely and the scar to disappear.

SCHIZOPHRENIA

At one time a woman with schizophrenia would come into my office trying to get a reading from me. She had developed a fascination with me, even though I had never met her before and had never spoken to her. She began to believe that I was her best friend and that she talked to me at night in her sleep. She would constantly write me letters, telling me that she believed the end of the world was coming and certain people were after her. She would write letters to another person, too, a man she was obsessed with. One day he came to my office to find out why she was after him. Apparently she had told him that I was her best friend. She would tell him in these letters that he was her boyfriend, but he told me he had never met her. You can imagine how surprised we both were when we discovered that neither of us knew her. These kind of delusional episodes are typical of schizophrenia.

Schizophrenia is a chronic, severe and disabling brain disorder that has been recognized throughout recorded history. People with schizophrenia may hear voices other people do not hear or may believe that others are reading their minds, controlling their thoughts or plotting to harm them. These experiences are terrifying and can cause fearfulness, withdrawal or extreme agitation. People with schizophrenia may not make sense when they talk, may sit for hours without moving or talking much, or may seem perfectly fine until they talk about what they are really thinking. Because many people with schizophrenia have difficulty holding a job or caring for themselves, the burden on their families and society is significant.

Available treatments can relieve many of the disorder's symptoms, but most people who have schizophrenia must cope with some residual symptoms as long as they live. Nevertheless, this is a time of hope for people with schizophrenia and their families. Researchers are developing more effective forms of medication and using new research tools to understand the causes of schizophrenia and find ways to prevent and treat it, and many people with the disorder now lead rewarding and meaningful lives in their communities.

Types

There are four basic types of schizophrenia:

- *Catatonic schizophrenia* is characterized by unusual postures and frenzied movement.

- *Disorganized schizophrenia* is characterized by a lack of normal regular motion, along with speech that displays a disorganized way of thinking.

- *Paranoid schizophrenia* is characterized by hallucinatory and delusional symptoms.

- *Undifferentiated schizophrenia* involves a mixture of symptoms.

Causes

The underlying cause of schizophrenia is not known. There are many theories, and some researchers believe that schizophrenia is hereditary. There is indeed evidence that in some cases it is the result of an inherited defect in body chemistry.

Others theorize that schizophrenia results from external factors such as complications during birth, a head injury, a reaction to a virus or environmental poisoning that damages the brain.

Yet another theory focuses on nutritional factors. There is some indication that schizophrenia may be associated with high copper levels in body tissues. Zinc deficiency may result in damage to the pineal gland and this can make an individual vulnerable to schizophrenia and other psychoses.

In general, men appear more likely to have schizophrenia than women. This may be due to the hormone oestrogen, which may protect the brain in women.

The levels of and balance between the neurotransmitters dopamine, epinephrine, norepinephrine and serotonin and the way in which the brain responds to these substances are thought to play a profound role in the development of schizophrenia.

Intuitive Insights

I believe that schizophrenia is caused by a virus about 50 percent of the time. This causes an energetic separation in the cerebrum, which makes a division in the brain and results in a person with two personalities and no filters between the imagination, the intuitive information that comes into the brain from the outside and the unfiltered information from the unconscious mind.

Schizophrenia can also be an inherited condition and due to the abuse of hallucinogenic drugs.

Additionally, it can be caused by too much dopamine being released in the brain.

Usually, with schizophrenia the clients don't find you. It is their mother, sister or aunt who drags them to you. To show the difference between schizophrenia and other forms of mental problems, a person with multiple personality disorder wants to change things and make things better. The schizophrenic, on the other hand, is usually quite happy being where and who they are. But they will have at least two distinct personalities, so you have to know which one you are dealing with. People who want to be healed from schizophrenia have to come on their own. Then you know they do want to be healed.

There are many things that can trigger a schizophrenic episode and one of them is drug use. People with schizophrenia have to be very careful with drugs or alcohol. For instance, a (married) lady in my area had the delusion that she was supposed to go off and marry Bruce Willis. She believed he was watching her, waiting to seize the moment! She saw him incognito, dressed up in disguise, coming in to see her as a customer when she was a waitress. She believed that when they were married, Danny De Vito and Arnold Schwarzenegger would come and sweep her up so that they could all build a school together. This school would be the last safe place on Earth and everything else would be destroyed! For many years, she actually believed this was going to happen. She believed her husband was going to die so that she could be with these people. I asked the Creator what would help her, and I was told that she should stop smoking marijuana. It is my belief that it was the marijuana use that was triggering her schizophrenic episodes.

The problem with delusions is that they can become dangerous. That woman might have put poison in the sugar bowl, for instance, to hasten her husband's demise.

Intuitive Remedies

Most of the time people with schizophrenia don't want to be healed. However, I have had good results with people who do want to be healed.

There are always waywards present, and it may seem that there are two or more spirits fighting for supremacy over the body. People who are on medication for schizophrenia have a tendency to pull wayward energy to them. When I work on schizophrenics, I sometimes see up to two or three different spirits inside them. Sometimes you can work on the person by commanding the spirits to leave their body. They will fight with you and say that there is an agreement between them and that they are supposed to share the same body. You need to ask the Creator if this is true, because usually it's not. Once the spirits have gone, the person will return to normal.

To heal schizophrenia, intuitively go into the brain to see if it is starting to separate. Connect to the Creator and witness the two halves of the brain coming together to work in harmony. Balance the brain chemicals. Balance the dopamine levels. Ask the Creator what is right for the person. Send any waywards to God's light.

To help a person with schizophrenia to heal themselves, have them visualize their consciousness moving over to the right side of the skull. This will stop the voices and restart the brain.

Do not take them off their medication. There is a reason why they are on it, and you can make them very ill if they discontinue it all at once. But if they begin to respond to the healings, work with a doctor who can lower their medication a little bit at a time. People with mental disorders such as schizophrenia use powerful drugs such as thorazine. These would cause harm to a normal person if they used them.

Belief and Feeling Work

You have to be very patient and persistent with this disorder. Make sure the person knows what it feels like to feel safe and how to keep control of their own space.

You have to realize that if they didn't come to you to be helped of their own accord, they are going to sit there and play with you. They are intelligent and they love to play head games. Don't buy into these games during a belief work session. They'll just make you go round in circles and they'll love it. They have learned how to manipulate people and this is part of the disorder.

Nevertheless, you need to do all the belief work that they will allow. If they won't allow it, don't put yourself in any physical danger by pushing them too hard! And remember that you still have to have their permission before you can work on them.

Schizophrenia can be complicated, and it is sometimes better to ask the Creator what feelings the person needs.

Download:

'I know the difference between my thoughts and those that are invading my head.' (If this applies to your client.)

'My mind is my own.'

'I know what the Creator feels like.'

'I know the difference between the energy of the Creator and any negative energies that surround me.'

'I know what it feels like to live without being paranoid.'

'My body gets stronger every day.'

'Every thought that I have is my own.'

'I know how to live without fighting my own thoughts.'

'Nothing can take over my mind.'

'I have won the battle.'

'It is safe to think my thoughts.'

'I am impervious to negative thoughts interfering with my life.'

'I am in control of my thoughts, mind and body.'

'I live without the fear of being persecuted.'

'I know what it feels like to live without being paranoid about things I cannot understand.'

'My body is safe.'

'I am one.'

'The energy that flows through all things works with me and I work with it.'

'I can easily tap into the Creator's energy.'

'Nothing stops me from creating my destiny.'

'I see my destiny as it truly is.'

'Through the Creator of All that Is, I can create my own destiny.'

'My definition of truth and the Creator's are the same.'

'I see the truth in situations and get validation.'

'I live without frightening other people.'

Supplements

Be aware that magnesium deficiency can cause schizophrenic-like symptoms. Many psychiatric disorders can be attributed to vitamin and mineral deficiencies. The following supplements may be beneficial:

- amino-acid complexes
- flaxseed oil
- folic acid
- glutathione
- Lecithin
- multivitamin and mineral complexes with calcium and magnesium
- raw thyroid glandular
- vitamin B complex

People with schizophrenia should avoid caffeine, alcohol and drugs.

SCHMIDT'S SYNDROME

See Adrenal Disorders.

SCOLIOSIS

Scoliosis is a condition that affects the spines of many children, teenagers and adults. The spine features many natural curves, which help us to move and be flexible. When a person has scoliosis, however, it begins to curve in ways that are unbeneficial.

Intuitive Remedies

Little by little, move the vertebrae and train the muscles to accept the new position. Follow the same remedies as broken or out of place bones (*see Bone Fractures*). It must all be done gradually, over as many sessions as the Creator needs.

Downloads

'My back is straight.'

'Every day in every way my back becomes straighter.'

'I walk with grace and ease.'

'I hold my body with pride.'

'I stand with pride in myself.'

'It's easy for me to stand tall.'

'I love myself.'

'I love those around me.'

'I am a reflection of how I feel about myself; therefore, it is easy for me to stand with pride.'

'I am supported by God.'

'Every day, in every way, I become stronger.'

SEPTIC SHOCK

Septic shock is a serious condition that occurs when an overwhelming infection leads to low blood pressure and low blood flow. The brain, heart, kidneys and liver may not work properly or may fail. People can die in as little as three days. Generally, people with compromised immune systems contract septic shock.

A client of mine was the longest survivor of sepsis her doctors had seen. Apparently, she got it from one of her feeding IV shunt tubes. I did a healing on her and told her to go to hospital. They did tests but were unable to find out what was wrong with her and sent her home. She went to her personal doctor, who also ran some tests. He did a test on her blood and found out she was septic. Apparently, she had been septic for almost nine days before it was diagnosed. The doctors did not understand how she could have septicaemia and still be functioning, let alone still be alive! They finally got her on antibiotics that took care of it. She attributes her survival to the healings that were done on her.

The bacteria she had were different from anything that I had seen before. The Creator told me to send her to the doctor. I was not offended by this and listened to what I was told.

To heal septic shock, ask the Creator to get rid of it and to show you. Instant healings are necessary here and the person should always consult a doctor as well.

THE SEXUAL SYSTEM

See the Reproductive System.

SEXUALLY TRANSMITTED DISEASES (STDS)

There are many diseases that are passed on through sexual contact.

Types

Types of sexually transmitted diseases include AIDS, chancroid, *Chlamydia*, genital herpes, gonorrhoea, *Granuloma inguinale*, hepatitis, *Lymphogranuloma vernereum*, syphilis and trichomoniasis.

- *For AIDs and Chlamydia, see pages 11 and 135.*
- *Gonorrhoea* is caused by a micro-organism called *Neirreria gonorrhoeae*. These bacteria are commonly referred to as gonococci. If left untreated, infection can travel through the bloodstream and go on to affect bones, joints and tendons, causing systemic illness. Symptoms of this stage of the illness are inflamed joints and occasionally skin lesions. The organism is difficult to detect and the condition is often misdiagnosed as simple osteoarthritis. If left untreated, gonorrhoea can cause sterility.
- *For Herpes, see page 216.*
- *Syphilis* is caused by a type of bacteria called *Treponema pallidum*. This disease is usually contracted through close physical contact such as kissing, as well as through sexual intercourse. If not treated, it progresses over the course of many years through three basic stages. Ten to 90 days after contact, a red painless ulcer appears on the spot where the bacteria entered the body. In the second stage, four to ten weeks after contact, a rash and patches of flaking tissue appear in the mouth, on the palms of the hands, the soles of the feet or the genital area. If the disease progresses to its third stage, a year or more after the initial infection, blindness, brain damage, hearing loss and/or heart disease can occur. This disease can remain dormant for up to 20 years.

Early Symptoms

Candidasis
Itching in the genital area, pain when urinating and a thick odourless genital discharge.

Genital Herpes

Itching, burning in the genital area, discomfort while urinating, a watery vaginal or urethral discharge, weeping fluid-filled eruptions in the vagina or on the penis. Herpes is contagious even if the person shows no outward signs of the virus.

Genital Warts

Cauliflower-like growths appearing either singly or in clusters in or around the vagina, penis, groin and/or scrotal area.

Gonorrhoea

Gonorrhoea often has no symptoms in women. When there are symptoms, they include abdominal menstrual bleeding, acute inflammation of the pelvic area, frequent or painful urination and vaginal discharge.

Men, on the other hand, usually experience symptoms, including a yellow discharge of pus or mucus from the penis and slow, difficult and painful urination.

Symptoms usually appear between 2 and 20 days after sexual contact.

Syphilis

A sore on the genitalia, fever, patches of flaking tissue, rash, sore throat and sores in the mouth or anus.

Trichomoniasis

For women, vaginal itching and pain with a foamy greenish or yellow foul-smelling discharge.

For men, a clear urethral discharge.

Conventional Treatment

For many of these ailments, antibiotics will clear the problem, but with others there is no known conventional cure.

Belief Work

The contraction of STDs cycles around worthiness issues. Work on the beliefs the person had when they contracted the disease. Download:

> 'I am worthy of a wonderful relationship.'
>
> 'I love myself.'
>
> 'I love the Creator of All That Is.'

'I feel good about myself.'

'I deserve good things.'

'My body becomes stronger every day.'

'I know how to leave the past behind.'

'I know what it feels like to be free of regrets.'

'I am happy and healthy.'

'I understand what it feels like to be loved by God.'

'Every day, in every way, I am worthy of God's love.'

'It is easy to be worthy of God's love.'

'I am secure in myself.'

'It is easy for people to love me.'

SHINGLES

Shingles is a disease caused by the varicella-zoster virus, which is the virus that causes chickenpox. It is a herpes virus. When you have had chickenpox, the virus stays in your body. It can remain dormant in the spinal cord and not cause problems for many years. However, as you get older, it may reappear as shingles.

Unlike chickenpox, shingles is not contagious.

Ninety percent of the people who have had chickenpox are at risk of developing shingles. The chance of an attack can be increased by many factors, including cancer, spinal cord injuries, stress and conditions that suppress the immune system. Shingles can be dangerous for people who have immune system deficiencies because it is capable of doing damage to the internal organs. Death can occur as a result of a secondary bacterial infection or viral pneumonia brought on by shingles.

Symptoms

Early signs of shingles include burning or shooting pain and tingling or itching, usually on one side of the body or face. The pain can be mild to severe. Blisters then form and last up to 14 days.

If shingles appears on the face, it may affect vision or hearing. The pain of shingles may last for weeks, months or even years after the blisters have healed.

Conventional Treatment

There is no known medical cure for shingles. Early treatment with medicines that fight the virus may help. These may also help prevent lingering pain. With some people the pain of shingles becomes so intense that they need narcotic pain medication.

A vaccine may prevent shingles or lessen its effects. This is for people aged 60 or over.

Intuitive Remedies

Look for the virus in the body. Herpes hides in the lower spine.

You have to work on the virus's attitude, which will require a lot of belief work. Sometimes, however, the removal of beliefs will be enough to be rid of the virus, so pull the beliefs on the virus and instil feelings as well. Ask the Creator to show you and witness the changes.

Check to see if the DNA of the body has changed because of the virus. If it has, then repair it.

See also Viruses (Prologue).

Belief Work

Viruses are smart enough to survive in the body until the associated beliefs are pulled. Beliefs will vary, but pull:

'I'm not good enough.'

'I'm not worthy.'

'God is punishing me.'

Since most shingles outbreaks are stress-induced, it is good to work on the beliefs that are causing the stress.

In many instances you can go back to find the emotions that were associated with the person when they had chickenpox and work on those beliefs. However, if they were too young, there may not be any beliefs associated with that time.

Make sure the person understands what it feels like to be worthy of love, forgiveness, joy and respect. Download:

'I know what it feels like to live without stress.'

'I know how to live my day-to-day life without allowing stress to affect how I think and how I feel.'

'I know how to live without reacting to stress in painful ways.'

'I know how to live without regret.'

'It is easy for me to become strong.'

'Every day, in every way, my body becomes stronger and stronger.'

'I know how to be happy.'

'I know life is good.'

Supplements

- acidophilus
- ALA
- bee pollen and propolis
- cayenne pepper
- DMSO to clear the skin
- milk thistle to clean the liver
- noni juice, both topically and internally
- omega 3s
- super salve topically
- vitamin A
- vitamin B complex
- vitamin E on the blisters
- zinc

SICKLE-CELL ANAEMIA

See Anaemia.

SINUS TROUBLE

Sinus trouble can be associated with being irritated by a person who is very close.

It is often also associated with teeth. Go up and ask the Creator if the person has any infected teeth.

Too much histamine can cause sinus problems, as can too much acetaldehyde in the system.

Downloads

'Every day, in every way, I feel stronger and stronger.'

'I know what it feels like to live without being exhausted.'

'I know how to find new strength.'

'I know what it feels like to know my adrenals have the strength they need.'

'Everything in my body works in harmony.'

'My hormones are balanced.'

'It is easy for me to breathe.'

'I know how to live without allowing others to irritate me.'

'I know how to live my day-to-day life without allowing others to take advantage of me.'

'I know how to react and interact with people in a good way.'

'I know what it feels like to say no in situations before drama begins.'

'I know what it feels like to be happy.'

'I know what it feels like to permit my body to relax.'

'Every day, my sinuses become clearer.'

Supplements and Other Nutritional Remedies

- If the sinus trouble is caused by too much acetaldehyde, you need to supplement with molybdenum to pull out the acetaldehyde and change the person's allergies.
- If it is caused by histamine, good muscle-building exercises will help create cortisone and block the histamines. CoQ10 and vitamin C will help.

THE SKELETAL SYSTEM

The skeletal system has many purposes:

- The backbone provides the structure that enables us to stand erect.
- The ribcage protects the delicate organs of the body.
- The skull protects the soft tissues of the brain.

- The vertebrae of the spinal column surround the spinal cord to encapsulate the complex bundle of nerves that sends messages to the whole of the body.

Without the skeletal system, we would slither around, unable to stand up or walk, merely a sack of tissue on the floor, limp like an amoeba.

We are born with 300 bones. Once we are an adult, some of these fuse together, resulting in a total of 206. They move with the synchronistic biology of the muscles to bring the skeletal system to life. In an incredible symphony, messages both conscious and unconscious are sent to enable the various body parts to move.

The joints are flexible connections between the bones. The body has different kinds of joints that pivot in different directions for different purposes.

The bones are not simply an inert framework of hard substances, they are alive. As with other cells in the body, the bone cells work closely with the blood and circulatory system. This is why a bone repairs itself in the event of a break. For example, when you break your toe, blood clots form to close up the space between the broken segments. Then your body mobilizes bone cells to recreate the interlacing framework that will mend the break.

Some bones are hollow, but in the centre of many bones the bone marrow makes new red and white blood cells. Red blood cells ensure that oxygen is distributed to all parts of the body and white blood cells enable us to fight germs and disease.

Intuitive Insights

The bones are the easiest thing to see when you first start doing body scans. The life force shines in, out and around them, making them teem with life. They are many colours, not just white. They love to show their magnificence to you. When you go inside them, they look like shimmering, incandescent, liquid light.

Since the bones hold us up, they think they are the most important part of the body (as do all the systems) and it is true that everything is based on them: the ligaments, muscles and nervous system. The bones are the core of all that we are. They are directly connected to the crown chakra and because of this they are the spiritual tuning fork, hence the saying 'I feel it in my bones.'

Intuitive Remedies

The skeletal system is extremely easy to heal and is happy to co-operate. The bones listen to what they are told in a healing and are obedient.

It is possible to heal a broken bone instantly. Simply go to the Creator and command that it be done by saying, 'Creator of All That Is, change it and show me. Thank you. It is done. It is done. It is done.' Witness the healing.

When doing a healing on bone, remember to bring in extra energy, otherwise the body will steal calcium from the other bones, especially from the hips.

Belief Work

Bone injury can be tied to subconscious beliefs.

You must be very tactful with the client when there are emotional issues in the bones, because they are generally about trust and having support in life.

Download:

'I know what it feels like to be loved by the Creator.'

'I know how to live without having to suffer.'

'I know how to live without struggling to be close to the Creator.'

'I know how to live without feeling abandoned by the Creator.'

'I know how to live without feeling rejected by the Creator.'

'I know how to live without feeling my life has been stolen from me.'

'I know how to live without feeling I must do it all by myself.'

'I know how to live without carrying the weight of the world on my shoulders.'

'I know how to live without feeling overburdened.'

'I know what it feels like to give.'

'I know what balance feels like.'

'I know what it feels like to be balanced physically, mentally, emotionally and spiritually.'

'I know how to live without being a martyr.'

'I understand the Creator's definition of money.'

'I know what it feels like to be close to the Creator at all times.'

'I know how to live without the fear of going forward.'
(For the leg bones.)

'I know what the Creator's love feels like.'

Supplements

When a healer connects to the Creator of All That Is with the crown chakra, magnesium and calcium are used up and need to be replaced with good supplements.

THE SKIN

The skin is an iridescent organ and is every colour of the rainbow. When we begin life as a baby *in vitro*, it is translucent. It is the largest organ in the body and is attached to all the nerve endings of the central nervous system, so it is a reflection of what is going on internally, physically, mentally and spiritually. If the liver is congested, for example, there are visible effects on the skin. The tighter and shinier the skin, then the healthier the inside of the body.

The skin is our shield, our outer defensive covering for the body. It not only breathes oxygen from the air, but draws the universal life force into the body from the Creator.

The skin is the first contact with feelings outside the body that are then felt inside the body. It holds a thin protective energy field around us. It is a major communicator of intuitive information. We can feel the presence of people, objects and emotions through it.

Intuitive Insights

When you work with someone, ask them if it's all right to touch them. The skin, like many other organs, locks abuse and trauma in its cells, and to touch a person may be overwhelming to them. If you reach out and get into their comfort zone without their permission, they will feel violated. So always ask permission before physically touching during a session.

When someone has a problem being touched on the legs, it may be an indicator that they have been abused.

All cultures have different beliefs about touch.

When you touch someone, your cells talk to their cells and your DNA sings and talks to their DNA. The DNA teaches and learns in seconds and, at times, is the best way of passing on psychic information.

Intuitive Remedies

When the skin experiences trauma, it is shocked by the fact that it is hurt, as it thinks it is impervious to injury. Tell it that it is OK to heal after trauma and reassure it that it is doing a good job. Release the trauma and stress.

When witnessing a healing on the skin, keep the affected area covered. For example, breast cancer can become an oozing, open sore. The eyes see the wound and may connect it with fear. If you cover the wound, your mind doesn't accept that it's there, so it is easier to heal. This is true in all cases of wounds and cuts: if you cover the wound and do a healing, the skin may grow back completely. Ask the Creator of All That Is how long it needs to be covered in order to heal. This may vary from person to person. It may take just 20 seconds. Remember, you may check the person's beliefs to see if it will take a long time to heal.

Belief Work

With skin problems there may be programmes concerning:

- change
- comfort zones
- discernment in touch
- feeling beautiful making you weak/strong
- how the world perceives you
- irritation
- loving and accepting your body
- receiving love back
- reflecting your beauty
- showing affection
- understanding other people's body language

Download:

'I know what it feels like to live without believing it is weak to show feelings.'

'I respect and understand people's boundaries.'

'I love my body.'

'I know how to live without hating my body.'

'It's OK to receive affection.'

'I have proper discernment about someone's touch.'

SORE THROAT

This is one of the most common of health complaints – a raw burning and/or scratchy feeling at the back of the throat.

Causes

Most sore throats are caused by viral infections or bacterial infections, especially the *Streptococcus* infection.

A sore throat can also be caused by anything that irritates the sensitive mucous membranes at the back of the throat and mouth. Irritants include dust, fumes, medication, radiation therapy, smoke, surgery and extremely hot food or drink.

Sore throats can signal a cold, the flu, mononucleosis, the Epstein-Barr virus and herpes simplex, as well as many childhood illnesses such as measles and chickenpox.

Intuitive Remedies

Small babies generally get exposed to streptococci while they're crawling around on the ground. Streptococci tend to breed behind and under refrigerators. Simply washing your hands and the hands of your children can prevent many infections such as streptococci from entering the system by about 70 percent.

There are some streptococci A types that can quickly destroy the body. In this instance, the person needs an immediate healing and immediate medical attention. Give the person a healing, but make sure that your fear does not interfere with it.

To do a healing on a sore throat, command that the bacteria are gone and witness the Creator scraping the throat clean and the problem disappearing. If it doesn't disappear, follow up with belief work.

Belief Work

I am not against a person using antibiotics if they have streptococci in the throat. However, people who have strep on a recurring basis do not know how to stand up for themselves in a proper way. They do not know how to verbalize how they feel. To prevent a person drawing recurring streptococci, use the belief and feeling work.

Supplements

The following can help prevent a sore throat:

- acidophilus
- bee pollen and propolis
- colloidal silver (only use it for a week or so, as too much can turn your skin blue)
- Echinacea (to build the immune system)
- multivitamins and minerals
- vitamin C – 2,000 mg at a time spread throughout the day, building up to 5,000 mg a day

See also Strep Throat.

STDs

See Sexually Transmitted Diseases.

STOMACH ULCERS

Long before conventional medicine figured out a cause for ulcers, I knew they were not caused by stress. For a long time, when I went into people's stomachs, I could see there were bacteria in there, but it took me a while to come up with a suggested remedy. Once the doctors found that ulcers were caused by *Helicobacter pylori* bacteria, they had to change all the prescribed medications for ulcers to antibiotics.

Symptoms

The major symptom of an ulcer is a burning or gnawing feeling in the stomach area that lasts between 30 minutes and three hours. This pain is often interpreted as heartburn, indigestion or hunger. It usually occurs in the upper abdomen, but may occur below the breastbone. In some individuals it occurs immediately after eating; in others, hours after eating. The pain frequently wakes the person at night. Weeks of pain may be followed by weeks of respite. The pain can be relieved by drinking milk, eating, resting or taking antacids.

Appetite and weight loss are other symptoms of ulcers. People with duodenal ulcers may experience weight gain, however, because they eat more to ease the discomfort.

Anaemia, blood in the stool and recurrent vomiting are other symptoms.

Causes

Infection with *Helicobacter pylori* is thought to play an important role in causing both gastric and duodenal ulcers. *Helicobacter pylori* may be transmitted from person to person through contaminated food and water.

Injury of the gastric mucosal lining and weakening of the mucous defences are also responsible for gastric ulcers.

Excess secretion of hydrochloric acid, genetic predisposition and psychological stress are important contributing factors in the formation and worsening of duodenal ulcers.

Another major cause of ulcers is the chronic use of anti-inflammatory medication such as aspirin.

Cigarette smoking is also an important cause of ulcer formation and ulcer treatment failure.

Intuitive Remedies

By going up to the Creator and saying, *'Show me what needs to be done,'* you can see the ulcer being completely cleared out of the stomach.

Since bacteria replace themselves every half-hour, you may have to do the healing more than once just to be sure.

Supplements

- *Aloe vera* juice and probiotics are good.
- Ginger is said to get rid of an ulcer, but you have to take it consistently. Most people aren't consistent with their herbs.
- Oregano can be used, but you may not want to take it because it might irritate the stomach a little bit.
- There are also a lot of good antibiotics that will kill the bacteria.

See also Peptic Ulcers.

STREP THROAT

Strep throat is an infection caused by the group of streptococcus bacteria. It is very common among kids and teenagers. The symptoms include fever, stomach pain and red swollen tonsils.

If our bodies were acid–alkaline balanced, things such as strep would never bother us. On entering the body, these viruses and bacteria would automatically change to something else.

Strep is interesting in that it will stay dormant in the system and come back again. The strep that infects the ears can be almost impossible to eradicate with antibiotics. If someone comes to you with strep and they are on antibiotics, don't take them off, otherwise the strep will build up a resistance to the antibiotic.

Children get strep all the time because of their direct contact with children who have it. So you can do a healing on the strep, but if they are in contact with others who have it, they can become reinfected.

The drip pans at the bottom of some refrigerators are a breeding ground for strep. Little kids that crawl around on the floor can get it this way.

Intuitive Remedies

You can do a healing on strep, but the bacteria multiply every 30 minutes, so it is best to do a follow-up healing. Also, people are often stuck in the mindset that they have to get an antibiotic. So what I do is, I do a healing on them, but I still suggest they use a Melaleuca oil gargle (for a throat infection).

Here's a secret: ginger will kill strep. If you take a piece of raw ginger and put it on the side of an infected baby's ear with a bandage over it, it will get rid of the ear infection. This will work on adults as well.

STROKE

A stroke is a medical emergency. It happens when blood flow to the brain stops. When this happens, brain cells begin to die within minutes.

A person who has suffered a stroke sometimes loses the mobility of certain body parts. This is because some of the neurons no longer exist or are not connected as they were before.

Types

There are two kinds of stroke:

- The more common kind, called *ischaemic stroke*, is caused by a blood clot that blocks or plugs a blood vessel in the brain.
- A blood vessel that breaks and bleeds into the brain causes the other kind, called *haemorrhagic stroke*.

'Mini-strokes', or transient ischemic attacks (TIAs), occur when the blood supply to the brain is briefly interrupted.

Intuitive Remedies

If you are working with a person who's about to have a stroke, clean out the aneurysm area, strengthen the vein walls and clear the veins.

When working with an adult who has had a stroke, witness the Creator go in and ask the body to wake up the fetal memory and change the things that are needed in the brain. Go in and say, *'Creator, show me.'* This is the fastest way for the brain to reproduce itself.

When I witness a healing on a stroke, I go in, wake up the brain cells and make sure that they can use all of the remaining neurons. I witness the new neurons being redirected to take the job of those that have been destroyed. Then I put my hands on them and witness that they remember how to function.

In cases of stroke, the brain has too many dead brain cells. It must recreate them and relearn. That's why, to heal a stroke, you connect to the Creator and command the fetal memory to wake up and the cells to remember and relearn. It is not necessary to know the mechanics of how this is done; all that you have to do is make the command for the Creator to take care of it and be the witness. Personally, I like to know what I am witnessing, so I ask the Creator what is going on when the person is being healed. In the instance of a stroke, I was told that I was watching cells waking up and relearning how to do things.

Young children can correct a stroke episode and become perfectly functioning adults simply because of the stem cells. When working with any child who has suffered a stroke, go in and command the body to totally replenish itself and work to activate the stem cells.

I usually expect results within two to three weeks and all the results within three months. Some people have results the day of the healing or the day after.

However, we must remember that it takes a person around a year to learn how to walk as a baby and it is likely to take a few months to relearn with healings. Sometimes relearning how to walk and how to move certain limbs takes some time, but overall, what we think of as 'some time' is really not that long. It may take you a month to recover movement in your arm where it took months to move it properly when you were a baby. So be patient when you work with people who've had a stroke. A stroke makes a person feel totally rejected.

Downloads

'I am happy, healthy and recovering each day.'

'Each day I recover more and become healthier.'

'My cells recover and relearn.'

'My body receives the breath of life.'

'My body remembers all it knew before.'

'I am a strong person.'

'I will continue forward.'

'Every day in every way continuing forward becomes easier.'

'I am grateful for my life.'

'I am grateful to be alive.'

'I know how to live without depression.'

'I know what it feels like to be happy.'

'I know what it feels like to live without despair.'

'I know how to live without despair.'

'It is easy for me to recover.'

Supplements

Stroke is commonly associated with a lack of basic minerals, like selenium. If the person who has had a stroke is over 18 years old, suggest:

- a multivitamin and mineral combination
- amino-acid complex
- selenium
- vitamin E

THE TEETH

Teeth are a very basic part of the skeletal system and are connected energetically to all other parts of the body. Teeth challenges create problems in the organs of the body. These hidden challenges are generally caused by cavities underneath the teeth in the jaws.

Intuitive Insights

The teeth, like the bones, are full of luminescent light, suffused with energy as they giggle with joy.

The feelings and programmes that were created as a child during visits to the dentist can prevent healings on the teeth, but you can command teeth to grow back and you can straighten teeth intuitively. Children's teeth in particular move easily because they are not embedded in the bones of the jaw yet.

Mercury amalgams in teeth act as receivers, picking up negative thought forms from other people.

Fluoride may cause Alzheimer's disease.

Root canals block the meridians of the body and can encapsulate infections.

Red meat and sugar in excess create cavities.

Remember, when it comes to healing teeth, practice makes perfect. Look for limiting beliefs connected to the teeth.

Supplements

- It is suggested that a person use chlorophyll and greens for the teeth. Chlorophyll is great for the skeletal system in general.
- Tea tree oil (with a little water on a toothbrush) will help your gums to recover and regrow.
- Use good minerals, calcium, magnesium, vitamin C and zinc to keep your gums healthy and strong.

See also the Skeletal System.

THROMBOSIS

Thrombosis is caused by not enough circulation to the legs and can also be caused by inactivity (when flying in planes, for example) resulting in blood clots. It is important to exercise and stretch the body to circulate the lymph system.

Intuitive Remedies

Always seek medical advice!

A short-term remedy is as follows: warm a pack of arnica oil and then immerse a cloth in it. Apply it and reapply it to the affected area until relief is obtained.

THYROID IMBALANCES

See Hyperthyroidism and Hypothyroidism.

TRANSPLANTS

Conventional medicine uses pig and human valves to repair the heart and can transplant a whole range of other body parts. Your body has the choice to accept or reject them. It knows that they are foreign substances (which in itself is proof of the intelligence of the cells in the body).

Every cell in your body has a special memory of everything that you have ever done, and each has its own special song. A transplant does not match these vibrations and memories. This means when you have a transplant, there are memories from the original owner in it. Sometimes the body is not willing to accept these memories, thoughts and energies, and will attack the transplant. If this happens, you can command balance in the body.

To balance the body for acceptance of the transplant, go up and command the person's body to find acceptance of the energy of the transplant. Ask the Creator to show you what has to be done and witness it change.

Downloads

'With each day, my body adjusts easily and effortlessly to the new organ transplants that are in my body.'

'I know what it feels like to accept my transplant.'

'I know how to accept all the new gifts the Creator has given me.'

'I know what it feels like to live without having to fight for everything I receive.'

'I know what it feels like to know when to fight and how to fight.'

'I know it's possible to live in harmony.'

'Every day in every way I am more in harmony.'

'Every day in every way my mind is at harmony.'

'Every day in every way my immune system is in harmony.'

'It is easy for me to be happy.'

'The Creator shows me how to be happy.'

'My body is strong and healthy.'

TUBERCULOSIS

Tuberculosis (TB) is a life-threatening infection that primarily affects the lungs. It has plagued human beings for millennia. Signs of it have been found in Egyptian mummies and in bones dating back 5,000 years. Doc Holliday, one of our more famous gunslingers in the Old West, died from it. They used to call it consumption. Today, despite advances in treatment, TB is a global pandemic, fuelled by the spread of HIV–AIDS, poverty, a lack of health services and the emergence of drug-resistant strains of the bacterium that cause the disease. It is a common disease; about one third of the human population is infected with it and nearly two million people die from it worldwide every year.

Mycobacterium tuberculosis, the bacterium that causes tuberculosis, spreads in microscopic droplets that are released into the air when someone with the active form of the disease coughs, speaks, laughs, sings or sneezes.

Although tuberculosis is contagious, it's not especially easy to catch. In general, you need long-term contact with an infected person to become infected yourself. Even then, symptoms may not show up until many years later. You are much more likely to contract tuberculosis from a family member or close co-worker than from a stranger on a bus or in a restaurant. A person with non-resistant active TB who has been treated for at least two weeks is generally no longer contagious.

Left untreated, tuberculosis can be fatal. However, with proper care, most cases can be treated, even those resistant to the antibiotic drugs commonly used against the disease.

Although your body may harbour the TB bacterium, your immune system can often prevent you from becoming ill. For that reason, doctors make a distinction between:

- *TB infection:* This condition, sometimes called latent TB, causes no symptoms and is not contagious.
- *Active TB:* This condition makes you ill and can spread to others. However, the infection may be asymptomatic for years, even though it is active and causing damage.

The immune system begins to attack the TB bacteria two to eight weeks after becoming infected. Sometimes the bacteria die and the infection clears completely. In other cases, the bacteria remain in the body in an inactive state and cause no tuberculosis symptoms. In still other cases, people develop active TB.

Symptoms

TB mainly affects the lungs (pulmonary tuberculosis) and coughing is often the only indication of infection at first. Symptoms of active pulmonary TB include:

- a cough lasting three or more weeks that may produce discoloured or bloody sputum
- chills
- fatigue
- loss of appetite
- night sweats
- pain with breathing or coughing (pleurisy)
- slight fever
- unintended weight loss

Tuberculosis also targets almost any part of the body, including the bone marrow, bones, central nervous system, joints, lymphatic system, muscles and urinary tract. It can spread through the entire body, simultaneously attacking many organ systems.

Inactive Infection

Approximately two to eight weeks after the lungs are infected with *M. tuberculosis*, the immune system springs into action. Macrophages, specialized white blood cells that ingest harmful organisms, begin to surround the tuberculosis bacteria in the lungs. If the macrophages are successful, the bacteria may remain within these walls for years in a dormant state. In this case, the person will test positive on the TB skin test, but will not have any symptoms and not be contagious.

Active TB

However, a number of factors can weaken the immune system, including aging, chemotherapy, diseases such as HIV/AIDS, drug or alcohol abuse, malnutrition and the prolonged use of prescription drugs such as corticosteroids, and about one in 10 people who have dormant TB go on to develop active TB some time in their life. The risk is greatest in the first year after infection, but the disease may not resurface for decades.

As the immune defences fail, the TB bacteria actually begin to exploit macrophages for their own survival, causing the white blood cells to form into tightly packed groups called granulomas. The bacteria multiply inside the granulomas, which eventually may enlarge into non-cancerous tumour-like nodules. The centres of these nodules have the consistency of soft, crumbly cheese. Over time, the centres can liquefy and break through the granulomatous wall surrounding them, spilling bacteria into the lungs' airways and causing large air spaces (cavities) to form (active TB). Filled with oxygen, the air spaces make an ideal breeding ground for the bacteria, which multiply in enormous numbers. They may then spread from the cavities to the rest of the lungs as well as to other parts of the body.

Without treatment, many of the people with active TB die. Those who survive either develop chronic debilitating symptoms, such as chest pain and a cough with bloody sputum, or their immune system recovers and the disease goes into remission.

The Spread of TB

Today, new infections and deaths from the disease are increasing. Hardest hit are sub-Saharan Africa and South East Asia. The leading cause is the spread of HIV. TB and HIV have a deadly relationship – each fuels the progress of the other.

Infection with HIV suppresses the immune system, making it difficult for the body to control TB bacteria. As a result, people with HIV are many times more likely to progress from dormant to active disease than are people who are not HIV-positive. TB is one of the leading causes of death among people living with AIDS – not only because they're more susceptible to TB, but also because TB can increase the rate at which the AIDS virus replicates. One of the first indications of HIV infection may be the sudden onset of TB.

Other factors contributing to the spread of TB include:

- an increase in the drug-resistant strains of TB
- crowded living conditions (TB spreads most easily in cramped, crowded, poorly ventilated spaces)
- increased immigration
- increased poverty and lack of access to medical care

Intuitive Remedies

I have worked with tuberculosis, and there are some important things to know. I am not afraid of tuberculosis, but I do take precautions. If you suspect someone has tuberculosis, make sure that they see their health provider, so that they can take advantage of all the options available to them. It also gives the health practitioner a heads-up that someone in the area has tuberculosis.

The basic healing works well with TB. Witness the lesions in the lungs being healed. Bacteria are easy to get rid of intuitively. Make the command: 'Creator, heal this and show me.' Witness the healing as done.

The majority of people who have come to me with tuberculosis have recovered successfully and are doing well.

Some recommendations for a person with TB:

- Avoid stress.
- Avoid the use of cortisone because of the immune-compromising problems associated with it.
- Avoid smoking.
- Tuberculosis has an incredible capacity for reproduction. Filtered air purification is a good suggestion.

Belief Work

When you work with tuberculosis, remember it is a bacterium, so the person will have issues pertaining to guilt and issues of the lungs, which are associated with sorrow.

Supplements

If the person is on antibiotics for TB, you must be careful with the supplements that you suggest for them, so that they do not conflict with the effects of the antibiotics.

Useful supplements:

- amino-acid complex
- flaxseed oil
- fresh pineapple juice
- multivitamins and minerals
- raw thymus glandular
- vitamin B complex
- vitamin C

ULCERATIVE COLITIS

Ulcerative colitis is an inflammatory bowel disease that causes chronic inflammation of the digestive tract. It is distinguished by abdominal pain and diarrhoea. Like Crohn's disease, it can be debilitating and sometimes lead to life-threatening problems. It usually affects only the innermost lining of the large intestine (colon) and rectum. It occurs only through continuous stretches of the colon, unlike Crohn's disease, which occurs in patches anywhere in the digestive tract and often spreads deep into the layers of bowel tissues.

There is no known cure for ulcerative colitis, but therapies are available that may dramatically reduce its symptoms and even bring about long-term remission.

Symptoms and Classifications

Ulcerative colitis symptoms can vary, depending on the severity of inflammation and where it occurs. For these reasons, doctors often classify it according to its location:

- *Fulminant colitis:* This rare, life-threatening form of colitis affects the entire colon. It causes profuse diarrhoea, severe pain and sometimes dehydration and shock.

- *Left-sided colitis:* As the name suggests, the inflammation extends from the rectum up the left side through the sigmoid and descending colon. Symptoms include abdominal cramping, bloody diarrhoea, pain and weight loss.

- *Pancolitis:* Pancolitis affects the entire colon. Symptoms include abdominal cramps, attacks of bloody diarrhoea that may be severe, fatigue, night sweats, pain and weight loss.

- *Ulcerative proctitis:* In this form, the inflammation is confined to the rectum, and for some people, rectal bleeding is a symptom.

There are times when the symptoms of ulcerative colitis lead to aches and pains in the joints that are similar to arthritis. Ulcerative colitis can also cause other disorders such as diverticulosis. People with this disorder have the tendency to be compulsive perfectionists.

Causes

No one is quite sure what triggers ulcerative colitis. Some scientists think a virus or bacterium may be the cause and that the digestive tract may become inflamed when the immune system tries to fight off the invading micro-organism (pathogen). It's also possible that the inflammation may stem from an auto-immune reaction in which the body mounts an immune response even though no pathogen is present.

Because you are more likely to develop ulcerative colitis if you have a parent or sibling with the disease, scientists suspect that a genetic predisposition plays a contributing role.

Ulcerative colitis affects about the same number of women as men. Risk factors may include:

- *Age:* Ulcerative colitis can strike at any age, but most people develop the condition when young. It often strikes people in their thirties, although a small number of people may not develop the disease until their fifties or sixties.
- *Family history:* You are at higher risk if you have a close relative such as a parent, sibling or child with the disease.
- *Inflamed bile ducts:* This condition, called primary sclerosing cholangitis, causes inflammation of the bile ducts of the liver and is associated with ulcerative colitis.
- *Isotretinoin (Accutane) use:* Isotretinoin (Accutane) is a powerful pharmaceutical drug sometimes used to treat scarring cystic acne or acne that does not respond to other treatments.
- *Where you live:* If you live in an urban area or in an industrialized country, you're more likely to develop ulcerative colitis. People living in northern climates also seem to be at greater risk.

Downloads

'I know how to live without being a compulsive perfectionist.'

'I know what it feels like to enjoy life.'

'I know what it feels like to know I am good enough.'

'I know what it feels like to live my life without finding fault in everything I do.'

'I know what it feels like to live my life without finding fault in everything others do.'

'I know how to live my life in harmony.'

'I know what it feels like to live without compulsive worry.'

'I know what it feels like to enjoy the many things life has to offer.'

'I know what it feels like to live without having to control others.'

'I know how to permit others to be who they are.'

'I know what it feels like to live without taking on the problems of the world.'

Supplements and Other Nutritional Recommendations

- acidophilus (to stimulate the good bacteria of the digestive tract)
- ALA
- *Aloe vera* juice (to soothe the intestinal tract)
- colon cleanses
- essential fatty acids
- Jerusalem artichoke (for the digestion)
- magnesium
- noni
- omega 3s, 6s and 9s
- stinging nettle
- vitamin B complex
- vitamin C

***

- Avoid carbonated soft drinks, spicy foods and caffeine.
- Avoid oranges and grapefruit.
- Avoid processed foods.
- Do not eat fruit on an empty stomach.
- Drink plenty of liquids.
- Eat foods that are broiled or baked and not fried.
- Have a high-fibre diet. Wholegrains that are well cooked can be beneficial.
- Have a low-carbohydrate high-protein diet. Baked or broiled fish, chicken and turkey (without the skin) are acceptable sources of protein.

- Keep fats and oils out of your diet, since they can cause the diarrhoea that comes with colitis.
- Vitamin K deficiencies can lead to ulcerative colitis, so eat foods high in vitamin K such as dark green leafy vegetables that are well steamed.

URINARY TRACT INFECTION

A urinary tract infection (UTI) is an infection that begins in the urinary system.

The urinary system is composed of the kidneys, ureters, bladder and urethra. All play a role in removing waste from the body. The kidneys filter waste from the blood. Tubes called ureters carry urine from the kidneys to the bladder, where it is stored until it exits the body through the urethra. All of these components can become infected, but most infections involve the lower tract, the urethra and the bladder. Generally, the infection is limited to the bladder. Serious consequences can occur if it spreads to the kidneys.

Women are more at risk of developing a urinary tract infection. In fact, half of all women will develop a UTI during their lifetimes and many will experience more than one. These infections can be painful and annoying.

Antibiotics are the conventional treatment.

Symptoms

Symptoms depend on which part of the urinary tract is infected and include:

- a strong, persistent urge to urinate
- a burning sensation when urinating
- blood in the urine (haematuria) or cloudy, strong-smelling urine
- passing frequent small amounts of urine

Types

- *Acute pyelonephritis:* This is an infection of the kidneys and may occur after spreading from the bladder. Kidney infection can cause a high fever, chills, nausea, shaking, upper back and flank pain, and vomiting.
- *Cystitis:* Inflammation or infection of the bladder may result in frequent painful urination, lower abdomen discomfort, pelvic pressure and strong-smelling urine.

• *Urethritis:* This is inflammation or infection of the urethra, which leads to burning on urination. In men, it may cause penile discharge.

Urinary tract infections happen when bacteria enter the urinary tract through the urethra. The urinary system has infection-fighting capabilities that reduce the growth of unbeneficial bacteria. However, certain factors increase the odds that bacteria will enter the urinary tract and multiply into a full-blown infection.

Cystitis may occur in women after sexual intercourse. However, even girls and women who aren't sexually active are susceptible to lower urinary tract infections because the anus is so close to the female urethra. Most cases of cystitis are caused by *Escherichia coli* (*E. coli*), a species of bacteria commonly found in the gastrointestinal tract.

In urethritis, the same organisms that infect the kidney and bladder can infect the urethra. In addition, because of the female urethra's proximity to the vagina, sexually transmitted diseases (STDs) such as herpes simplex virus and *Chlamydia* are also possible causes. In men, urethritis often is the result of bacteria acquired through sexual contact. The majority of such infections are caused by gonorrhoea and *Chlamydia*.

Intuitive Insights

In my experience, urinary tract infections are usually exacerbated if someone is angry with another person or if there are buried resentments that are awakened into negative emotion. When you don't work on these issues, a urinary tract infection can be the result, and it can recur until the bottom issues are dealt with and released.

Intuitive Remedies

Go up out of your space and command all the unhealthy bacteria to go to God's light. Watch them all leave until they have completely gone from the body. This will heal a urinary infection nine times out of ten.

If the person is not better within a half an hour, start the belief work.

Belief Work

If the person needs belief work, the first thing you ask is, 'Who are you angry with?' When they tell you, ask them, 'Would you like to get rid of that anger?'

If you do not get rid of the anger and the issues, it is not likely that the infection will go away.

ThetaHealing® Diseases & Disorders

I have seen people who are on heavy-duty antibiotics for a urinary infection and still it will not go away until the anger is released and the bottom belief found.

Download:

'I know what it feels like to forgive the person I am angry and upset with.'

'I know what it feels like to live my day-to-day life without resentment and anger.'

'I know the energy that I give away while angry and upset can be used for a higher purpose.'

'I know what it feels like to forgive myself and others.'

'Every day, in every way, I become healthier and healthier.'

'My body responds.'

'I am happy.'

Supplements

- Cranberry juice can be used to flush the system.
- Juniper berry and ulva ursi (also called bearberry) should not be used with antibiotics that have been prescribed for a urinary infection.

See also Bladder Infections.

VIRUSES

See Prologue.

WARTS

I have bought warts from children. I'll pay them a quarter and they'll disappear. This seems to work because you've bought the wart, therefore it must go away.

Warts are caused by viruses and you can also go in and see the virus in the body and ask the Creator to take care of it.

WILSON'S DISEASE

Wilson's disease is an inherited disorder that causes too much copper to accumulate in the vital organs. The disease shows up in many different ways, but can remain dormant for years. Left untreated, it can be fatal. When diagnosed early, however, it is treatable and many people with the disorder live normal lives.

Copper plays a key role in the development of healthy bones, collagen, nerves and the skin pigment melanin. Normally, it is absorbed from the food and any excess is excreted through bile, a substance produced in the liver. Wilson's disease is a genetic mutation of chromosome 13, affecting ATP7B, a protein that helps transport copper into bile. ATP7B is also involved in incorporating copper into ceruloplasmin, a protein that carries the mineral through the bloodstream. The defects in the ATP7B gene cause improper elimination of copper. Instead, it builds up in the liver, where it can cause damage. In time, excess copper spills out of the liver and begins accumulating in other organs, especially the brain, eyes, kidneys and joints. This can damage the organs and tissues. The liver and central nervous system are most often affected.

Wilson's disease is inherited as an autosomal recessive characteristic, which means that to develop the disease two copies of the defective gene must be inherited, one from each parent. If both parents are carriers of one abnormal Wilson's gene, they have a 25 percent chance of having a child with two normal genes, a 50 percent chance of having a child who also is a carrier and a 25 percent chance of having a child with two recessive genes who will develop the disease. For this reason, it is recommended that all children and siblings of people with Wilson's be tested for the disease.

Symptoms

In people with Wilson's disease, copper begins accumulating in the liver directly after birth, but symptoms rarely occur before the age of five or six. The disease usually becomes apparent before the age of 30, but the symptoms can appear later in life.

The Liver

Because the liver is the filter for the body, copper accumulates in this vital organ and most people with Wilson's disease show signs of liver damage, including abdominal pain and yellowing of the skin (jaundice), and anaemia or the vomiting of blood can occur. Cirrhosis of the liver can develop – irreversible scarring of the liver that affects its ability to carry out its vital roles. Symptoms of cirrhosis include swelling in the abdomen or legs and an enlarged spleen.

Neurological Symptoms

One third of people with Wilson's disease have neurological symptoms, such as an unsteady walk, difficulty speaking, drooling, muscle spasms and tremors.

Behavioural and Psychological Issues

Wilson's disease can cause sudden personality changes and improper behaviour. Children with the disease can be misdiagnosed as having behavioural problems because they behave erratically.

Eyes, Kidneys and Bones

Many people with Wilson's disease, even those who do not have other symptoms, develop a golden-brown pigmentation around the cornea called a Kayser-Fleischer ring. This is caused by the build-up of copper deposits.

Wilson's disease can also interfere with the filtering function of the kidneys and lead to osteoporosis.

Intuitive Insights

Most of the people who come to me with Wilson's disease have already been diagnosed. However, one woman who had an appointment with me was different – she had no idea what was wrong with her. From the moment that I got on the phone with her, I knew that she had Wilson's disease. Once you have felt the energy of the disease, you cannot mistake it. When I began to converse with her, I found that she was completely psychotic, believing that no one could help her and everyone was trying to either kill her or do something to her. I did my best to get her to go to the doctor to be tested for Wilson's disease and she refused, because she was so psychotic she did not believe anything I told her. The disease had progressed to the point where she was badly unbalanced.

I have watched many young people in my area die from Wilson's disease and I have also watched people heal from it.

Gene Work

The best way to work on Wilson's disease is through gene work.

Go to the person's space and ask the Creator to change the gene that is causing the problem through the following process:

The Process for Gene Work

1   Centre yourself in your heart and visualize going down into Mother Earth, which is a part of All That Is.

2   Go beyond the universe, past the white lights, past the dark light, past the white light, past the jelly-like substance that is the Laws, into a pearly iridescent white light, into the Seventh Plane of Existence.

3   Make the command, *'Creator of All That Is, I command that the genetic flaw in* [name the person] *be healed. Show me. Thank you! It is done. It is done. It is done.'*

4   Go into the person's space and witness the change. It may happen so quickly that you may only see a flash of light.

Downloads

'I know it is possible to make changes in my life.'

'I have a life to live.'

'I have the ability to go forward.'

Supplements and Other Nutritional Recommendations

A number of foods, especially avocados, eggs, liver, mushrooms, nuts and shellfish, contain abundant amounts of copper, so are best avoided. Also:

- Avoid alcohol and coffee.
- Eat onions because they have sulphur in them, which will pull out the excess copper.
- Have your water tested to check for levels of copper in it.
- If you are taking a multivitamin, check for the levels of copper in it.

WILSON'S SYNDROME

See Hypothyroidism.

WORMS

See Prologue.

YEAST

See Prologue.

Vitamins and Minerals

There is an abundance of information available on vitamins and minerals. You can find hundreds of books filled with information on the subject. This short overview is intended to give you some ideas of the problems that can be caused by the lack of certain vitamins and minerals.

When you look into a person's body and see deficiencies, the person can usually correct this by using the proper vitamins and minerals. You must train yourself to ask the body and the Creator what specific vitamins or minerals are needed. Eventually you will be able to recognize these deficiencies at a glance.

We know that a lack of vitamins and minerals can create diseases in the body. However, with a proper balance of these vital supplements, the body creates health. The cells have an incredible way of absorbing and distributing vitamins and minerals for the body's myriad needs. There are, however, many ways in which this absorption is blocked.

What people overlook is the emotional and mental component in the absorption of vitamins and minerals. Depending on our beliefs, we may not get all the nutrition from vitamins and minerals because of energetic blocks held there by emotions and programmes. If we train the cells to accept anger and frustration and to reject love and joy, we may also be training them to reject the substances that will give us the ability to create the feelings of love and joy.

Download:

'I understand how to accept vitamins and minerals in my body in the highest and best way.'

'I know what it feels like to absorb the essence of life from vitamins and minerals.'

'I know that vitamins and minerals are a gift from the Creator of All That Is to make my body strong.'

Also remember that thoughts are real things. They have essence. They can create anything in the planes of existence. Your beliefs can create the same energy as a vitamin. The more that you clear your mind, the more you can access the Seventh Plane easily to bring the body into balance. Illness is not your enemy, it is a sign of imbalance. You have to have many negative beliefs to create a disease. I once pulled the hatred that a little boy held for his father, and his colon cancer went away, just like that. Download your clients with everything in the *Advanced ThetaHealing* book, if possible, then they can let go of everything that doesn't serve them easily and quickly.

VITAMINS

For dosages of vitamins, refer to *The Real Vitamin and Mineral Book* by Shari Lieberman (Avery, 2007).

VITAMIN A

Vitamin A is required for reproduction, DNA maintenance and tissues. It is beneficial for the treatment of acne, psoriasis and skin disorders and for use with chronic ulcers. It helps the immune system and is used in the treatment of cancer. It is used for the absorption of beta-carotene and is beneficial for the lungs.

Deficiencies of vitamin A show up in the glands, the mucous membranes and the skin and in the form of gastritis.

Vitamin A is safe for use by people who have frequent bronchitis, cold sores, flu, respiratory infections and sore throats. Most fish products are high in vitamin A. It is also found in beef, chicken, eggs and liver.

VITAMIN BS

Vitamin B should always be taken in a B-complex form. By taking it this way, your body can break it down much more easily. Vitamin B is used to produce energy for the body.

Vitamin B1

Vitamin B1 is also called thiamine. It has to do with the metabolism of carbohydrates in the body. It is effective in helping with conditions such as anxiety, it helps when you are on a diet and it is used for emotional and physical stress.

A classic kind of vitamin B1 deficiency is beriberi. It has also been determined that people who are schizophrenic are very low in this vitamin.

Vitamin B2

Vitamin B2 is called riboflavin. It is used as a protein metabolism for enzymes and for tissue repair during stress. It is necessary to transport oxygen to cells. It promotes healthy eyes and is found in the pigment of the retina.

Major medical problems such as burns, fever, injuries, surgery and tuberculosis create a higher demand for vitamin B2. People who have anaemia have a shortage of it.

Some of the diseases treated with vitamin B2 are anxiety, carpal tunnel syndrome, depression and stress. It is also used for cataract prevention.

Vitamin B3

Vitamin B3, known as niacin, is one of the very few things that will pull out radiation. In several studies, it appears that it is effective against more than one type of carcinogen. So it is associated with the prevention of many types of cancer.

Deficiencies of niacin are a major factor in the development of anxiety, circulation problems, depression and high cholesterol.

Excellent food sources for niacin are broccoli, carrots, cheese, eggs, fish, milk, potatoes, sweetcorn, tomatoes and wholewheat. However, it is often presented in food in a form that is not absorbable. It can be lost when overcooking vegetables. Steaming vegetables will help prevent this.

Vitamin B6

Vitamin B6 is known as pyridoxine. It is one of the most essential, widely utilized vitamins in the body. It is a co-enzyme that is used in over 60 enzymatic reactions involved in the metabolism of the amino acids, the essential fatty acids. Therefore, it is needed for proper growth and the maintenance of body functions.

Deficiencies in pyridoxine bring forth an astonishing variety of symptoms, usually affecting the nervous system or the skin. Typical problems are confusion, depression, dizziness, insomnia, irritability, nervousness, the feeling of pins and needles in the feet and hands and even a slowing in the brain's functions. Carpal tunnel syndrome is usually caused by the lack of B6.

Food sources for pyridoxine are carrots, chicken, eggs, fish, meat, peas and spinach.

Many people who have muscular sclerosis have done quite well while being treated with B6. PMS (premenstrual syndrome) is often eliminated with B6. It helps with asthma and kidney stones and can also be used as a diuretic.

Vitamin B12

Vitamin B12 is cobalamin. Deficiencies of it show up as anaemia and fatigue. Most alcoholics are short of it.

B12 can be given to pregnant women who are having problems with morning sickness.

The chief food sources are beef, kidney, lamb and veal. Other good sources are cheese, clams, crab, herring, mackerel, oysters, salmon and sardines. There are no known toxicity effects from taking too much of this vitamin.

VITAMIN D

It is important to have sufficient amounts of vitamin D so you can metabolize the calcium and phosphorus in your body.

Symptoms of vitamin D deficiencies in children are irreversible bone deformities, stunted growth, tooth decay and weakness. Rickets is caused by a deficiency of vitamin D. In adults, vitamin D deficiency can cause difficulty in labour. Hypoglycaemia is associated with low calcium in the blood, as is osteoporosis. These maladies can be directly related to vitamin D deficiency because it is essential in the absorption of calcium.

One source of vitamin D is sunlight. It is also found in many supplements such as calcium.

A thousand units per day of vitamin D appears to be safe. However, overdosing on vitamin D is not advised. Too much vitamin D can make you sick to your stomach and cause other symptoms such as diarrhoea, fatigue, headache, loss of appetite, restlessness or worse.

VITAMIN E

Vitamin E consists of four substances called: alpha, beta, delta and gamma. Another name for it is tocopherol.

This particular vitamin is an anti-aging aid – the daily requirement may help slow the process of aging. It is phenomenal when working on cancer and is a vital component in cancer prevention. It also has amazing powers to increase muscular regeneration. It helps the cells in the blood, heart, liver and lungs. It is unbelievable for helping your sex life. It is a very important supplement for the blood, helping platelets to stick together. It is an aid in healing wounds and vital in minimizing scar tissue. It is wonderful for cardiovascular disease prevention, core circulation, menopausal hot flushes, premenstrual syndrome and the prevention of excessive bleeding.

VITAMIN K

Vitamin K is assimilated from food and the bacteria in the intestines naturally create it. It has an important role in helping blood to clot when we have open wounds. Red blood cells die more quickly than usual, however, if they have too much vitamin K.

Good sources of vitamin K are green cabbage, lean meat, liver, spinach and tomatoes. Other sources are egg yolks, strawberries and whole wheat.

FOLIC ACID

Folic acid is closely related to vitamin B12 in the body. It is involved in the metabolism of amino acids. Many aspects of the immune system are affected by a deficiency of folic acid.

Anaemia, anxiety and depression can be treated with folic acid. Take it with molybdenum for *Candida*.

Folic acid has no known toxic effects; however, women who are using contraceptives are at risk if they are taking folic-acid supplements.

PANTOTHENIC ACID

Pantothenic acid converts into a co-enzyme that is used during the metabolism of fats. It is used for anxiety, arthritis, depression and joint inflammation. It has no known toxicity effects. It has helped those with rheumatoid arthritis and sinus problems.

It is important to note that if you are eating a high-fibre breakfast and then immediately take your vitamins, the fibre is digested first and the vitamins are often flushed away. So if fibre is a part of your everyday diet, take your vitamins at least two hours after eating it.

MINERALS

I believe that mineral deficiency is an underlying cause of many modern illnesses. Due to the depletion of our soils, minerals are no longer as available to us as they once were.

A suggestion for the proper absorption of supplemental minerals is to take a chelated mineral. It is easier for chelated minerals to get into the bloodstream and be absorbed through the walls of the cells than it is for non-chelated minerals. Finding a chelated mineral is extremely important.

BORON

Boron is an essential mineral. It helps in the absorption of calcium, magnesium and zinc and increases bone density.

CALCIUM

Calcium is needed to help heal and maintain the bones. It builds the bones while at the same time giving vitality and endurance to the body. It helps maintain mental stability and keeps the muscles fit. It should be used with vitamin D and magnesium for proper absorption.

Very few people when I have looked at actually have enough calcium in their bodies. People who have healing and intuitive abilities seem to be particularly low on it. It appears that quantities of calcium are consumed in making connections of an electromagnetic nature; therefore I tell anyone who is going to do healing work to be sure they take plenty of calcium.

If you do not have enough calcium, you can develop osteoporosis. High blood pressure can also be associated with a lack of calcium.

Some forms of calcium, such as oyster-shell calcium, cannot be absorbed by the body and become a toxin in the system. Some kidney dysfunctions are associated with the lack of the correct form of calcium.

An interesting fact is that we actually absorb as little as 20 to 40 percent of the calcium from our food. We have found that milk products do not carry as much calcium as they used to because milk is now pasteurized and homogenized. Whole milk is much more beneficial than skimmed milk. Carrots are also a good source of calcium.

Tips for increasing calcium absorption:

- Avoid excessive calcium inhibitors: chard, cranberries and spinach.
- Calcium supplements should be used with mineral-rich foods such as alfalfa/kelp or with a mineral formula.
- Chlorophyll-rich foods are essential to get enough vitamin D.
- Dairy foods: the fermented kinds, such as buttermilk, cottage cheese, kefir and yoghurt, are digested more readily.
- Eat calcium-, magnesium-, chlorophyll- and mineral-rich foods: leafy greens, legumes and seaweed.
- Exercise regularly but moderately to halt calcium loss and increase bone mass.
- Get sufficient vitamin D from sunshine: ideally, 20 percent of the body should be exposed for 30 minutes daily or full-spectrum lighting should be employed.
- Pre-soak grains and legumes before cooking to neutralize the phytic acid content.

CHROMIUM

It is interesting to note that chromium has been used in a variety of studies for the treatment of diabetes. It has also been used to treat high cholesterol, especially in cases of related diabetes, and can be used to treat hypoglycaemia.

CO-ENZYME Q10

CoQ10 supplies energy for the heart's pumping action. Without a sufficient supply of it, the heart simply fails. A cell's energy is also derived in part from CoQ10.

People who have MS are usually deficient in CoQ10. CoQ10 will benefit everyone who has MS.

People who have been exposed to radiation also need to be taking CoQ10.

COPPER

Copper is an interesting trace mineral. Organic copper will pull out other copper that is in the system as a toxin. Certain diseases are caused by the toxicity of copper. You can identify the toxicity from the inability to get 'that metallic taste' out of your mouth. Too much copper can cause abdominal pain, headaches and nausea.

Be careful when taking copper. You should never take too much if you have Wilson's disease.

IODINE

The function of the thyroid is aided by the use of iodine. Good sources are fish, shellfish and most seafood. Most bland vegetables are rather low in iodine. One of the biggest sources of iodine is iodized salt.

Iodine has a toxic effect if you use over 1,000 micrograms a day. If you take in too much iodine, an iodized goitre can form in the body.

IRON

Iron is needed for the red blood cells in the body. Approximately 75 percent of the haemoglobin in our red blood cells is responsible for carrying the oxygen through our lungs. Major deficiencies in iron can cause inconsistencies in this vital process. Difficulties with anaemia only occur after the body's store of iron is depleted. Iron deficiency is also associated with some types of asthma.

There are several good food sources of iron, including eggs, fruit, green vegetables and milk. Iron is also found in a large variety of plants.

Inorganic iron is extremely hard to absorb, which unfortunately is most of the iron that is sold in healthfood stores and otherwise. When you purchase an iron supplement, ensure it is chelated iron so your body can absorb it.

MAGNESIUM

Magnesium is necessary to relax the nerves. It is used as a motor stimulant for the brain and relieves 'brain lag'. It also keeps the intestines functioning and is beneficial as a laxative.

Low magnesium is associated with angina, heart problems and high blood pressure.

POTASSIUM

Potassium is vital in maintaining the fluid balance in the cells. It is also vital for the heart. It exists in balance with the sodium in the body.

Potassium deficiency usually causes terrible cramps, muscle spasms, nausea, rapid heartbeat, vomiting, weakness and sometimes heart failure.

Potassium is readily available in fresh fruit and other fresh foods, for example, bananas, cream of tartar, oranges, potatoes, tomatoes and watermelon.

More than 18 grams of potassium a day could cause kidney failure. Common sense is the best advice in the use of supplements.

SELENIUM

Selenium is vital for the absorption of vitamin E. It is remarkable in the treatment of cancer. It pulls out the toxicity effects of heavy metals that are carcinogenic, such as mercury. It is used for arthritis, cancer, the heart and mercury accumulations. In high doses, it is toxic.

ZINC

Without the proper amounts of zinc, there can be a decrease in your sense of smell and taste. It is a phenomenal mineral used in pulling heavy-metal toxins out of the body. It should be taken in a chelated form.

Lack of zinc in your system can cause you to have poor night vision. Your immune system will not function to full capacity and you will find you are a prime candidate for some immunological disorders.

MINERAL DEFICIENCIES

With the advent of modern farming, the manner in which crops are grown has changed dramatically. At one time the soil was replenished with natural fertilizer (manure), creating humus, a mineral-rich soil for plants to grow in. Today, most farmers use only three basic minerals for most ground crops: nitrogen, potassium and phosphorous. Without a full complement of trace minerals to draw on from the soil, a plant does not transfer them to us. This means that every slice of bread, every tomato and every ear of corn has a little less trace mineral in it. Each year, the earth becomes more depleted of the essential trace minerals we need to maintain health and prevent disease.

Here are some of the possible side-effects of a lack of dietary minerals:

Acne: sulphur, zinc

Anaemia: cobalt, copper, iron, selenium

Arthritis: boron, calcium, copper, magnesium, potassium

Asthma: manganese, potassium, zinc

Birth defects: cobalt, copper, magnesium, manganese, selenium, zinc

Brittle nails: iron, zinc

Cancer: germanium, selenium

Candida: chromium, selenium, zinc

Cardiovascular disease: calcium, copper, magnesium, manganese, potassium, selenium

Chronic fatigue syndrome: chromium, selenium, vanadium, zinc

Constipation: iron, magnesium, potassium

Cramps: calcium, sodium

Depression: calcium, chromium, copper, iron, sodium, zinc

Diabetes: chromium, vanadium, zinc

Digestive problems: chlorine, chromium, zinc

Eczema: Zinc

Gingivitis (bleeding and receding gums) and peritonitis: boron, calcium, magnesium, potassium

Goitre (low thyroid): copper, iodine

Greying hair: copper

Hair loss: copper, zinc

Hyperactivity: chromium, lithium, magnesium, zinc

Hypoglycaemia (low blood sugar): chromium, vanadium, zinc

Hypothermia: magnesium

Immune system weakness: chromium, selenium, zinc

Impotence: calcium, chromium, manganese, selenium, zinc

Liver dysfunction: chromium, cobalt, selenium, zinc

Memory loss: manganese

Muscular dystrophy/muscular weakness (also cystic fibrosis):
manganese, potassium, selenium

Nervousness: magnesium

Oedema: potassium

Osteoporosis: boron, calcium, magnesium

PMS: chromium, selenium, zinc

Sexual dysfunction: manganese, selenium, zinc

Wrinkles and sagging (facial aging): copper

Note: This is not a diagnostic chart and should not be used in place of a
health professional to determine a recovery programme.

MINERAL-RICH FORMULA

Here is a mineral-rich formula to boost your intake of vital minerals. It is a
good idea to take this for one season each year (wintertime is ideal).

> 1 part horsetail
> 1 part oatstraw
> 1 part kombu or kelp
> ½ part lobelia
> Simmer 1 oz of formula in 1 pint water for 25 minutes. Drink ½ cup
> two to three times a day.
> At the end of three weeks, stop using the formula for 1 week.

AMINO ACIDS

Problems can also arise when your body is lacking certain amino acids.
Certain amino acids actually help to stimulate what is called the 'growth
hormone' in the body.

The following is a list of the amino acids that the body uses:

alanine

arginine

asparagines

aspartic acid

cysteine

glutamic acid

glutamine

glycine

histidin

isoleucine

leucine

lysine

methionine

phenylalanine

praline

serine

threonine

tryptophan

tyrosine

valine

Supplementation for amino-acid complexes should have the proper balance of these amino acids.

HERBS

In this section, I will cover the herbs that you should not use in certain situations and how they interact with pharmaceutical drugs and contradict each other. Many herbal companies out there are creating combinations that could give people reactions. Not everyone can safely use some herbal combinations and not everyone who makes these products knows what they are doing.

The body works best with one or two herbs at a time. If you add more than this, the chance of an allergic reaction is increased by 72 percent. There is also the additional concern that one of the herbs may cause an adverse reaction if prescription medicine is being used.

The following are some herbs that are often misused:

- *Gingko biloba:* Gingko expands the capillaries to help blood flow and should not be used with high blood pressure medicine. It is also not good to suddenly discontinue the use of gingko, because the capillaries will restrict, causing a stroke.

- *Goldenseal:* Goldenseal should not be used if you are nursing or are diabetic.

- *Guarana:* Guarana is one of the most perfect forms of caffeine on the planet. It should not be used with high blood pressure or heart medicine.

- *Liquorice root:* Liquorice root should not be used with prescription cortisone. If a person has Addison's disease or Cushing's, they must be very careful using liquorice root.

- *St John's wort:* St John's wort should not be taken with antidepressants or if you are a diabetic.

Let's take this discussion one step further. For instance, you might go into a herbal shop and buy a product called ginseng. You also might expect that it is going to help you the way it is supposed to. However, what you don't know is that out of 100 different products called ginseng that were tested, only 10 actually had the herb in them. This is why so many authorities want to regulate herbal medicines.

In ThetaHealing, we never diagnose or prescribe. We merely suggest that certain supplements might be something to consider. I have had people come to me as clients who are misusing vitamins and supplements, and these are doing them more harm than good. I suggest the clients reconsider their use of them.

Taking certain herbs, vitamins and minerals as supplements does, however, give a person psychological control over their own illness. It shows the subconscious that they truly want to get better. I have found that recommending ways in which people can help themselves can motivate them as much as any healing that I have ever done.

Healers using the Second Plane of Existence understand how to use herbs and vitamins in order to achieve health. Healing from the Second Plane takes persistent use and requires time to take effect. Healers working with this plane require extensive knowledge of plants and their reactions to medicines. Without this knowledge, there is a risk to the client. As with minerals, there is an organic combination of plants for every illness.

Remember, unless you are qualified to practise medicine, you cannot advise someone to use any drug or herbal product whatsoever. It is not advisable to tell a person to change or discontinue their medication. Remember that Theta healers only pray for people. It is the Creator who is the healer!

Blessing Food and Herbs

When buying herbs, vitamins or even food, ask the Creator of All That Is if what you are buying is for your highest good. You can determine this by connecting to the Creator while holding the product and simply asking if it is for your highest good and, if so, if the potency is correct. Energy testing and pendulums are often not useful here, because the unconscious mind has a tendency to interfere with the answer. Always ask the Creator.

Once the substance has passed the test, it should be blessed before use to ensure maximum potency, effectiveness and quality. Since everything has a consciousness and we absorb this essence when we consume it, we need to bless all the food and herbs we eat! If these substances have not been treated with the respect they deserve, the benefits will be reduced. Genetically altered food, especially corn and soya, has a consciousness that is perhaps not for our best. If there is a question about the essence of the food, go back and bless it from its origin.

HERBS AND SUPPLEMENTS LIST

Acidophilus: Aids the digestion of milk products, lowers cholesterol, maintains normal bacterial balance in the intestines.

Aloe vera: High in vitamin C, useful for arthritis, constipation, stomach disorders and ulcers.

Apple juice: The pectin found contained in apple juice removes toxins and metals, lowers cholesterol and is beneficial for heart disease and gallstones.

Bay berry: Helps menstrual cramps, tones the female organs, strengthens the uterus during pregnancy. Stimulates the intestinal movement, slows breathing and can be used for bronchial constriction.

Bee pollen: Good source of vitamin C, amino acids, fatty acids, calcium, magnesium, potassium, so useful for allergies, cancer (keep in mind that if you are counselling cancer patients or are giving someone a protein supplement, bee pollen contains high amounts of protein), colon disorders, depression and fatigue.

Bilberry: Antiviral, benefits capillaries, aids in the function of the eye and the circulation in varicose veins. There are many people who are allergic to this herb.

Black cohosh: Contains natural oestrogen (synthetic oestrogen has been known to cause cancer). Good for hot flushes during menopause, regulates menstrual flow, acts as tonic for mucous and serous tissues, good for childbirth pain, menstrual cramps and menopausal symptoms, lowers blood pressure and cholesterol levels, reduces mucus. This herbal should not be used by people who have breast or other oestrogen-related cancers.

Black walnut: Clears parasites and fungal infections. Should not be used by diabetics.

Burdock root: Blood and gall bladder purifier, good for gout symptoms.

Camu: A very potent antidepressant, anti-migraine and antiviral.

Carrot juice: Good overall source of vitamins and cancer fighter.

Cascara sagrada: Cleans the valves, acts as a laxative for constipation and parasites.

Cat's claw: An antioxidant, cleans the intestinal tract, good for cancer and intestinal problems.

Catnip: Nature's own Alka-Seltzer, has a mild sedative effect on the nervous system, helps prevent miscarriage, acts as a pain-reliever, is good for the nerves and worms.

Cayenne pepper: Used for arthritis, bleeding ulcers and poor circulation.

Chamomile: A gentle pain-reliever that can be given to infants and is also good for relaxation.

Chinese Angelica: An immune-enhancer.

Chinese Ma Huang (commonly referred to as Ephedra in the United States): Used for asthma, colds, respiratory problems and heart disorders. When given with Guarana it becomes a strong stimulant that can be dangerous. Should never be taken with heart medication.

Chlorella: An excellent source of carbohydrates, chlorophyll, protein, vitamin C and vitamin E. Used for asthma, bleeding gums, burns and infections. One of the best ways of pulling mercury from the body (start with small doses and increase slowly).

CoQ10: A stimulant useful for anti-aging, cellular energies and the heart.

Damiana: An excellent hormone regulator. Increases fertility in both males and females. Do not use if you have had oestrogen-related cancers!

Dandelion root: Acts as a diuretic, cleanses the bloodstream and liver, helps age spots, the kidneys, pancreas, spleen and stomach. You should only use this herb for short periods of time, because it will affect the blood sugar and can have adverse effects on the liver.

Echinacea: An immune stimulant that flushes the lymph system by enhancing macrophages in the blood, promotes T-cell activation and stimulates white blood cells. An anti-inflammatory for colds, the flu and general infections.

Fenugreek: An anti-inflammatory that helps the lungs and lymphatic system.

Feverfew: Good for arthritis, fever, headaches and muscle tension, acts as a pain-reliever, increases blood platelets and is an anti-inflammatory.

Flaxseed oil: An excellent source of fibre, magnesium, protein, potassium, vitamin B and vitamin C. Used as a pain-reducer and for arthritis, inflammation and the liver.

Garlic powder: Antibiotic, anti-fungal, antioxidant and lowers blood pressure.

Ginger root: An antioxidant that cleanses the colon and reduces spasms.

Ginkgo biloba: Good for brain function, Alzheimer's disease and Parkinson's disease, also pulls toxins.

Goldenseal: An anti-bacterial and anti-inflammatory useful for strengthening the immune system. Do not use if there is diabetes or hypoglycaemia. Do not give to small children.

Grapeseed extract: Grapeseed extract has been well studied in the treatment of micro-vascular disorders. It has been used for capillary fragility, muscular degeneration and varicose veins. It is an antioxidant that helps cancer treatment, toxin removal and visual function.

Green tea: An antioxidant useful in cancer prevention, it lowers cholesterol, reduces clotting, regulates blood sugar and is good for weight loss.

Guarana: A pure form of caffeine often used with Chinese Ma Hung. This is not a good combination and should not be used, so beware when buying.

Irish moss: Will eliminate dead tissue in the body. It is an excellent source of iodine that is compatible with the body.

Kava kava: Useful for depression, insomnia, stress and urinary infections.

Liquorice root: Good for the adrenals, allergic reactions, asthma, a colon cleanse, depression, fever and stomach problems, and helps the bowels. Should not be used by those who are using cortisone or have breast cancer.

Maca: For women: useful for extra energy, healthy bones, menopausal symptoms, PMS, post-menopausal symptoms, the 'blues' and vaginal dryness. Do not use with oestrogen-related cancers. For men: useful for enhanced energy, fertility, libido, sexual potency and stamina.

Marshmallow: Helps bladder infections, kidney problems and the skin.

Milk thistle: A liver cleanse. Not to be given in the spring because the liver is purging itself during springtime.

Mistletoe: Used to aid lymph-gland function. It has some uses in cancer treatment too, but must be administered by a registered herbalist due to the inherently strong nature of the herb.

Olive-leaf extract: Used to treat parasites and yeast infections and enhance the immune system.

Oregano: A cleanse for tapeworms and other parasites.

Parsley: A stimulant useful for bladder function, kidney function, the lungs, parasites and the thyroid.

Peppermint leaves: Good for chills, diarrhoea, headaches and nausea.

Pumpkin seeds: A cleanse for tapeworms and other parasites.

Red clover: An antibiotic and blood purifier, good for cleaning the lungs, HIV, liver diseases, valve disorders and strengthening a weakened immune system.

Red raspberry: Use five weeks before the delivery of a baby to tone the uterus and other organs and ease childbirth.

Safflower powder: Aids the colon, cleanses the blood and neutralizes uric acid.

Saw palmetto: This herb has a good effect on all diseases of the reproductive system. It has been known to enlarge the breasts of under-developed females. It benefits all glandular tissue and rids the body of excess mucus from the head, lungs and sinuses. Good for prostate enlargement, some prostate cancers; useful as an appetite stimulant, diuretic and urinary antiseptic.

Siberian ginseng: Strengthens the adrenal-reproduction glands and immune system, stimulates the appetite. Useful for bronchitis, circulatory problems, diabetes, infertility and stress. Not to be given to small children because of the high numbers of hormones.

Slippery elm: Good for the lungs, mucus membranes, throat and urinary tract. A good nutrient builder that aids the digestive system.

Spirulina: A concentrated source of amino acids, iron and proteins and a source of chlorophyll. Pulls diseases and toxins and strengthens the immune system.

Stinging nettle: Good for allergies. The Russians have researched the use of the root in cancer of the prostate, with some positive results.

Valerian root: Acts as a sedative. Clears the mucus from colds. Provides the trace minerals required for blood and nerve functions and body fluids. Useful for blood pressure, fatigue, irritable bowel syndrome and the circulation.

White oak bark: Good as an antibacterial and for nasal polyps.

White willow bark: Nature's aspirin – performs all the functions of aspirin.

Yellow dock root: A cleanser and purifier that improves colon and liver functions.

Yucca root: A liver cleanse that is also good for arthritis, blood purification and osteoporosis. Helps the body produce its own cortisone.

NERVINE HERBS

Blue cohosh: A relaxant.

Catnip: A relaxant.

Chamomile: A relaxant useful for drug withdrawal.

Hops: Calm the nerves and nerve disorders.

Lobelia tincture: Used for hyperactivity, insomnia, migraine, nerves, pain and palpitations of the heart.

Melatonin: Good for inner-clock disorders, SAD and sleep disorders.

Passion flower: A sedative used for alcohol withdrawals, headaches and nerves.

Skullcap: A sleep aid also useful for muscle twitch and neuritis.

Thyme: Useful for alcohol withdrawal, hangovers and headaches.

Valerian root: A nervine and relaxant.

RECOMMENDED READING

Anatomy and Physiology Made Incredibly Easy, Springhouse Publishing Company, 2004

Steven Bratman, *Physicians' Desk Reference for Nutritional Supplements*, PDR, PO Box 10689, Des Moines, IA 50336

Alma E. Guinness (ed.), *ABCs of the Human Body*, Reader's Digest, 1987

Richard Harness, Pham., FASCP, *Drug-Herb-Vitamin Interactions Bible*, Prima, 2000

ThetaHealing Classes

ThetaHealing® is an energy-healing modality founded by Vianna Stibal, based in Ammon, Idaho, with certified instructors around the world. The classes and books of ThetaHealing® are designed as therapeutic self-help guides to develop the ability of the mind to heal. ThetaHealing® includes the following books, manuals and classes:

Classes taught by Vianna and certified ThetaHealing® instructors:

Vianna's DNA 2 Course

Vianna's DNA 2 Advanced Course: The Planes of Existence

Vianna's Intuitive Anatomy Course

Vianna's Children of the Rainbow Course

ThetaHealing Manifesting and Abundance Course

ThetaHealing Diseases and Disorders Class

ThetaHealing World Relations Class

Certification classes taught exclusively by Vianna at the ThetaHealing Institute of Knowledge:

Vianna's Children of the Rainbow Teacher's Course

Vianna's DNA 2 Teacher's Course

Vianna's DNA 2 Advanced Teacher's Course

Vianna's Intuitive Anatomy Teacher's Course

ThetaHealing Diseases and Disorders Certification Class

ThetaHealing World Relations Certification Class

DNA 3

BOOKS

Titles currently available:

ThetaHealing (Hay House, 2010)

Advanced ThetaHealing (Hay House, 2011)

Class manuals:

ThetaHealing® Practitioner Manual

Vianna's Teacher's Manual

Vianna's DNA 2 Advanced Manual

Vianna's DNA 2 Advanced Teacher's Manual

Vianna's Intuitive Anatomy Manual

Vianna's Intuitive Anatomy Teacher's Manual

Vianna's Rainbow Children's Young Children's Manual

Vianna's Rainbow Children's Young Adult's Manual

Vianna's Rainbow Children's Teacher's Manual

ThetaHealing® Manifesting and Abundance Manual

For further information about schedules for ThetaHealing® classes, call (1) 208 524-0808 at the ThetaHealing Institute of Knowledge, Ammon, Idaho 83406, USA; email: vianna@thetahealing.com; website: www.thetahealing. com

ABOUT THE AUTHOR

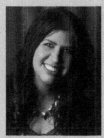

Starshots

Vianna Stibal is a young grandmother, an artist and a writer. Her natural charisma and compassion for those in need of help have also led to her being known as a healer, intuitive and teacher.

After being taught how to connect with the Creator to co-create and facilitate the unique process called ThetaHealing, Vianna knew that she must share this gift with as many people as she could. It was this love and appreciation for the Creator and humanity that allowed her to develop the ability to see clearly into the human body and witness many instant healings.

Her encyclopaedic knowledge of the body's systems and deep understanding of the human psyche, based on her own experience, as well as the insight given to her by the Creator, make Vianna the perfect practitioner of this amazing technique. She has successfully worked with such medical challenges as hepatitis C, Epstein-Barr virus, AIDS, herpes, various types of cancers and many other disorders, diseases and genetic defects.

Vianna knows that the ThetaHealing technique is teachable, but beyond that she knows that it *needs* to be taught. She conducts seminars all over the world to teach people of all races, beliefs and religions. She has trained teachers and practitioners who are working in 14 countries, but her work will not stop there! She is committed to spreading this healing paradigm throughout the world.

www.thetahealing.com